Learning Radiology

Learning Radiology: Recognizing the Basics

William Herring, MD, FACR

Vice Chairman and Program Director
Department of Radiology
Albert Einstein Medical Center
Philadelphia, Pennsylvania

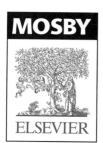

MOSBY

ELSEVIER

1600 John F. Kennedy Blvd.
Ste 1800
Philadelphia, PA 19103–2899

LEARNING RADIOLOGY: RECOGNIZING THE BASICS   ISBN: 978-0-323-04317-5

Library of Congress Cataloging-in-Publication Data

Herring, William.
   Learning radiology : recognizing the basics / William Herring – 1st ed.
      p. ; cm.
   Includes bibliographical references.
   ISBN-13: 978-0-323-04317-5   ISBN-10: 978-0-323-04317-5
   1. Radiology, Medical—Study and teaching.   I. Title.
   [DNLM: 1. Radiography—methods.   2. Diagnosis, Differential. WN 200 H567L 2007]
   R899.H472 2007
   616.07′57071—dc22

                                                                    2006046715

ISBN: 978-0-323-04317-5

Acquisitions Editor: Jim Merritt
Developmental Editor: Andrea Deis
Project Manager: David Saltzberg
Design Direction: Steve Stave

Printed in the United States of America

Last digit is the print number: 9 8 7 6 5 4 3 2

To Pat, Sharon, Debbie, Alex, and Sam

For reminding me to recognize the basics in life

Preface

If you're the kind of person, like I am, who reads the preface after you've read the book, I hope you enjoyed it. If you're the kind of person who reads the preface before reading the book, then you're in for a real treat.

Suppose for a moment that you wanted to know what kind of bird with a red beak just landed on your window sill (don't ask why). You could get a book on birds that listed all of them alphabetically from albatross to woodpecker and spend time looking at hundreds of bird pictures. Or you could get a book that lists birds by the colors of their beaks and thumb through a much shorter list to find that it was a cardinal.

This is a red beak book. Where possible, groups of diseases are first described by the way they *look* rather than by what they're *called*. Imaging diagnoses frequently, but not always, rest on a recognition of a reproducible visual picture of that abnormality. That is called the *pattern recognition approach* to identifying abnormalities, and the more experience you have and more proficient you become at looking at imaging studies, the more comfortable and confident you'll be with that approach.

Before diagnostic images can help you decide what disease the patient may have, you must first be able to differentiate between what is normal and what is not. That isn't as easy as it may sound. Recognizing the difference between normal and abnormal probably takes as much, if not more, practice than deciding what disease the person has.

In fact, it takes so much practice, some people—I believe they are called *radiologists*—have actually been known to spend their entire life doing it. You won't be a radiologist after you've completed this book, but you should be able to recognize abnormalities and interpret images better. By so doing, perhaps you can participate in the care of patients with more assurance and confidence.

In this text, you'll spend time in each section learning how to recognize what is normal so that you can differentiate between such things as a skin fold and a pneumothorax or so that you can recognize whether that fuzzy white stuff at the lung bases is pneumonia or the patient simply hasn't taken a deep breath.

Where pattern recognition doesn't work, we'll try whenever possible to give you a logical *approach* to reaching a diagnosis based on simple yet effective decision trees. These will be little decision trees—saplings with only a few branches—so that they are relatively easy to remember.

By learning an approach, you'll have a method you can apply to similar problems again and again. Have you ever heard the saying "Give a man a fish; you have fed him for today. Teach a man to fish, and you have fed him for a lifetime"? Learning an imaging approach is like learning how to fish, except a lot less smelly. An approach will enable you to apply a rational solution to diagnostic imaging problems.

This text was written, in part, to make complementary use of the medium for which radiologic images are ideally suited: the computer screen. The web is ideal for accessing and displaying images, but many people do not want to read large volumes of text from their computer screens. So we've joined the text in the printed book with photos, quizzes, and tutorials available online at StudentConsult.com in a series of *web enhancements* that accompany every chapter.

This text is not intended to be encyclopedic. There are many wonderful radiology reference texts available, some of which contain thousands of pages and weigh slightly less than a Volkswagen. This text is oriented more towards students, interns, and residents or residents-to-be.

Not every imaging modality is covered equally in this book, and some are not covered at all. This book emphasizes conventional radiography because that is the type of study most patients have first and because the same imaging principles that apply to recognizing the diagnosis on conventional radiographs can be applied to making the diagnosis on more complex modalities.

With a better appreciation and understanding of why images look the way they do, you'll soon be recognizing abnormalities and making diagnoses that will impress your mentors and peers and astound your friends and relatives.

Let's get started.

Acknowledgments

I owe a special debt of gratitude to the hundreds of radiology residents and medical students who, over the years, have made it so enjoyable to be their instructor and who have provided me with an audience of motivated learners without whom no teacher could teach.

I am also grateful to the many, many thousands of people I have never met but who found a website called Learning Radiology really helpful and who told me how much they appreciated it by the volume and frequency of their visits.

For their help and suggestions, I want to thank my colleagues Morrie Kricun, MD, Mindy Horrow, MD, Adam Guttentag, MD, and Susan Summerton, MD, who agreed to read and critique several chapters and who helped supply some much needed photographs without once asking for a percentage of the royalties.

I have had many wonderful teachers and mentors, and I thank all of them for their guidance both by training and example, as well as my associates and chairs for their support. I especially want to thank Bernard Ostrum, MD, Morrie Kricun, MD, and Michael Love, MD, who helped me learn how to teach better.

Janet Birkmann, our Academic Coordinator, helped me write this book by doing all of the things she does every day related to resident education in our department. By so doing she made—and continues to make—my real job that much easier.

I want to acknowledge my wife Pat, daughters Debbie and Sharon, son-in-law Alex, and grandson Sam, who probably would have found this book a lot more interesting if I somehow managed to make everything rhyme and included a few bears in each chapter. I'll try that next time.

And I certainly want to thank Jim Merritt and Andrea Deis from Elsevier for first recognizing that I might have something to say that could help folks like yourself in learning radiology and then for checking that the pages were numbered correctly, the photographs were labeled correctly, the words were spelled correctly, and for making sure the arrows—and I—were pointing in the right direction.

Contents

1 Recognizing Anything

The "Colorful" World of Radiology
- It helps to think of radiologic images in **"color."**
- The colors of radiologic images, in most cases, will be **black, white,** and **varying shades of gray,** but nonetheless they are still colors.
- The denser an object is, the more x-rays it absorbs, and the "whiter" it appears on radiographic images.
  - **Bone is the densest naturally occurring tissue.**
    - It absorbs the greatest amount of x-ray and appears white on radiographs.
  - **Metal is even denser** (whiter) than bone and essentially absorbs all x-rays, **but metal does not occur naturally in humans.**
    - Things like bullets or artificial hip replacements are metal density and will appear whiter than any other object on a conventional image (Fig. 1-1).
- **The less dense an object is, the fewer x-rays it absorbs, and the "blacker" it will appear on radiographs.**
  - Air absorbs few or no x-rays and appears the blackest on a radiograph.
- In conventional radiography, the terms *opaque, nonopaque, dense,* and *lucent* are used to describe the density of a structure *relative to its surrounding tissue.*
- These terms do not specifically identify any particular disease (hundreds of diseases may produce lucencies and many hundreds more produce opacities) but rather define a lesion's density relative to its surroundings.
- Here are some examples of how different densities are described:
  - A **hole in a bone** (remember, the bone itself is white) will appear **blacker** than the rest of the bone and is said to represent a **lucency** in the bone (see Fig. 21-21).
  - A **fracture** through a bone is usually **blacker** than the surrounding bone and is said to represent a **lucency** in the bone (see Fig. 22-7).
  - A **large pneumothorax** will contain no lung markings and may make the affected hemithorax appear **blacker** or more **lucent** relative to the normal hemithorax (see Fig. 9-10).
  - A **large pleural effusion** will absorb more x-rays than normally aerated lung and will make the affected hemithorax appear **whiter** or more **opaque** than the normal hemithorax (see Fig. 7-9).
  - **Calcified gallstones** visible on a conventional radiograph of the abdomen will be **whiter** than their surrounding tissues and are said to be **opaque** calculi (Fig. 1-2).

A Systematic Approach: The "Truth" About Systems
- Some look at imaging studies such as chest radiographs from the outside of the image to the inside of the image; others look at them from the inside out or from top to bottom.

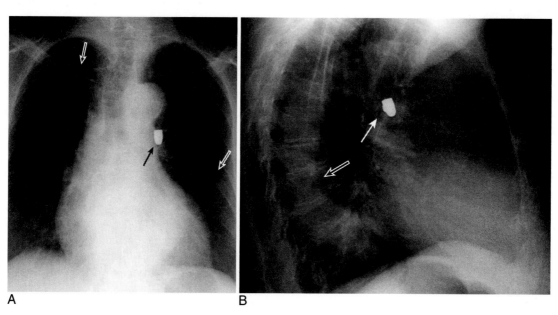

A   B

Figure 1-1. **Bullet in the chest.** *The dense (white) metallic foreign body in the region of the aortopulmonary window resembles a bullet because it is a bullet (black and white closed arrows). It is much denser (whiter) than the bones, represented by the ribs, clavicles, and spine (open white arrows). Two views at 90° angles to each other, such as these frontal* **(A)** *and lateral* **(B)** *chest radiographs, are called orthogonal views (see Chapter 2). With only one view, it would be impossible to know the location of the bullet. Orthogonal views are used throughout conventional radiography to localize structures in all parts of the body.*

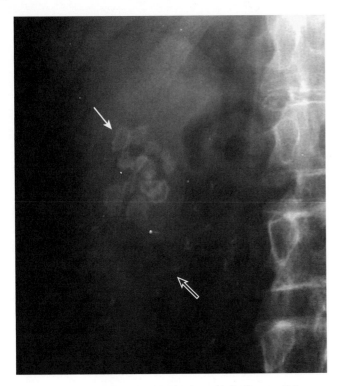

Figure 1-2. **Gallstones.** *Multiple laminar, calcific densities (whiter than surrounding soft tissue) are seen in the right upper quadrant (closed white arrow) with flattened edges where they rub against each other in the lumen of the gallbladder (perhaps to stay warm). These are called faceted gallstones. The numerous small opacities (open white arrow) represent radiopaque metallic sutures from prior surgery.*

- Some systems for reminding you to examine every part of an image have catchy acronyms and mnemonics.
- **Truth one: it doesn't matter what system you use as long as you look at everything on the image.**
  - So, **use whatever system works for you** but be sure to look at everything.
  - "Looking at everything," by the way, includes looking at **all of the views available in a given study,** not just everything on *one* view.
    - Some beginners examining frontal and lateral chest studies never even glance at the lateral radiograph—not even once; this is a common beginner's mistake (more on that as we get to "Truth four").
- **Truth two: Experienced radiologists usually have no system at all.**
  - "Burned-in" images are bad for computer monitors and television screens but they're great for radiologists.
  - "Burned" into the neurons of a radiologist's brain are mental images of what a normal frontal chest radiograph looks like, what thoracic sarcoidosis looks like, and so on.
  - They frequently use a "gestalt" impression of a study which they see in their mind's eye within seconds of looking at an image.
    - If the image does or does not correspond to the mental image that resides in their brains, **then** they systematically study the images.

- This is not magic; this ability comes only with experience and one other very important factor.
- **Truth three: You are not an experienced radiologist, so you are not quite ready to use the "gestalt" approach.**
- **Truth four** (this is the last one): The "one other very important factor" is ***knowledge.***
  - If you don't know what you are looking for, you can stare at a radiograph for hours or even days or, in the case of the lateral chest radiograph, you can ignore an image entirely and the end result will be: you won't see the findings.
    - There is an axiom in radiology: **You only see what you look for and you only look for what you know.**
    - So, if you don't know what to look for, you will never recognize the finding no matter what system you use or how long you stare at it.
  - **That's why you're reading this book** (isn't it?): **so you know what to look for and so that you'll recognize it when you see it. Knowledge!**

Terminology

- "Oh no," you say, "not the terminology section. Let me skip to the good parts."
  - You can do that: just remember where this section is because you may have to refer to it later.
- Like politics, all terminology is local.
  - Follow the terminology conventions used in your hospital or, alternatively, the person rendering your course grade, even if those conventions are different from what is described here.
- **Here are the terminology conventions used in this book:**
- **Image:** a good, all-around term that can be **used to describe any type of rendering of a radiologic examination.**
  - It works for all modalities; use it freely.
  - You could say you were looking at an "***image*** of the abdomen on a conventional radiograph," or a "CT (computed tomographic) ***image*** of the abdomen," or an "ultrasound ***image*** of the abdomen," and so on.
  - Try not to use the word *picture* in radiology: ***image*** will make you sound much smarter.
- **X-ray:** seems like an easy enough term, but its use is the subject of some controversy among terminology toughies
  - Technically, an "x-ray" is the invisible form of energy that helps produce the image.
  - The image you are looking at or holding in your hand is technically not an "x-ray"-you can't see or hold x-rays.
  - **Fact:** Many people (including us) use the term ***x-ray*** to refer to the actual image and not just the invisible rays and we have not been struck down by lightning for doing so.
  - In this book, we will usually use the term ***radiograph*** to refer to the actual image you are viewing, but we all know that when someone says they are going to "look at the chest x-rays on Mr. Jones" they are not intending to conjure up Roentgen's mysterious rays but the radiographic images of Mr. Jones' chest.

- **Film:** once the only way to view an image was on a piece of film which was then placed on a lightbox or viewbox (almost always backward or upside-down if the film placement was being done as part of a movie or TV show).
  - Film is still the viewing medium in many clinics and departments of radiology.
  - If you are using film to view your images, **remember that when you place the film on the viewbox, you and the patient are always looking at each other face to face.**
    - That is, **the patient's right side,** whether it is on conventional radiographs or a CT scan, **is on your left side and the patient's left side should be on your right side.**
    - This is the convention by which radiographs are viewed **no matter what position the patient was in when the image was exposed.**
  - With the advent of *PACS* (see below), the computer monitor replaces film.
- **Cassette:** a cassette is the flat device that looks like a huge iPod that **holds either a piece of film or a special digital plate** in which x-rays and light combine to **produce a latent image** that will become visible when it is *processed* in one of two ways, depending on whether the cassette contains **film** or contains a **digital phosphor plate** without film.
  - **If the cassette contains film,** the film will be removed from the cassette in a **darkroom** (or by something called a *daylight loader* that simulates a darkroom) and **sent through an automatic processor** that contains a series of chemicals **that will develop the image,** make it visible to the human eye, and fix it permanently on the film.
    - A new, unexposed piece of film will then be loaded into the cassette and the cassette will be ready for the next exposure.
  - **If it is a digital cassette and contains no film,** it will be **processed through an electronic reader** that will decipher the electronic image stored on the phosphor plate in the cassette and transmit that digital image to another system to store it.
    - The electronic image in the cassette is then "erased" and the cassette is used again and again.
- **Computed radiography (CR) and PACS:** uses the kind of digital cassettes described above.
  - Computed radiography uses the same x-ray equipment that film-based cassettes use except that a digital cassette is substituted for one containing film.
  - The electronic images so obtained are almost always viewed on and interpreted from computer monitors and stored in a large database archived by patient name, date of birth, type and date of study, etc. for future retrieval.
  - The **computer-based system that archives and stores the images for later retrieval** is called a **picture archiving, communications, and storage system,** known by the acronym **PACS.**
    - In this case, using the term *picture* probably seemed like a good idea since using the word *image* or *x-ray*

would have resulted in acronyms that were impossible to pronounce *(XACS?).*
- **Radiograph:** technically the physical representation of the image x-rays help produce, as in **chest radiograph.**
  - But we all know that the term **chest x-ray** transmits the same meaning to most people, and even though many radiographs today are viewed electronically and not on film, most people use the terms **radiograph** and **film** and **x-ray** interchangeably to refer to the image we view, as in **chest radiograph** or **chest film** or **chest x-ray.** Confused yet?
- **Plain films** are images produced through the use of x-rays but without added contrast material like barium or iodine
  - We may substitute the term **conventional radiographs** for the term **plain films** and, even though their meanings are technically slightly different, if you don't tell anyone, we won't either.
    - Besides, the term **conventional radiographs** makes them sound more exotic and difficult to interpret than does the term **plain films.**
- **Study** or **examination:** used interchangeably, they refer to a **collection of images that examine a particular part of the body or system,** as in "double contrast **study** of the colon" (a series of images of the colon using air and barium and produced through the use of x-rays); or, an "MRI (magnetic resonance imaging) **examination** of the brain" (a collection of images of the brain using MRI to produce the images).
- **Contrast material:** usually something that is administered to a patient in order to make certain structures more easily visible (frequently referred to as **contrast**)
  - The **most widely used examples of radiologic contrast materials** include liquid **barium,** which is administered orally for upper gastrointestinal (UGI) examinations and rectally for barium enema (BE) examinations, and **iodine,** which is administered intravenously for contrast-enhanced CT scans of the body.
  - There are also contrast agents used for MRI and ultrasound.
- **Dye:** the lay term for contrast, as in "they gave me dye for my kidney x-ray and I thought I would die."
  - Although *contrast* is the better term, many patients, and some radiologists in explaining tests to patients, use the term *dye.*
    - Don't use the word dye unless you are talking to a patient explaining a test: use the term *contrast* or *contrast agent.*
- **Flat plate:** an archaic, but still used, term meaning a conventional radiograph or plain film of the abdomen, almost always obtained with the patient lying supine
  - This term is left over from the pioneer days of radiology before film was used as the recording medium and the image was produced on a flat, glass plate.
- **Wet reading:** another archaic term **still used sometimes to refer to an immediate or "stat" interpretation of a study.**
  - The term derives from the manner in which radiographs were originally processed—by manually moving the

radiograph through a series of tanks containing photographic chemicals.

- A *wet reading* was one that was done more quickly, before the liquids on the radiograph actually dried.
- **White and black:** these are not radiologic terms, but almost every modality displays its images in white, black, and various shades of gray (see "The 'Colorful' World of Radiology" earlier in this chapter).
  - Unfortunately, the specific terms used to describe what appears as *white* on an image and what appears as *black* on an image change from one modality to another.
  - Table 1-1 is a handy chart that describes the interpretations of black and white in various modalities.
- **"En face" and "in profile":** used primarily in conventional radiography and barium studies.
  - When you look at a lesion directly "head-on," you are seeing it *en face.*
  - A lesion seen tangentially (from the side) is seen *in profile.*
  - Only a sphere, which, by definition, is perfectly round in every dimension, will appear exactly the same shape no matter what plane in which it is viewed (e.g., a nodule in the lung) (Fig. 1-3).
  - Naturally occurring structures, whether normal or abnormal, of any shape other than a sphere will appear slightly different in shape if viewed *en face* or *in profile.*

- This is not an easy concept to grasp because it **involves making a mental reconstruction of a three-dimensional object from the two-dimensional projections** conventional radiographs provide.
- For example, a disk-shaped object (one that looks like a playing piece used in the game of checkers), such as an ingested coin, will appear circular when viewed *en face* but rectangular when viewed in perfect *profile* (Fig. 1-4).
- **Extravasated** and **extraluminal:** often used in radiology to describe any substance that is outside the vessel

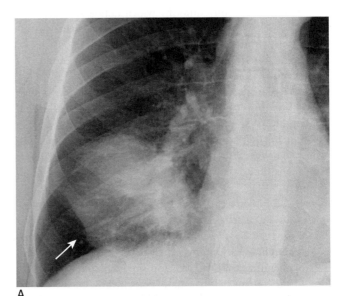

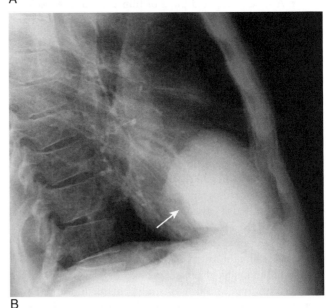

Figure 1-3. **Right lower lobe bronchogenic carcinoma.** *There is a nearly spherical mass in the right middle lobe of the lung (white closed arrows) seen on the frontal (**A**) and lateral (**B**) radiographs of this patient. Because the mass is nearly spherical, it has relatively the same shape when viewed **en face** and **in profile**.*

Table 1-1

WHITE AND BLACK—TERMS FOR EACH MODALITY

Modality	Terms Used for "White"	Terms Used for "Black"
Conventional radiographs	Increased density; opaque	Decreased density; lucent
Computed tomography (CT)	Increased attenuation; hyperintense or hyperdense	Decreased attenuation; hypodense
Magnetic resonance imaging (MRI)	Increased signal intensity	Decreased signal intensity
Ultrasound (US)	Increased echogenicity; sonodense	Decreased echogenicity; sonolucent
Nuclear medicine	Increased tracer uptake	Decreased tracer uptake; photopenic
Barium studies	Radiopaque	Nonopaque; radiolucent

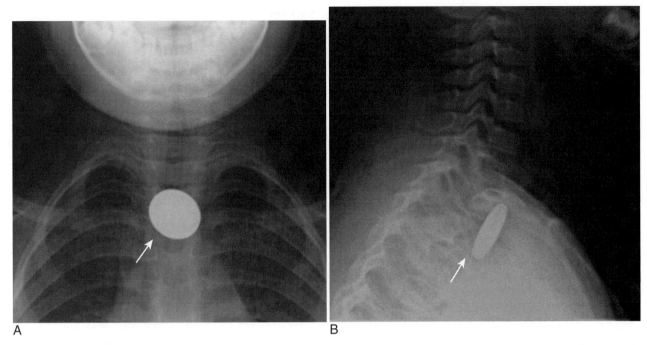

A   B

Figure 1-4. **Coin in the esophagus.** *Both the frontal* **(A)** *and the lateral* **(B)** *images of this child's upper thorax demonstrate a radiopaque (white) metallic density in the region of the upper esophagus (white closed arrows). The child swallowed a quarter, which is temporarily lodged in the esophagus just above the aortic arch. Notice how different the coin looks when viewed* en face *in* **(A)** *where it is seen as a circle and in profile* **(B)** *where it is seen on end.*

(*extravasated*) or other luminal structure (*extraluminal*) that originally contained it.

- For example, a ruptured urinary bladder is often said to demonstrate *extravasated* urine, although the correct term to use here is actually *extraluminal.*
- *Extravasation,* according to its original definition, should refer to **blood that escapes from the vessel that contained it.**
- So, there may be *extraluminal contrast* seen arising from a ruptured urinary bladder or *extraluminal barium* seen arising from a ruptured duodenal ulcer or *extravasation of contrast* arising from a torn renal artery.
- **Hemidiaphragm:** although anatomically we only have one diaphragm that separates the thorax from the abdomen, radiographically we don't normally see the diaphragm from one side to the other, so radiologists divide the diaphragm into a right hemidiaphragm and a left hemidiaphragm.
- **Horizontal versus vertical x-ray beams:** terms that describe orientation of x-ray beams.
  - Horizontal and vertical orientation is a very important concept to understand because it will help you in interpreting all kinds of conventional radiographic studies and in understanding their limitations, which may, in turn, prevent you from falling for a diagnostic pitfall.
  - An x-ray beam is usually directed either *horizontally* between the tube and the cassette (as in an erect chest examination in which the patient is standing up) or

vertically between the tube and the cassette (as in a supine radiograph of the abdomen with the patient lying on the examining table).

- **Horizontal x-ray beams are usually parallel to the floor** of the examining room (unless the room was built by do-it-yourselfers on weekends).
- In conventional radiography, **an air-fluid or fat-fluid level will be visible only if the x-ray beam is horizontal,** *regardless of the position of the patient.*
  - Therefore, **you will never see an air-fluid level** no matter what the position of the patient **unless the conventional radiographic exposure is made using a horizontal x-ray beam.**
  - An air-fluid or fat-fluid level is an interface between two substances of different density in which the lighter substance rises above and forms a straight-edge interface with the heavier substance below.
- **You** usually **don't have to specify whether you want the x-ray beam to be horizontal or vertical when ordering a study;** by convention, certain studies are always done using one method or the other (Table 1-2).
  - In general, any study with the terms *erect, cross-table,* or *decubitus* is always **done with a horizontal beam.**
  - **You can see fluid levels (if present) with any of these types of studies, no matter how the patient is positioned.**
- You should be aware of the limitations inherent in vertical beam examinations.

Table 1-2

HORIZONTAL VERSUS VERTICAL X-RAY BEAM

Examples of Types of Studies	Orientation of Beam	Implications
Erect view of the abdomen	Horizontal	Air-fluid levels will be visible; free air will rise to diaphragm
Left lateral decubitus view of the abdomen	Horizontal	Air-fluid levels will be visible; free air will rise over liver
Supine abdomen	Vertical	Air-fluid levels will not be visible: free air will rise to undersurface of anterior abdominal wall and may not be visible until large amounts are present
Erect chest	Horizontal	Pneumothorax, if present, will usually be visible at apex of lung; air-fluid levels (e.g., in cavities) will be visible
Supine chest	Vertical	Requires much larger pneumothorax to be visible; air-fluid levels will not be visible
Cross-table lateral examination of the knee	Horizontal	Fat-fluid levels (lipohemarthrosis), if present, will be visible
Supine examination of the knee	Vertical	Fat-fluid levels will not be visible

Conventions Used in this Book
- **Bold type** is used liberally throughout this text to **highlight important points, and** because this is a book overflowing with important points, **there is much bold type.**
- **Diagnostic pitfalls** (translation: watch your step here or you may fall into a false-negative or false-positive trap) are signaled by this icon:
- **Really, really important points** (even more important than the important points in **boldface** type) are signaled by this icon:
- The weblink symbol means there is additional instructional material available on the StudentConsult.com website for registered users:

"Take-home" points at the end of chapters are signaled by this icon:

- You may use these points in any location, not only your home.
- Don't look for them at the end of this chapter because once the word "terminology" was mentioned earlier, you probably skipped ahead to the remainder of the chapters that do have take-home points.

WebLink

More information on recognizing the basics of radiology is available to registered users on StudentConsult.com.

2 Recognizing a Technically Adequate Chest Radiograph

- You need to do **three things** to feel more comfortable interpreting chest radiographs:
  - **First, you have to be able to quickly determine if a study is technically adequate** so that you don't mistake technical deficiencies for abnormalities.
  - **Second, you need to be able to recognize the difference between normal and abnormal.**
  - **Third,** if you decide the finding is abnormal, **you need to have some strategy for deciding what the abnormality is.**
- **First things first:** This chapter will enable you to make a quick evaluation of the technical adequacy of the chest radiograph by helping you become more familiar with the diagnostic pitfalls technical artifacts can introduce.
  - Throughout this text, **this icon** **will alert you to a diagnostic pitfall** and how to avoid it.
- Evaluating **five technical factors** will help you to determine if a chest radiograph is **adequate** for interpretation:
  - **Penetration**
  - **Inspiration**
  - **Rotation**
  - **Magnification**
  - **Angulation**

Penetration
- Unless the body part being studied is adequately penetrated by x-rays, you may not visualize everything possible on the image produced.
  - To determine if a frontal chest radiograph is adequately penetrated, **you should be able to faintly see the thoracic spine through the heart shadow** (Fig. 2-1).
- **Pitfalls of underpenetration (inadequate penetration)**
  - You can tell **if a frontal chest radiograph is underpenetrated** (too light) because **you will not be able to see the spine through the heart.**
  - At least **two errors** can be introduced into your interpretation as a result of underpenetration:
    - First, **the left hemidiaphragm may not be visible on the frontal film** because the **left lung base may appear opaque** (Fig. 2-2).
      - Such underpenetration could either **mimic** or **hide** true disease in the left lower lung field (e.g., left lower lobe pneumonia or left pleural effusion).
    - **Solution**
      - Look at the lateral chest radiograph to confirm the presence of disease at the left base (see "The Lateral Chest" in this chapter).

- Second, the **pulmonary markings, i.e., the blood vessels in the lung, may appear more prominent** than they really are.
  - You may mistakenly think the patient is in congestive heart failure or has pulmonary fibrosis.
  - **Solutions**
    - Look for other radiologic signs of congestive heart failure (Chapter 11).
    - Look at the lateral chest film to confirm the presence of increased markings you suspected from the frontal radiograph.
- **Pitfall of overpenetration**
  - If the study is **overpenetrated** (too dark), the **lung markings may seem decreased or absent** (Fig. 2-3).
    - You could mistakenly think the patient has emphysema or a pneumothorax, or the degree of

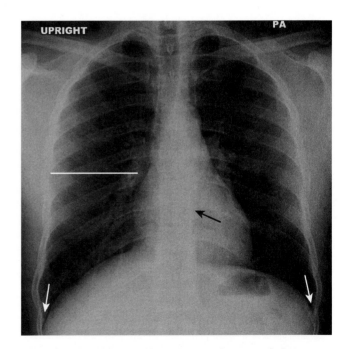

Figure 2-1. **Well-exposed frontal view of a normal chest.** *Notice how the spine (closed black arrow) is just visible through the heart shadow. Both the right and left lateral costophrenic angles are sharply and acutely angled (closed white arrows). The white line demarcates the approximate level of the minor or horizontal fissure. There is no minor fissure on the left side. The major or oblique fissures are oriented in a diagonal plane such that they are generally not visible on the frontal radiograph.*

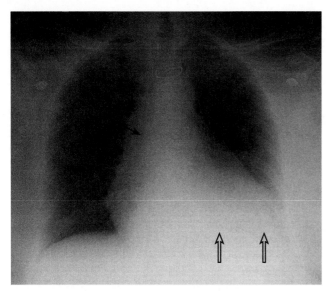

*Figure 2-2. **Underpenetrated frontal chest radiograph.** The spine (closed black arrow) is not visible through the cardiac shadow. The left hemidiaphragm is also not visible (open black arrows) and the degree of underpenetration makes it impossible to differentiate between actual disease at the left base versus nonvisualization of the left hemidiaphragm from underpenetration. A lateral radiograph of the chest would help to differentiate between artifact of technique and true disease.*

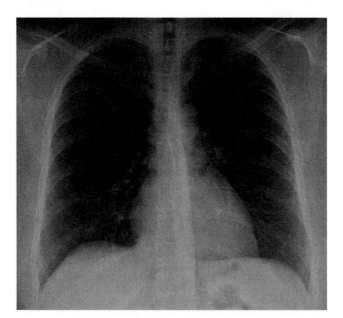

*Figure 2-3. **Overpenetrated frontal chest radiograph.** The overpenetration makes lung markings difficult to see, mimicking some of the findings in emphysema or possibly suggesting a pneumothorax. How lucent (dark) the lungs appear on a radiograph is a poor way of evaluating for the presence of emphysema because of artifacts introduced by technique. In emphysema, the lungs are frequently hyperinflated and the diaphragm flattened (see Chapter 14). In order to diagnose a pneumothorax, you should see the pleural white line (see Chapter 9).*

overpenetration could render findings like a pulmonary nodule almost invisible.
- **Solutions**
  - Look for other radiographic signs of emphysema (Chapter 14) or pneumothorax (Chapter 9).
  - Ask the radiologist if the film should be repeated.

Inspiration
- A full inspiration ensures a reproducible radiograph from one time to the next and eliminates artifacts that may be confused for, or obscure, disease.
  - The **degree of inspiration can be assessed by counting the number of posterior ribs visible** above the diaphragm on the frontal chest radiograph.
    - To help in differentiating the **anterior** from the **posterior ribs,** consult Box 2-1.
  - **If 10 posterior ribs are visible, it is an excellent inspiration** (Fig. 2-4).
  - In many **hospitalized patients, visualization of eight to nine posterior ribs** signals a degree of inspiration **adequate** for accurate interpretation of the image.
- **Pitfall: Poor inspiration**
  - A **poor inspiratory effort will compress and crowd the lung markings,** especially at the bases of the lungs near the diaphragm (Fig. 2-5).
  - This may lead you to mistakenly think the study shows lower lobe pneumonia.
    - **Solution**
      - Look at the lateral chest radiograph to confirm the presence of pneumonia (see "The Lateral Chest" in this chapter and Chapter 8).

Rotation
- **Significant rotation** (the patient turns the body to one side or the other) **may alter the expected contours of the heart and great vessels, the hila, and hemidiaphragms.**
- The easiest way to assess whether the patient is rotated toward the left or right is by studying **the position of the medial ends of each clavicle relative to the spinous process** of the thoracic vertebral body between the clavicles (Fig. 2-6).

Box 2-1

Differentiating Between Anterior and Posterior Ribs

Posterior ribs are immediately more apparent to the eye on frontal chest radiographs.

The posterior ribs are oriented more or less horizontally.

Each pair of posterior ribs attaches to a thoracic vertebral body.

Anterior ribs are visible—but are more difficult to see—on the frontal chest radiograph.

Anterior ribs are oriented downward toward the feet.

Anterior ribs attach to the sternum or each other with cartilage that is usually not visible until later in life when the cartilage may calcify.

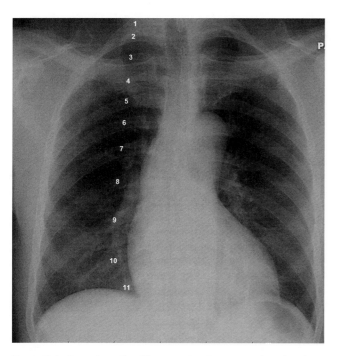

Figure 2-4. **Counting ribs.** *The posterior ribs are numbered in this photograph. Ten posterior ribs are visible above the right hemidiaphragm, an excellent inspiration. In most hospitalized patients, eight to nine visible posterior ribs in the frontal projection is an inspiration that is adequate for accurate interpretation of the image. When counting ribs, make sure you don't miss counting the second posterior rib, which frequently overlaps the first rib.*

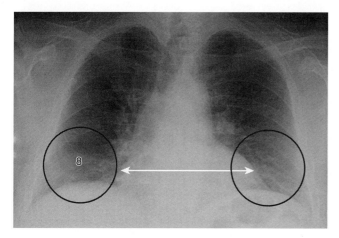

Figure 2-5. **Poor inspiration.** *Only eight posterior ribs are visible on this frontal chest radiograph. A poor inspiration may "crowd" and therefore accentuate the lung markings at the bases (black circles) and will make the heart seem larger than it actually is (white double arrow). The crowded lung markings may mimic the appearance of aspiration or pneumonia. A lateral chest radiograph should help in eliminating the possibility, or confirming the presence, of basilar airspace disease suspected from the frontal radiograph.*

- The **medial ends of the clavicles are anterior structures.**
- The **spinous process is a posterior structure.**
- On the frontal chest radiograph, **if the spinous process appears to lie equidistant from the**

medial ends of each clavicle, there is no rotation (Fig. 2-7A).
- If the spinous process appears **closer to the medial end of the left clavicle,** the patient is **rotated toward his own right side** (Fig. 2-7B).
- If the spinous process appears **closer to the medial end of the right clavicle,** the patient is **rotated toward his own left side** (Fig. 2-7C).
- These relationships hold true regardless of whether the patient was facing the x-ray tube or facing the cassette at the time of exposure.
- **Pitfalls of excessive rotation**
  - Even minor degrees of rotation can distort the normal anatomic appearance of the heart and great vessels, the hila, and hemidiaphragms.
  - **Marked rotation can introduce errors in interpretation:**
    - **The hilum may appear larger** on the side rotated farther away from the imaging cassette because objects farther from the imaging cassette tend to be more magnified than objects closer to the cassette.
      - **Solutions**
        - **Look at the hilum on the lateral chest view** to see if that view confirms hilar enlargement (see "The Hilum" in this chapter).
        - Compare the current study to a previous study of the same patient to assess for change.
    - There may be a distorted appearance of the normal contours of the heart and hila.
    - The **hemidiaphragm may appear higher** on the side rotated away from the imaging cassette (Fig. 2-8).
      - **Solution**
        - Compare the current study to a previous study of the same patient.

Magnification
- Depending on the position of the patient relative to the imaging cassette, magnification can play a role in assessing the size of the heart.
- **The closer any object is to the surface on which it is being imaged, the more true to its actual size the resultant image will be.**
  - As a corollary, **the farther any object is from the surface on which it is being imaged, the more magnified that object will appear.**
- In the standard *PA* chest radiograph, i.e., one obtained in the **posteroanterior projection,** the **heart, being an anterior structure, is closer** to the imaging surface and thus **truer to its actual size.**
  - In a PA study, the x-ray beam enters at "P" (posterior) and exits at "A" (anterior).
    - The **standard frontal chest radiograph is** usually a **PA** exposure.
- In an *AP* image, i.e., one obtained in the **anteroposterior projection,** the **heart is farther** from the imaging cassette and is therefore **slightly magnified.**

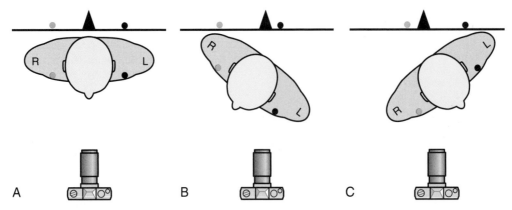

Figure 2-6. **How to determine if the patient is rotated.** In **A**, the patient is not rotated and the medial ends of the right (orange dot) and left (black dot) clavicles are projected on the radiograph (black line) equidistant from the spinous process (black triangle). In **B**, the patient is rotated toward his own right. Notice how the medial end of the left clavicle (black dot) is projected closer to the spinous process than is the medial end of the right clavicle (orange dot). In **C**, the patient is rotated toward his own left. The medial end of the right clavicle (orange dot) is projected closer to the spinous process than is the medial end of the left clavicle (black dot). The camera icon depicts this as an AP projection, but the same relationships would be true for a PA projection as well. Figure 2-7 shows how this applies to radiographs.

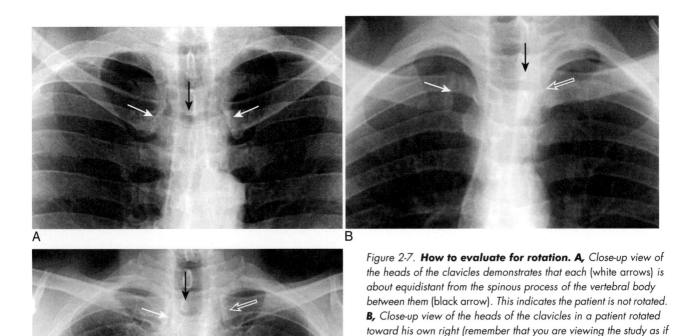

Figure 2-7. **How to evaluate for rotation. A,** Close-up view of the heads of the clavicles demonstrates that each (white arrows) is about equidistant from the spinous process of the vertebral body between them (black arrow). This indicates the patient is not rotated. **B,** Close-up view of the heads of the clavicles in a patient rotated toward his own right (remember that you are viewing the study as if the patient were facing you). The spinous process (black arrow) is much closer to the left clavicular head (open white arrow) than it is to the right clavicular head (closed white arrow). **C,** Close-up view of the heads of the clavicles in a patient rotated toward his own left. The spinous process (black arrow) is much closer to the right clavicular head (closed white arrow) than it is to the left (open white arrow).

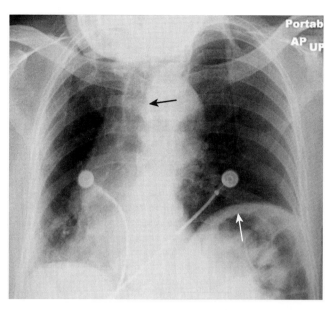

Figure 2-8. **Distorted appearance due to severe rotation.**
Frontal chest radiograph of a patient markedly rotated toward her own right. Notice how the left hemidiaphragm, being farther from the cassette than the right hemidiaphragm because of the rotation, appears higher than it normally would (closed white arrow). The heart and the trachea (closed black arrow) appear displaced into the right hemithorax because of the rotation.

- In an AP study, the x-ray beam enters at "A" (anterior) and exits at "P" (posterior).
  - **Portable, bedside chest radiographs are almost always AP.**
- Therefore, **the heart will appear slightly larger on an AP image,** like a portable chest study, **than will the same heart on a PA image,** the standard chest radiograph in the department (Fig. 2-9).
- There's another reason the heart looks larger on a portable AP chest image than a standard PA chest radiograph:
  - The **distance between the x-ray tube and the patient is shorter when a portable AP image is obtained** (about 40 inches) **than when a standard PA chest radiograph** is exposed (taken by convention at 72 inches).
  - The greater the distance the x-ray source is from the patient, the less the degree of magnification.
- **To learn how to determine if the heart is really enlarged on an AP chest radiograph, see Chapter 3.**

Angulation

- Normally, the x-ray beam passes **horizontally (parallel to the floor) for an erect chest** study and, with the patient upright, the **plane of the thorax is perpendicular** to the x-ray beam.
- **Hospitalized patients,** in particular, may not be able to sit completely upright in bed so that **the x-ray beam may enter the thorax with the patient's head and thorax tilted backward.**
  - This **has the effect of angling the x-ray beam toward the patient's head,** and the image so obtained is called an *apical lordotic view* of the chest.
  - On apical lordotic views, **anterior structures in the chest** (such as the clavicles) are projected **higher** on the radiograph **than posterior structures** in the chest, which are projected lower (Fig. 2-10).
- **Pitfall of excessive angulation**
  - You can recognize an apical lordotic chest study when you see the **clavicles project at or above the posterior first ribs on the frontal image** (Fig. 2-11).

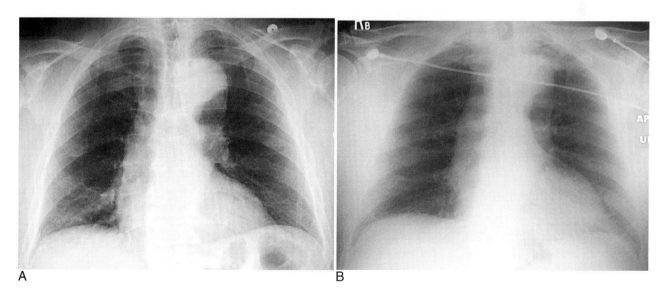

A   B

Figure 2-9. **Effect of positioning on magnification of the heart.** *Frontal chest radiograph done in the PA projection (A) shows the heart to be slightly smaller than in B, which is the same patient's chest exposed minutes earlier in the AP projection. Because the heart lies anteriorly in the chest, it is closer to the imaging surface in A and is therefore magnified less than in B, in which the heart is slightly farther from the imaging surface. In actual practice, there is very little difference in the heart size between an AP and PA exposure so long as the patient has taken an equal inspiration on both.*

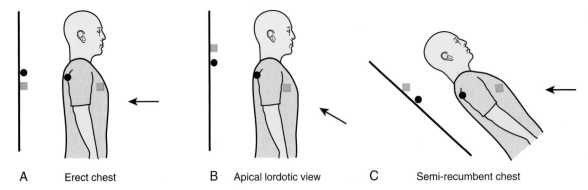

A   Erect chest   B   Apical lordotic view   C   Semi-recumbent chest

Figure 2-10. **Diagram of apical lordotic effect.** *In* **A,** *the x-ray beam (black arrow) is correctly oriented perpendicular to the plane of the cassette (black line). The orange square symbolizes an anterior structure (like the clavicles) and the black circle a posterior structure (like the spine). In* **B,** *the x-ray beam is angled upward, which is the manner in which an apical lordotic view of the chest is obtained. The x-ray beam is no longer perpendicular to the cassette, which has the effect of projecting anterior structures higher on the radiograph than posterior structures. The position of the x-ray beam and patient in* **C** *leads to the exact same end result as* **B** *and is how semirecumbent, bedside studies are frequently obtained on patients who are not able to sit or stand upright. Anterior structures in* **C** *are projected higher than posterior structures.*

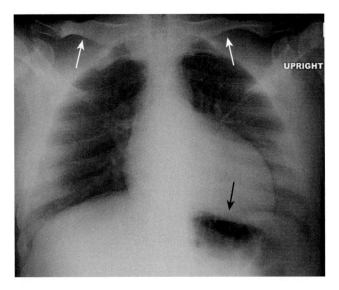

Figure 2-11. **Apical lordotic chest radiograph.** *An apical lordotic view of the chest is now most frequently obtained inadvertently in patients who are semirecumbent at the time of the study. Notice how the clavicles are projected above the first ribs and their usual "S" shape is now straight (closed white arrows). The lordotic view also distorts the shape of the heart and produces spurious obscuration of the left hemidiaphragm (closed black arrow). Unless the artifacts of technique are understood, these findings could be mistaken for disease that doesn't exist.*

Table 2-1

WHAT DEFINES A TECHNICALLY ADEQUATE CHEST RADIOGRAPH?

Factor	What You Should See
Penetration	Should be able to see spine through the heart
Inspiration	Should see at least eight to nine posterior ribs
Rotation	Spinous process should fall equidistant between the medial ends of the clavicles
Magnification	AP films (mostly portable chest x-rays) will magnify the heart slightly
Angulation	Clavicle normally has an "S" shape and superimposes on the third or fourth rib

- An apical lordotic view distorts the appearance of the clavicles, making their normal "S" shape appear straightened.
- Apical lordotic views may also distort the appearance of other structures in the thorax.
  - The **heart may have an unusual shape,** which sometimes mimics cardiomegaly or gives the appearance of a heart with an enlarged left atrium.

- The **sharp border of the left hemidiaphragm may be lost,** which could be mistaken as a sign of a left pleural effusion or left lower lobe pneumonia.
- **Solutions**
  - Know how to recognize technical artifacts and understand how they can distort normal anatomy (Table 2-1).
  - Consult with a radiologist about confusing images.

The Lateral Chest Radiograph

- As part of the standard two-view chest examination, patients usually have an upright PA frontal chest radiograph and an erect, left lateral view of the chest.
- A **left lateral chest x-ray** (the patient's left side is against the cassette) is of **great diagnostic value** but is **frequently ignored by beginners** because of their lack of familiarity with the findings that can be seen in that projection.

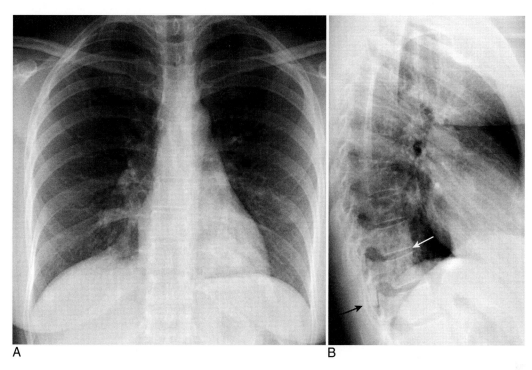

A   B

Figure 2-12. **The spine sign.** *Frontal **(A)** and lateral **(B)** views of the chest demonstrate airspace disease on the lateral film **(B)** in the left lower lobe that may not be immediately apparent on the frontal film (look closely at **A** and you can see the pneumonia in the left lower lobe behind the heart). Normally, the thoracic spine appears to get "blacker" as you view it from the neck to the diaphragm because there is less dense tissue for the x-ray beam to traverse just above the diaphragm than in the region of the shoulder girdle (see also Fig. 2-13). In this case, a left lower lobe pneumonia superimposed on the lower spine in the lateral view (closed white arrow) makes the spine appear "whiter" (more dense) just above the diaphragm. This is called the **spine sign.** Note that on a well-positioned lateral projection, the right and left posterior ribs almost superimpose on each other (closed black arrow), a sign of a true lateral.*

- **Why look at the lateral chest?**
  - It can help you determine the **location** of disease you already identified as being present on the frontal image (see Fig. 1-1).
  - It can **confirm the presence of disease** you may be unsure of on the basis of the frontal image alone, such as a mass or pneumonia.
  - It can **demonstrate disease not visible on the frontal image** (Fig. 2-12).
- **Five key areas to look for on the lateral chest x-ray** (Fig. 2-13 and Table 2-2):
  - **The retrosternal clear space**
  - **The hilar region**
  - **The fissures**
  - **The thoracic spine**
  - **The diaphragm and posterior costophrenic sulci**

THE RETROSTERNAL CLEAR SPACE
- Normally, there is a relatively lucent crescent just behind the sternum and anterior to the shadow of the ascending aorta.
  - **Look for this clear space to "fill in"** with soft tissue density when there is an **anterior mediastinal mass** present (Fig. 2-14).
  - Be careful not to mistake the soft tissue of the patient's superimposed arms for "filling in" of the clear space.

- Although patients are asked to hold their arms over their head for a lateral chest exposure, many are too weak to raise their arms.
- You should be able to identify the patient's arm by spotting the humerus (Fig. 2-15).

THE HILAR REGION
- Normally, it is difficult to identify the hila as discrete structures on the lateral view.
- When there is a hilar mass, such as would occur with enlargement of hilar lymph nodes, the hilum (or hila) will cast a distinct, mass-like shadow on the lateral radiograph (Fig. 2-16).

THE FISSURES
- On the **lateral film**, both the **major (oblique) and minor (horizontal) fissures may be visible** as fine white lines (about as thick as a line made with the point of a sharpened pencil).
  - The **major fissures** course obliquely, roughly **from the level of the fifth thoracic vertebra to** a point on the diaphragm **a few centimeters behind the sternum.**
  - The **minor fissure lies at the level of the fourth anterior rib** on the right side only and is **horizontally** oriented (see Fig. 2-13).
  - Both the major and minor fissures may be visible on the lateral view but because of the oblique plane of the major

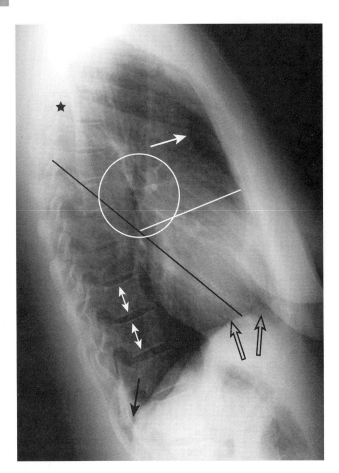

Figure 2-13. **Normal left lateral chest radiograph.** There is a clear space behind the sternum (closed white arrow). The hila produce no discrete shadow (white circle). The vertebral bodies are approximately of equal height and their end plates are parallel to each other (double white arrows). The posterior costophrenic angles (closed black arrow) are sharp. Notice how the thoracic spine appears to become blacker (darker) from the shoulder girdle (black star) to the diaphragm because there is less dense tissue for the x-ray beam to traverse at the level of the diaphragm. The heart normally touches the anterior aspect of the left hemidiaphragm and usually obscures (silhouettes) it. The right hemidiaphragm is frequently seen from the back all the way to the sternum (open black arrows) because it is not obscured by the heart. Notice the normal space posterior to the heart and anterior to the spine; this will be important in assessing cardiomegaly (Chapter 3). The black line represents the approximate location of the major or oblique fissure; the white line is the approximate location of the minor or horizontal fissure.

Table 2-2

THE LATERAL CHEST—A QUICK GUIDE OF WHAT TO LOOK FOR	
Region	**What You Should See**
Retrosternal clear space	Lucent crescent between sternum and ascending aorta
Hilar region	No discrete mass present
Fissures	Major and minor fissures should be pencil point–thin, if visible at all
Thoracic spine	Rectangular vertebral bodies with parallel end plates; disk spaces maintain height from top to bottom of thoracic spine
Diaphragm and posterior costophrenic sulci	Right hemidiaphragm slightly higher than left; sharp posterior costophrenic sulci

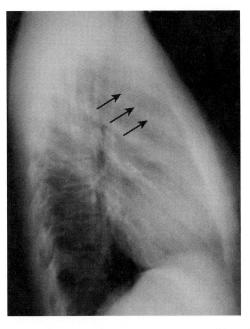

Figure 2-14. **Anterior mediastinal adenopathy.** Left lateral view of the chest demonstrates soft tissue filling in the normal clear space behind the sternum (closed black arrows). This represents anterior mediastinal lymphadenopathy in a patient with lymphoma. Adenopathy is probably the most frequent reason the retrosternal clear space is obscured. Thymoma, teratoma, and substernal thyroid enlargement also can produce anterior mediastinal masses but do not usually produce exactly this appearance.

fissure, **only the minor fissure is usually visible on the frontal view.**

- The fissures help demarcate the upper and lower lobes on the left and the upper, middle, and lower lobes on the right.
- **When a fissure contains fluid or develops fibrosis from a chronic process, it will become thickened** such that it will be thicker than a line that can be drawn with the point of a sharpened pencil (Fig. 2-17).
  - **Thickening of the fissure by fluid is almost always associated with other signs of fluid in the chest,** such as Kerley B lines and pleural effusions (see Chapter 11).
  - **Thickening of the fissure by fibrosis** is the more likely cause if there are **no other signs of fluid in the chest.**

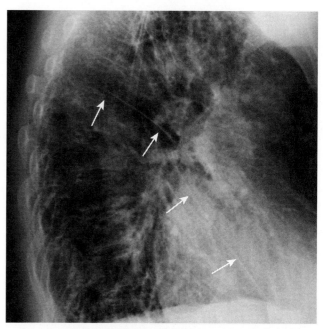

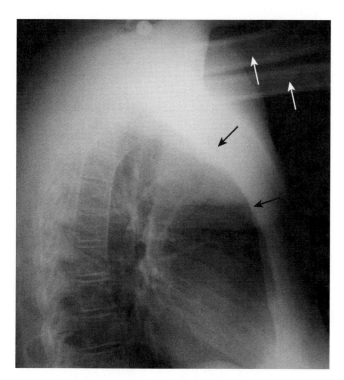

Figure 2-15. **Arms obscure retrosternal clear space.** In this example, the patient was not able to hold her arms over her head for the lateral chest examination, as patients are instructed to do in order to eliminate the shadows of the arms from overlapping the lateral chest. The humeri are clearly visible (closed white arrows) so even though the soft tissue of the patient's arms appears to fill in the retrosternal clear space (closed black arrows), this should not be mistaken for an abnormality such as anterior mediastinal adenopathy (see Fig. 2-14).

Figure 2-17. **Fluid in the major fissures.** Left lateral view of the chest shows thickening of both the right and left major fissures (closed white arrows). This patient was in congestive heart failure and this thickening represents fluid in the fissures. Normally, the fissures are either invisible or, if visible, they are fine, white lines of uniform thickness no larger than a line made with the point of a sharpened pencil. The major or oblique fissure runs from the level of the fifth thoracic vertebral body to a point on the anterior diaphragm about 2 cm behind the sternum. Notice the increased interstitial markings that are visible throughout the lungs and are due to fluid in the interstitial tissues of the lung.

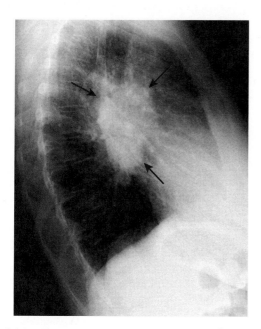

Figure 2-16. **Hilar mass on lateral radiograph.** Left lateral view of the chest shows a discrete mass in the region of the hila (closed black arrows). Normally, the hila do not cast a shadow that is easily detectable on the lateral projection. This patient had bilateral hilar adenopathy from sarcoidosis but any cause of hilar adenopathy or a mass in the hilum would have a similar appearance.

THE THORACIC SPINE

- Normally, the **thoracic vertebral bodies are** somewhat **rectangular** and **each** vertebral body's **end plate parallels the end plate of the vertebral body above and below it.**
- **Each intervertebral disk space becomes slightly taller than or remains about the same height as the one above it** throughout the thoracic spine.
- Degeneration of the disk can lead to narrowing of the disk space and the development of small, bony spurs (osteophytes) at the margins of the vertebral bodies.
- When there is a compression fracture, most often from osteoporosis, the vertebral body loses height.
  - Compression fractures very commonly involve depression of the superior end plate of the vertebral body (Fig. 2-18).
- **Don't forget to look at the thoracic spine when studying the lateral chest radiograph** for valuable clues about systemic disorders (see Chapter 24).

THE DIAPHRAGM AND POSTERIOR COSTOPHRENIC SULCI

- Because the diaphragm is composed of soft tissue (muscle) and has soft tissue structures below it, only the upper border of the diaphragm, abutting air-filled lung, is usually visible on conventional radiographs.

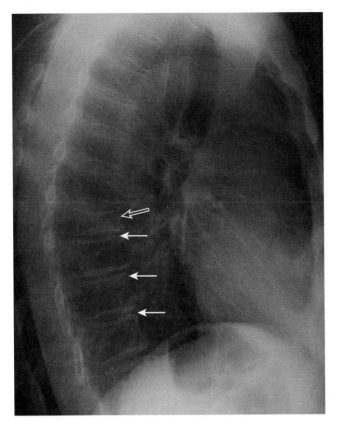

Figure 2-18. **Osteoporotic compression fracture and degenerative disk disease.** *Don't forget to look at the thoracic spine when studying the lateral chest radiograph for valuable information about a host of systemic diseases (see Chapter 24). In this study, there is loss of stature of the eighth thoracic vertebral body due to osteoporosis (open white arrow). Compression fractures frequently involve the superior end plate first. There are small osteophytes present at multiple levels from degenerative disk disease (closed white arrows).*

- Even though we have one diaphragm that separates the thorax from the abdomen, we do not normally see the entire diaphragm from side to side on conventional radiographs.
    - Therefore, we refer to the right half of the diaphragm as the **right hemidiaphragm** and the left half of the diaphragm as the **left hemidiaphragm.**
- **How to tell the right from the left hemidiaphragm on the lateral radiograph:**
    - The **right hemidiaphragm is usually visible for its entire length from front to back.**
    - The **left hemidiaphragm** is seen sharply posteriorly but **is silhouetted by the muscle of the heart anteriorly** (i.e., its edge disappears anteriorly) (Fig. 2-19).
    - **Air in the stomach or splenic flexure appears immediately below the left hemidiaphragm.**
        - The liver lies below the right hemidiaphragm and bowel gas is usually not seen between the liver and the right hemidiaphragm.
    - Normally, the **right hemidiaphragm is slightly higher than the left,** a relationship that tends to hold true on the lateral radiograph as well as the frontal.

- **The posterior costophrenic angles (posterior costophrenic sulci)**
    - Each hemidiaphragm produces a rounded dome that indents the central portion of the base of each lung, like the bottom of a wine bottle.
        - This produces a depression or **sulcus** that surrounds the periphery of each lung and represents the lowest point of the pleural space when the patient is upright.
    - On the conventional frontal chest radiograph, this sulcus is viewed in profile most easily at the outer edge of the lung as the **lateral costophrenic sulcus** (also called the *lateral costophrenic angle*) and on the lateral radiograph as the **posterior costophrenic sulcus** (also known as the *posterior costophrenic angle*) (see Figs. 2-1 and 2-13).
    - **Normally,** all of the **costophrenic sulci are sharp and acutely angled.**
    - When the patient is upright and there is pleural fluid present, the fluid accumulates in the deep recesses of the costophrenic sulci, filling in their acute angles.
        - This is called **blunting of the costophrenic angles** (see Chapter 7).

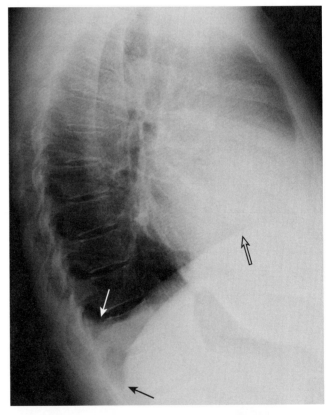

Figure 2-19. **Blunting of the posterior costophrenic sulcus by a small pleural effusion.** *Left lateral view of the chest shows fluid blunting the posterior costophrenic sulcus (closed white arrow). The other posterior costophrenic angle (closed black arrow) is sharp. The pleural effusion is on the right side because the hemidiaphragm involved can be traced anteriorly farther forward (open black arrow) than the other hemidiaphragm (the left), which is normally silhouetted by the heart and not visible anteriorly.*

- It takes only about **75 mL** of fluid (or less) to **blunt the posterior costophrenic angle** on the lateral film, but it takes about **250 to 300 mL** to **blunt the lateral costophrenic angles** on the frontal film (see Fig. 2-19).

WebLink
More information on how to recognize a technically adequate chest radiograph is available to registered users on StudentConsult.com.

TAKE-HOME POINTS: Recognizing a Technically Adequate Chest Radiograph

There are five parameters that define an adequate chest examination, and recognition of them is important to accurately differentiate abnormalities from technically produced artifacts.

If the chest is adequately penetrated, you should be able to see spine through the heart. Underpenetrated (too light) studies obscure the left lung base and tend to spuriously accentuate the lung markings; overpenetrated studies (too dark) may mimic emphysema or pneumothorax.

If the patient has taken an adequate inspiration, you should see at least eight to nine posterior ribs above the diaphragm; poor inspiratory efforts may mimic basilar lung disease and may make the heart appear larger.

The spinous process should fall equidistant between the medial ends of the clavicles to indicate the patient is not rotated; rotation can introduce numerous artifactual anomalies affecting the contour of the heart and the appearance of the hila and diaphragm.

AP films (mostly portable chest x-rays) will magnify the heart slightly compared to the standard PA chest radiograph (usually done in the radiology department).

Frontal images of the chest obtained with the patient semi-upright in bed (tilted backwards) may produce apical lordotic images that distort normal anatomy.

The lateral chest radiograph can provide invaluable information and should always be studied when available.

Five key areas to examine on the lateral chest radiograph are the retrosternal clear space, the hilar regions, the major and minor fissures, the thoracic spine, and the diaphragm including the posterior costophrenic sulci.

3 Recognizing Cardiomegaly

The Cardiothoracic Ratio

- Estimating the size of the heart is one of the simplest assessments to make on a frontal chest radiograph.
- You can make this evaluation using the *cardiothoracic ratio*, which is a measurement of the **widest transverse diameter of the heart** compared to the **widest internal diameter of the rib cage** (from inside of rib to inside of rib) on the frontal chest radiograph (Fig. 3-1).
  - The widest internal diameter of the rib cage usually is found at the level of the diaphragm.
  - **In most normal adults at full inspiration, the cardiothoracic ratio is less than 50%.**
    - That is, **the size of the heart is usually less than half of the internal diameter of the thoracic rib cage.**
- Although the cardiothoracic ratio provides a handy way of assessing heart size, it does have its pitfalls.

Extracardiac Causes of Apparent Cardiac Enlargement

- **Sometimes,** the cardiothoracic ratio can be greater than 50%, **but the heart itself may actually be normal.**
- This occurs when there is an *extracardiac* cause of apparent cardiac enlargement (Table 3-1).
  - **The most common cause of apparent cardiomegaly is the portable anteroposterior (AP) supine chest radiograph,** usually performed at the bedside (see Chapter 2).
    - A combination of magnification, rotation, and a poor inspiratory effort in very ill patients may make the heart appear larger than it really is.
  - Other causes of apparent cardiomegaly are conditions that **inhibit the patient's ability to take a deep inspiration** at the time of the chest exposure. These conditions include:
  - **Obesity**
  - **Pregnancy**
  - **Massive ascites**
  - Other causes of spurious cardiomegaly are **chest wall abnormalities** in which the **heart may be compressed** between the sternum and the spine, making the heart appear larger than it actually is. These conditions include:
  - **Straight back syndrome**
    - Loss of the normal kyphosis of the thoracic spine and a decreased distance between the sternum and thoracic spine can produce apparent cardiomegaly and has been called *straight back syndrome.*
  - **Pectus excavatum deformity**
    - Sometimes a congenital deformity of the lowermost section of the sternum causes it to bow inward and compress the heart against the thoracic spine (Fig. 3-2).

- **Rotation** of the patient, especially toward the patient's left, may make the heart appear larger than it actually is (see Chapter 2).
- Finally, what looks like an enlarged heart may, in fact, represent enlargement of the *cardiac silhouette* caused by the **accumulation of fluid in the pericardial sac** *(pericardial effusion).*
  - On conventional radiographs, pericardial fluid has the same radiographic density as the muscle of the heart and its contained blood.

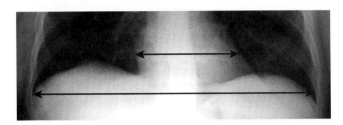

Figure 3-1. **The cardiothoracic ratio.** To estimate the cardiothoracic ratio, the widest diameter of the heart (upper double arrow) is compared to the widest internal diameter of the thoracic cage (inside of rib to inside of rib) (lower double arrow). The widest internal diameter of the thorax is usually at the level of the diaphragm. The cardiothoracic ratio should be less than 50% in most normal adults on a standard PA frontal radiograph taken with an adequate inspiration (nine posterior ribs).

Table 3-1

EXTRACARDIAC CAUSES OF APPARENT CARDIOMEGALY	
Cause	**Reason for Enlarged Appearance**
AP portable supine chest	Magnification due to AP projection
Obesity, pregnancy, ascites	Conditions prevent an adequate inspiration
Straight back syndrome, pectus excavatum deformity	Heart is compressed between the sternum and the spine
Rotation	Especially when it occurs to the patient's left, rotation may make the heart appear larger
Pericardial effusion	Other imaging modalities (most commonly ultrasound) or electrocardiographic findings will help to identify pericardial fluid

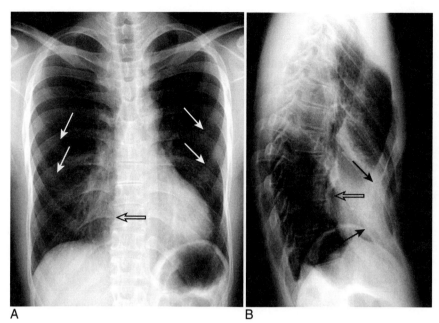

Figure 3-2. **Pectus excavatum deformity.**
Clues to the presence of a pectus excavatum deformity on the frontal radiograph (A) include a greater than usual downward orientation of the anterior ribs (closed white arrows) and displacement of the right heart border such that it no longer extends to the right beyond the thoracic spine (open black arrow). In the lateral projection (B), it's clear that the lower sternal segments are bowed inward, compressing the heart between the sternum (closed black arrows) and the thoracic spine (open black arrow). As a result, the heart appears spuriously enlarged in the frontal projection.

- **Differentiating cardiomegaly from pericardial effusion,** in which the heart may actually be normal in size, **frequently requires** the use of modalities besides conventional radiographs, most commonly **ultrasound** (see Chapter 10).

Effect of Projection and Inspiration on Perception of Heart Size
- **Effect of projection on apparent heart size**
  - The **heart resides anteriorly in the chest.**
  - On a **PA (posteroanterior) chest radiograph** (the standard frontal chest study in which the x-ray beam enters posteriorly and exits anteriorly where the cassette is positioned), **the heart appears truer to its actual size** because it is near the imaging surface.
  - On an **AP (anteroposterior) chest film** (the usual bedside, portable chest radiograph in which the x-ray beam enters anteriorly and exits posteriorly where the cassette is positioned), **the heart is slightly magnified** because it is farther from the imaging surface.
  - Therefore, **the heart will appear slightly larger on an AP chest radiograph** (e.g., a portable chest) **than will the same heart on a PA chest radiograph** (the standard chest x-ray in the department) (see Fig. 2-9).
- **Identifying cardiac enlargement on an AP chest radiograph**
  - So, you may ask, how do you estimate the size of the heart on a portable chest radiograph (Table 3-2)?
  - If the **left heart border is touching the left lateral chest wall,** the heart **is enlarged.**
  - If the **left heart border is very close to the left chest wall,** the heart is **probably enlarged.**
  - If the **heart is borderline enlarged on a portable AP film,** it is probably **normal** in size.

Table 3-2

RECOGNIZING CARDIOMEGALY ON AN AP CHEST RADIOGRAPH	
Heart Appearance On AP Study	**Likely Heart Size**
Borderline enlarged	Normal size
Significantly enlarged	Enlarged
Touching, or almost touching, the left lateral chest wall	Definitely enlarged

- In actual practice, there is usually **little difference in the size of the heart between a well-inspired AP versus a well-inspired PA chest radiograph.**
- The **degree of inspiration has a larger effect on the apparent heart size** than does whether the study was done AP versus PA.
- A good rule of thumb: If the heart appears enlarged on a well-inspired, portable chest radiograph, it probably is enlarged.

- **Effect of degree of inspiration on apparent heart size**
  - **In expiration,** the diaphragm moves upward and compresses the heart, making the **heart appear larger** than it would in full inspiration.
  - **Pregnant** patients, those with **ascites,** and **obese** patients **might not be able to take a full inspiration,** thus causing the heart to look larger than it actually is.

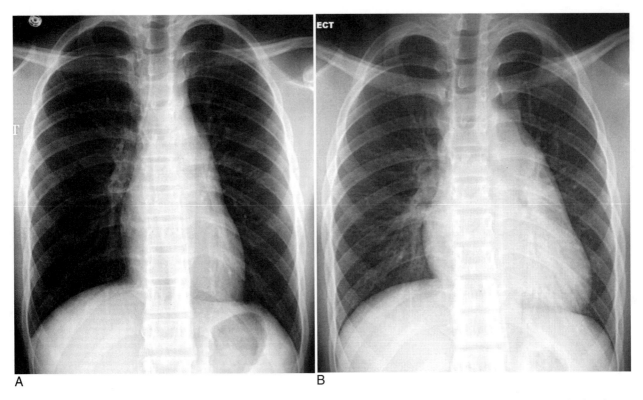

A B

Figure 3-3. **Effect of degree of inspiration on cardiac size.** *Two studies done on the same patient several minutes apart, both with an adequate inspiration, demonstrate how a difference of even one interspace can change the apparent size of the heart. The exposure in (A) has almost 11 posterior ribs visible, but that in (B) demonstrates about 10 posterior ribs. Even though both of these radiographs are technically acceptable, even a slight change in the degree of inspiration can affect the apparent size of the heart.*

- **If there are eight to nine posterior ribs visible on a frontal chest radiograph, then the inspiration is adequate for interpretation** (Fig. 3-3).
- **Recognizing an enlarged cardiac silhouette on the lateral chest radiograph**
  - Generally speaking, evaluation of cardiac size is best made on the frontal chest radiograph.
  - To evaluate for the presence of enlargement of the cardiac silhouette on the lateral projection, **look at the space posterior to the heart and anterior to the spine at the level of the diaphragm.**
  - In a **normal** person, the **cardiac silhouette will usually not extend posteriorly over the spine** or obliterate the clear space posterior to the heart (see Fig. 2-13).
  - As the **heart enlarges,** whether that enlargement is due to the left or right ventricle, the **posterior border of the heart may extend to, or overlap, the anterior border of the thoracic spine.**

- This is useful as a confirmatory sign of cardiac enlargement first suspected on the frontal projection (Fig. 3-4).
- **Both** pericardial effusions **and** true cardiomegaly **will cause the cardiac silhouette to overlap the spine on the lateral view.**

Recognizing Cardiomegaly in Infants

In newborns and infants, the heart will normally appear larger, relative to the size of the thorax, than it does in adults.

- Whereas a cardiothoracic ratio greater than 50% is considered abnormal in adults, the **cardiothoracic ratio may reach up to 65% in infants and still be normal** (Fig. 3-5).
- Newborns cannot take as deep an inspiration as adults and the relative proportions in size of their abdomen to chest are not the same as for adults.
- **Any assessment of cardiac enlargement in an infant** should **take into account other factors** such as the appearance of the **pulmonary vasculature** and any

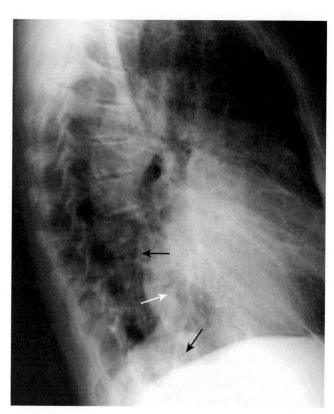

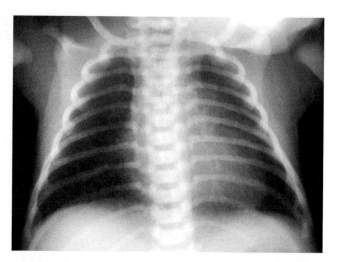

Figure 3-5. **Normal infant chest.** *In the normal infant, the cardiothoracic ratio may be as large as 65% (compared to 50% in adults). Any assessment of cardiac enlargement in an infant should take into account other factors such as the appearance of the pulmonary vasculature and any associated clinical signs or symptoms (such as a murmur, tachycardia, or cyanosis).*

Figure 3-4. **Enlargement of the cardiac silhouette in the lateral projection.** *In most normal patients, the posterior border of the heart does not overlap the thoracic spine. In this patient with cardiomegaly, the posterior border of the heart (closed black arrows) overlaps the anterior border of the spine (closed white arrow). Estimation of cardiac size is best made on the frontal projection but the lateral projection can be used for a confirmatory sign of enlargement of the cardiac silhouette.*

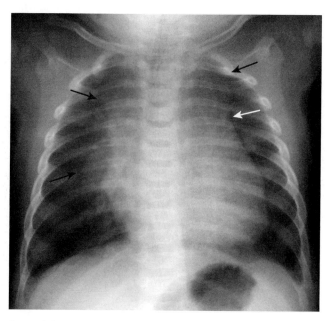

associated clinical signs or symptoms (for example, a murmur, tachycardia, or cyanosis).

- In a child, **the thymus gland may overlap portions of the heart** and thereby present a confusing picture.
  - The **normal thymus** gland **has a somewhat lobulated appearance,** especially where it is indented by the ribs (Fig. 3-6).
- The **normal thymus may be seen** on conventional chest radiographs **up to 3 years of age and sometimes may be seen as late as 8 years of age.**

 WebLink
More information on recognizing cardiomegaly is available to registered users on StudentConsult.com.

Figure 3-6. **Normal thymus gland.** *The thymus gland may overlap the upper portion of the cardiac silhouette and can be mistaken for cardiomegaly in a child. As in this example, the thymus gland is frequently lobulated (closed black arrows) and there may be an indentation on the left side between the heart and the thymus (closed white arrow). Although the thymus gland will usually involute by age 3, it may still be normally visible in children as old as 8 years of age.*

TAKE-HOME POINTS: Recognizing Cardiomegaly

In adults, a quick assessment of heart size can be made using the cardiothoracic ratio, which is the ratio of the widest transverse diameter of the heart compared to the widest internal diameter of the rib cage.

In normal adults, the cardiothoracic ratio is usually less than 50%.

Certain extracardiac causes can make the heart appear to be enlarged, even if it is normal in size.

The extracardiac causes include AP portable studies, factors that inhibit a deep inspiration, abnormalities of the bony thorax, and the presence of a pericardial effusion.

The heart will appear slightly larger on an AP projection than a PA projection of the chest because the heart is closer to the imaging surface on a PA exposure.

Guidelines for estimating the actual heart size on an AP chest examination closely follow the same guidelines as for a PA chest study.

On the lateral projection, the heart usually does extend posteriorly to overlap the spine unless it is enlarged or there is a pericardial effusion.

In an infant, the heart may normally be up to 65% of the cardiothoracic ratio; other factors should be assessed in an infant with apparent cardiomegaly, such as the pulmonary vasculature and the clinical signs and symptoms.

The thymus gland is usually seen in infants superimposed on the upper portion of the cardiac silhouette and can mimic cardiac enlargement.

4 Recognizing Airspace versus Interstitial Lung Disease

Normal Lung Markings
- **Vessels and bronchi—normal lung markings**
  - **Virtually all of the "white lines"** you see in the lungs on a chest radiograph are blood vessels.
    - Blood vessels characteristically branch and taper gradually from the hila centrally to the peripheral margins of the lung.
    - You cannot easily differentiate between pulmonary arteries and pulmonary veins on a conventional radiograph.
  - **Bronchi are mostly invisible** on a normal chest radiograph.
    - That's because they are normally very thin-walled; they contain air and are surrounded by air.

Classifying Lung Disease
- **Diseases** that affect the lung **can be arbitrarily divided into two main categories** based in part on their pathology and in part on the pattern they typically produce on a chest imaging study (Table 4-1):
  - **Airspace (alveolar) disease**
  - **Interstitial (infiltrative) disease**
- Why learn the difference?
  - Although many diseases produce abnormalities that display both patterns, recognition of these patterns frequently helps narrow the disease possibilities so that you can form a reasonable differential diagnosis.

Characteristics of Airspace Disease
- Airspace disease characteristically produces opacities in the lung which can be described as **fluffy, cloudlike, or hazy** (Fig. 4-1).
- These fluffy opacities tend to be **confluent,** meaning they blend into one another with imperceptible margins.
- The **margins of airspace disease are indistinct,** meaning it is frequently difficult to identify a clear demarcation point between the disease and the adjacent normal lung.
- Airspace disease may be **distributed throughout the lungs,** as in pulmonary edema, **or** it may **appear to be more localized** as in a segmental or lobar pneumonia (Fig. 4-2).
- Airspace disease may contain **air bronchograms.**
  - The **visibility of air in the bronchus because of surrounding airspace disease** is called an *air bronchogram.*
  - An air bronchogram is a **sign of airspace disease.**
    - Remember that bronchi are not usually visible because their walls are very thin, they contain air, and they are surrounded by air.

Table 4-1

CLASSIFICATION OF LUNG DISEASES
Airspace Diseases
Acute
Pneumonia
Pulmonary alveolar edema
Hemorrhage
Aspiration
Near-drowning
Chronic
Bronchoalveolar cell carcinoma
Alveolar cell proteinosis
Sarcoidosis
Lymphoma
Interstitial Diseases
Reticular
Idiopathic pulmonary fibrosis
Pulmonary interstitial edema
Rheumatoid lung
Scleroderma
Sarcoid
Nodular
Bronchogenic carcinoma
Metastases
Silicosis
Miliary tuberculosis
Sarcoid

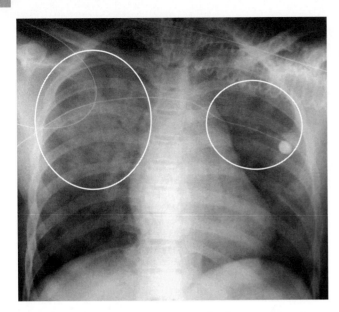

Figure 4-1. **Diffuse airspace disease of pulmonary alveolar edema.** *There are opacities throughout both lungs, primarily involving the upper lobes (white circles), that can be described as fluffy, hazy, or cloudlike and are confluent and poorly marginated, all pointing to airspace disease. This is an typical example of pulmonary alveolar edema (due to a heroin overdose in this patient).*

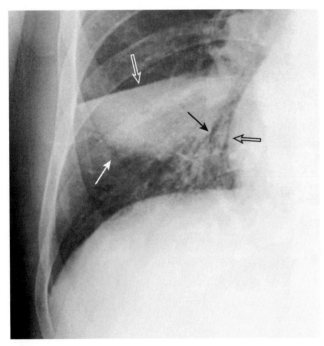

Figure 4-2. **Right middle lobe pneumonia.** *There is an area of increased opacification in the right lower lung field that has indistinct inferior margins (closed white arrow) and several black branching structures that represent air bronchograms (closed black arrow). These findings are consistent with airspace disease. Notice the sharp superior border of the disease (open white arrow), a sign that the airspace disease is abutting the minor fissure and establishing its location in the right middle lobe. The right heart border (open black arrow) is still visible because the disease involves a segment that is not in anatomic contact with the right heart border.*

- When something like fluid or soft tissue replaces the air normally surrounding the bronchus, then the air inside the bronchus becomes visible as **a series of black, branching tubular structures**—this is the ***air bronchogram*** (Fig. 4-3).
  - What can fill the airspaces besides air?
    - **Fluid,** such as occurs in pulmonary edema
    - **Blood,** e.g., pulmonary hemorrhage
    - **Gastric juices,** e.g., aspiration
    - **Inflammatory exudate,** e.g., pneumonia
    - **Water,** e.g., near-drowning
- Airspace disease may demonstrate a ***silhouette sign*** (Fig. 4-4).

  - If two objects **of the same radiographic density touch each other, the edge or margin between them disappears** and it will be impossible to tell where one object begins and the other ends.
  - **Conventional radiography is limited to demonstrating five basic densities** (Table 4-2):
    - **Air,** which appears the blackest on a radiograph
    - **Fat**
    - **Soft tissue or fluid** (because both soft tissue and fluid appear the same on conventional radiographs you can't differentiate between heart muscle and the blood inside the heart on a chest radiograph).
    - **Calcium** (usually contained within bones).
    - **Metal,** which appears the whitest on a radiograph

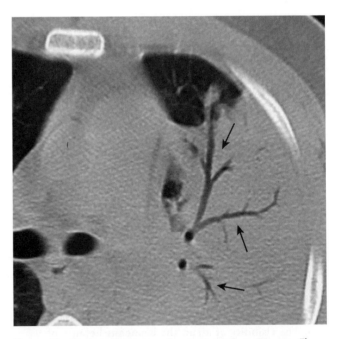

Figure 4-3. **Air bronchograms demonstrated on CT scan.** *There are numerous black, branching structures (closed black arrows) representing air that is now visible inside the bronchi because the surrounding airspaces are filled with inflammatory exudate in this patient with an obstructive pneumonia from a bronchogenic carcinoma. Normally, on conventional radiographs, air inside bronchi is not visible because the bronchial walls are very thin, they contain air, and they are surrounded by air.*

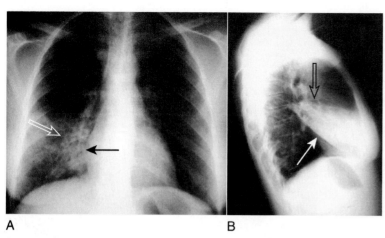

Figure 4-4. **Silhouette sign, right middle lobe pneumonia.** *Fluffy, indistinctly marginated airspace disease is seen (**A**) to the right of the heart (open white arrow), which partially obscures a small margin of the right heart border (closed black arrow). This is called the* **silhouette sign** *and establishes that the disease (1) is in contact with the right heart border (which lies anteriorly in the chest) and (2) that the disease is the same radiographic density as the heart (fluid or soft tissue). Pneumonia fills the airspaces with an inflammatory exudate of fluid density.* **B,** *The area of the consolidation is indeed anterior, located in the right middle lobe, which is bound by the major fissure below (closed white arrow) and the minor fissure above (open black arrow).*

Table 4-2

FIVE BASIC DENSITIES SEEN ON CONVENTIONAL RADIOGRAPHY

Density	Appearance
Air	Absorbs the least x-ray and appears "blackest"
Fat	Gray, somewhat darker (blacker) than soft tissue
Fluid or soft tissue	Both fluid (e.g., blood) and soft tissue (e.g., muscle) have the same density
Calcium	The most dense naturally occurring material (e.g., bones), absorbs most x-rays
Metal	Usually absorbs all x-rays and appears the "whitest" (e.g., barium)

- Objects of metal density do not occur in the body normally.
- Radiologic **contrast media** and **foreign bodies** are **examples of metal densities** artificially placed in the body.
- One of the major values of CT scanning is its ability to *expand the gray scale*, which enables us to differentiate many more than these five basic densities.
- **The silhouette sign is valuable not only in the chest but as an aid in the analysis of imaging studies throughout the body.**
  - Remember: **two conditions** must exist in order **to have** a positive **silhouette sign:**
    - **The two objects** in question **must be in contact** with each other.
    - **They must be the same radiographic density** (e.g., fat and fat, soft tissue and soft tissue).

- The characteristics of airspace disease are summarized in Box 4-1.

Some Causes of Airspace Disease
- Summarized in tabular form are three of the more common acute airspace diseases seen in clinical practice.
- Several characteristics of **pneumonia** (Fig. 4-5) are summarized in Box 4-2 (see also Chapter 8).
- Several characteristics of **acute alveolar pulmonary edema** (Fig. 4-6) are summarized in Box 4-3 (see also Chapter 11).
- Several characteristics of **aspiration** (Fig. 4-7) are summarized in Box 4-4 (see also Chapter 8).

Characteristics of Interstitial Lung Disease
- Sometimes referred to as *infiltrative lung disease,* interstitial lung disease has the following characteristics:
- Interstitial lung disease produces what can be thought of as **discrete "particles" of disease** that develop in the abundant interstitial network of the lung (Fig. 4-8).
  - These "particles" of disease can be further characterized as having **three patterns of presentation:**
    - **Reticular interstitial disease** appears as a network of lines (see Fig. 4-8A).
    - **Nodular interstitial disease** appears as an assortment of dots (see Fig. 4-8B).
    - **Reticulonodular interstitial disease** contains both lines and dots (see Fig. 4-8C).

Box 4-1

Characteristics of Airspace Disease

Opacities in the lung can be described as fluffy, cloudlike, and hazy.

The opacities tend to be confluent, merging into one another.

The margins of airspace disease are fuzzy and indistinct.

Air bronchograms or the silhouette sign may be present.

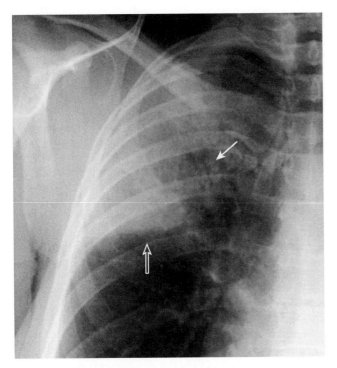

Figure 4-5. Right upper lobe pneumococcal pneumonia. *Close-up view of the right upper lobe demonstrates confluent airspace disease with several air bronchograms (closed white arrow). The inferior margin of the pneumonia is more sharply demarcated because it is in contact with the minor fissure (open white arrow). This patient had* Streptococcus pneumoniae *cultured from the sputum.*

Box 4-2

Pneumonia

About 90% of the time, community-acquired lobar or segmental pneumonia is caused by *Streptococcus pneumoniae* (formerly known as *Diplococcus pneumoniae*).

Pneumonia usually manifests as patchy, segmental, or lobar airspace disease.

Air bronchograms may be seen.

There may be little or no shift of the heart or mediastinal structures (see Chapter 5).

Clearing usually occurs in less than 10 days (pneumococcal pneumonia may clear within 48 hours).

- These "particles" or "packets" of interstitial disease tend to be **inhomogeneous,** separated from each other by visible areas of normal lung.
- The **margins of the "particles" of interstitial lung disease are sharper** than are the margins of airspace disease, whose boundaries tend to be indistinct.

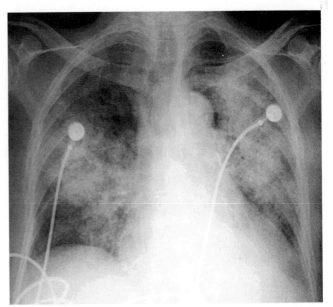

Figure 4-6. Acute pulmonary alveolar edema. *Fluffy, bilateral, perihilar airspace disease with indistinct margins sometimes described as a* **bat-wing** *or* **angel-wing configuration.** *No air bronchograms are present. The heart is enlarged. This represents pulmonary alveolar edema secondary to congestive heart failure.*

Box 4-3

Pulmonary Alveolar Edema

Acute, alveolar pulmonary edema classically produces bilateral, perihilar airspace disease sometimes described as having a **bat-wing** or **angel-wing configuration.**

Edema may be asymmetrical but is usually not unilateral.

Pulmonary edema that is cardiac in origin is frequently associated with pleural effusions and fluid that thickens the major and minor fissures.

Because fluid fills not only the airspaces but the bronchi themselves, there are usually no air bronchograms seen in alveolar pulmonary edema.

Classically, pulmonary edema clears rapidly after treatment (< 48 hours).

- Interstitial lung disease **can be focal** (as in a solitary pulmonary nodule) **or diffusely distributed** in the lungs (Fig. 4-9).
- There are **usually no air bronchograms present,** as there may be with airspace disease.
- **Pitfall:** Sometimes there is so much interstitial disease present that the overlapping "packets" of disease may superimpose and mimic airspace disease on conventional chest radiographs.
- **Solution: Look at the periphery** of such confluent shadows in the lung to help in determining whether they

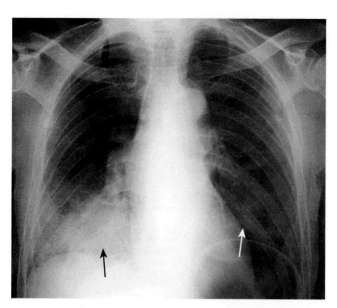

*Figure 4-7. **Aspiration, right and left lower lobes.** An area of opacification in the right lower lobe is fluffy and confluent with indistinct margins characteristic of airspace disease (closed black arrow). To a much lesser extent, there is a similar density in the left lower lobe (closed white arrow). The bibasilar distribution of this disease should raise the suspicion of aspiration as an etiologic factor. This patient had a recent stroke and aspiration was demonstrated on a video swallowing study.*

Box 4-4

Aspiration

Aspiration tends to affect whatever part of the lung is most dependent at the time the patient aspirates, and its manifestations depend on the substance(s) aspirated.

For most bedridden patients, aspiration usually occurs in either the lower lobes or the posterior portions of the upper lobes.

Because of the course and caliber of the right main bronchus, aspiration occurs more often in the right lower lobe than in the left lower lobe.

The material that is aspirated and the presence of infection will determine the radiographic appearance of aspiration and how quickly the airspace disease resolves.

Aspiration of bland (neutralized) gastric juice or water usually clears rapidly within 24 to 48 hours.

Aspiration of undiluted gastric acid (known as ***Mendelson's syndrome***) will produce a chemical pneumonitis or pulmonary edema that may appear very quickly and take days to weeks to clear.

If the aspirate is or becomes infected (usually with anaerobic organisms), the ensuing bacterial pneumonia may cavitate and take weeks or longer to resolve.

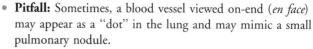

are, in fact, caused by airspace disease or a superimposition of numerous reticular and nodular densities (see Fig. 4-9).

- **Pitfall:** Sometimes, a blood vessel viewed on-end (*en face*) may appear as a "dot" in the lung and may mimic a small pulmonary nodule.
  - **Solutions:** The vessel feeding the vessel seen on-end will produce a "line" leading up to the "dot."
    - A small nodule will produce a "dot" with no such "line" leading into it.
    - A blood vessel viewed as a "dot" on-end in one projection will not appear as a "dot" on-end in the orthogonal view.
    - In other words, a blood vessel producing an on-end "dot" in the frontal view will "disappear" on the lateral view; a nodule will appear as a "dot" on both orthogonal views.
    - The size of a blood vessel viewed on-end will be about equal in size to other blood vessels in that part of the lung; real nodules may appear disproportionately large for the size of the blood vessels that surround them (Fig. 4-10).
- The characteristics of interstitial lung disease are summarized in Box 4-5.

Some Causes of Interstitial Lung Disease

- Summarized in tabular form are several diseases that typically produce an interstitial pattern, divided into those that are predominantly reticular and those that are predominantly nodular.
  - Keep in mind that **many diseases have patterns that overlap and many interstitial lung diseases have mixtures of both nodular and reticular changes (reticulonodular disease).**
- **Predominantly reticular interstitial lung diseases**
  - Several characteristics of **pulmonary interstitial edema** (Fig. 4-11) are summarized in Box 4-6 (see Chapter 11).
  - Several characteristics of **idiopathic pulmonary fibrosis** (Fig. 4-12) are summarized in Box 4-7.
  - Several characteristics of **rheumatoid lung** (Fig. 4-13) are summarized in Box 4-8.
- **Predominantly nodular interstitial lung diseases**
  - Several characteristics of **bronchogenic carcinoma** (Fig. 4-14) are summarized in Box 4-9 (see Chapter 13).
  - Several characteristics of **metastases to the lung** (Fig. 4-15) are summarized in Box 4-10 (see Chapter 13).
- **Mixed reticular and nodular interstitial disease (reticulonodular disease)**
  - Several characteristics of **sarcoidosis** (Fig. 4-16) are summarized in Box 4-11.

WebLink

More information on recognizing airspace and interstitial lung disease is available to registered users on StudentConsult.com.

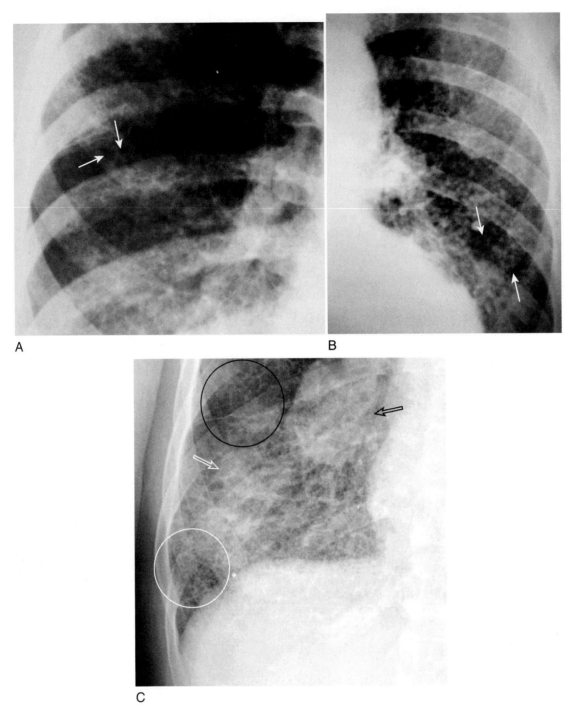

A

B

C

Figure 4-8. **A,** Interstitial lung disease, predominantly reticular. Close-up view of the right upper lung field shows a prominence of the markings that, on close inspection, represents a diffuse network of interwoven lines. Between the well-demarcated lines are numerous small areas of normal lung (closed white arrows). This pattern is characteristic of reticular interstitial disease. The patient had sarcoidosis. **B,** Interstitial lung disease, predominantly nodular. Close-up view of the left upper lung field demonstrates a prominence of the lung markings that has a small, nodular (dot-like) appearance. Interspersed between the sharply demarcated nodules are multiple zones of normal-appearing lung (closed white arrows). This pattern is typical for nodular interstitial lung disease, sometimes referred to as **micronodular lung disease** because of the small size of the nodules. The patient was known to have thyroid carcinoma, and these nodules represent innumerable small metastatic foci in the lungs. **C,** Interstitial disease of the lung, reticulonodular. Most interstitial diseases of the lung have a mixture of both a reticular (lines) and nodular (dots) pattern, as does this case, which is a close-up view of the right lower lobe in a patient with sarcoidosis. The disease in the white circle consists predominantly of an intersecting, lacy network of lines. There are also a few small nodules seen (black circle). The inferior margin of markedly enlarged hilar lymph nodes is seen (open black arrow). Notice how a portion of this disease appears confluent, like airspace disease (open white arrow). Always look at the peripheral margins of parenchymal lung disease to best determine the nature of the "packets" of abnormality and to help in differentiating airspace disease from interstitial disease.

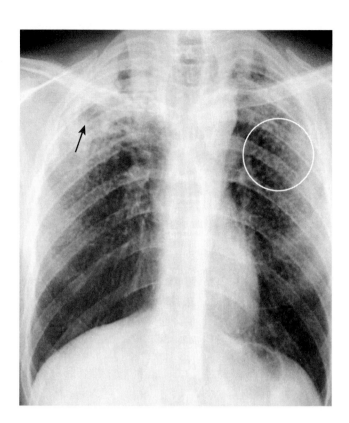

Figure 4-9. **Silicosis.** *The patient was a sandblaster with a long-term exposure to silica particles. Innumerable, small nodular densities are seen on the frontal radiograph most prominent in the upper lobes (white circle). The appearance and distribution are characteristic of silicosis. More confluent disease in this patient's right upper lobe includes cavity formation (closed black arrow). On further study, the disease in the right upper lobe was proved to represent tuberculosis. Silicosis is a predisposing factor in tuberculosis.*

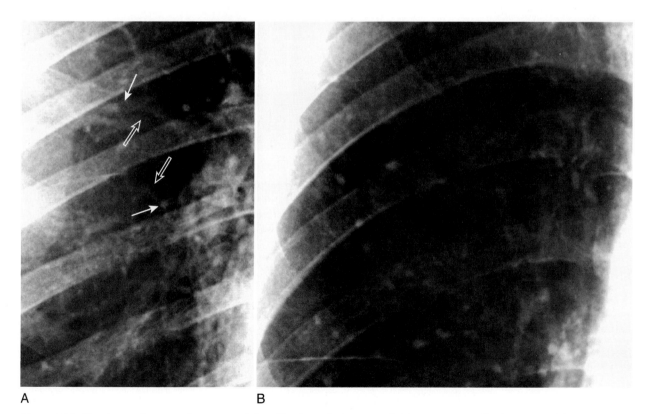

A   B

Figure 4-10. **Blood vessels on-end versus nodules.** *Blood vessels seen on-end **(A)** may mimic small pulmonary nodules **(B)**. To differentiate the two, always look for a "line" (open white arrows) leading up to the "dot" (closed white arrows). If one is present, the chances are good that you are looking at a vessel on-end. The "line" is the feeding vessel. Also, blood vessels seen on-end in one projection will "disappear" (they will no longer be on-end) on the orthogonal view. Nodules will appear the same on both orthogonal views. Finally, nodules **(B)** may be disproportionately large compared to the size of other blood vessels in the region (closed black arrows). These nodules are residual calcifications from a previous episode of varicella pneumonia.*

Box 4-5

Characteristics of Interstitial Lung Disease

Disease has discrete reticular, nodular, or reticulonodular pattern.

"Packets" of disease are separated by normal-appearing lung.

Margins of "packets" of interstitial disease are usually sharp and discrete.

Disease may be focal or diffusely distributed in the lungs.

Usually no air bronchograms are present.

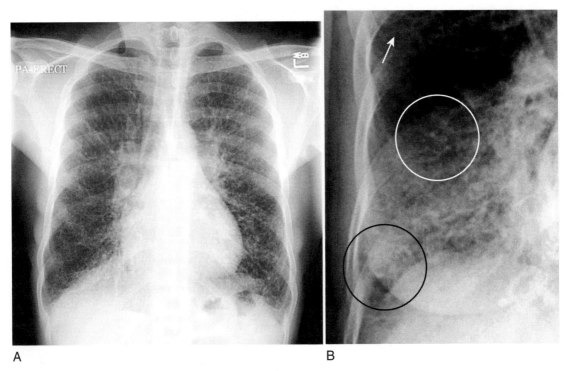

A   B

Figure 4-11. **Pulmonary interstitial edema secondary to congestive heart failure.** *A diffuse accentuation of the pulmonary interstitial markings is evident in the frontal radiograph* **(A)**. *A close-up view of another patient with the same disease* **(B)** *demonstrates multiple Kerley B lines (black circle) representing fluid in thickened interlobular septa. There is a network of crossing lines in the lung (white circle) that represent Kerley A lines. Peribronchial cuffing is present (closed white arrow) representing bronchial walls that are now visible because they are fluid-filled and dilated.*

Box 4-6

Pulmonary Interstitial Edema

Pulmonary interstitial edema can occur because of increased capillary pressure (congestive heart failure), increased capillary permeability (allergic reactions), or decreased fluid absorption (lymphangitic blockade from metastatic disease).

Considered the precursor of alveolar edema, pulmonary interstitial edema classically manifests four key radiologic findings: fluid in the fissures (major and minor), peribronchial cuffing (from fluid in the walls of bronchioles), pleural effusions, and Kerley B lines.

Classically, the patient may have few physical findings in the lungs (rales), even though the chest radiograph demonstrates pulmonary interstitial edema, because almost all the fluid is in the interstitium of the lung, rather than in the airspaces.

With appropriate therapy, pulmonary interstitial edema usually clears rapidly (< 48 hours).

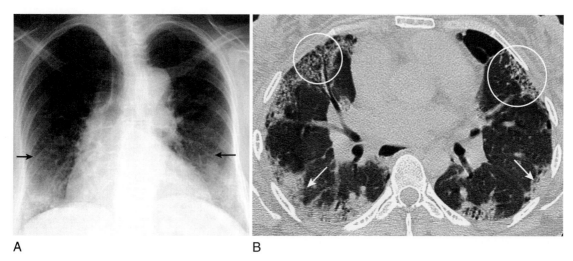

A   B

Figure 4-12. **Idiopathic pulmonary fibrosis.** *Idiopathic pulmonary fibrosis probably represents a spectrum of disease that may begin as* **desquamative interstitial pneumonia** *and lead to the findings here of* **usual interstitial pneumonia (UIP). A,** *Coarse reticular interstitial markings represent fibrosis, predominantly at the lung bases (closed black arrows). A high-resolution CT scan of the chest* **(B)** *shows abnormalities at the lung bases, peripherally in a subpleural location, the typical distribution for UIP. There are small cystic spaces called honeycombing (white circles) with hazy densities called ground-glass opacities (closed white arrows).*

Box 4-7

Idiopathic Pulmonary Fibrosis

This disease of unknown etiology usually occurs in older men who develop cough and shortness of breath.

Early stage is a milder form known as **desquamative interstitial pneumonia (DIP)** and its findings are usually seen best on high-resolution CT scans of the chest.

Later in the disease, it is called **usual interstitial pneumonia (UIP),** and there is marked thickening of the interstitium, bronchiectasis, and small cystic spaces in the lung called **honeycombing.**

UIP is also best demonstrated on high-resolution CT scans of the chest.

Conventional radiographs of the chest may show a fine or, later in the disease, a coarse reticular pattern that is bilaterally symmetrical, most prominent at the bases, subpleural in location, and frequently associated with volume loss.

Idiopathic pulmonary fibrosis is considered the end-stage of disease along the spectrum of these interstitial pneumonias.

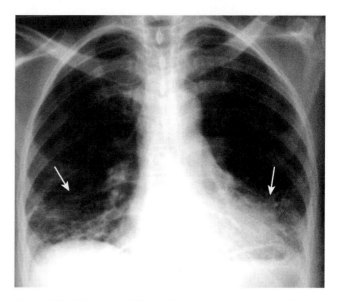

Figure 4-13. **Rheumatoid lung.** *Prominent markings at both lung bases have a predominantly reticular appearance (closed white arrows). Bibasilar interstitial disease can be found in numerous diseases including bronchiectasis, asbestosis, desquamative interstitial pneumonia (DIP), scleroderma, and sickle cell disease. This patient was known to have rheumatoid arthritis. Pleural effusion is the most common manifestation of rheumatoid lung disease. Pulmonary fibrosis, usually diffuse but more prominent at the bases, is seen second most commonly.*

Box 4-8

Rheumatoid Lung Disease

Rheumatoid lung disease is found in some patients with rheumatoid arthritis.

The three most common manifestations of rheumatoid lung disease are (in order of decreasing frequency) pleural effusions, interstitial lung disease, and nodules in the lung called **necrobiotic nodules**.

Pleural effusions are usually unilateral and characteristically remain unchanged in appearance for long periods of time.

The interstitial pattern of disease is usually reticular; it can be seen diffusely throughout the lung, but is usually most prominently seen at the lung bases.

Necrobiotic nodules are identical to subcutaneous rheumatoid nodules and occur mostly at the lung bases near the periphery of the lung; cavitation frequently occurs.

Unlike the joint findings of rheumatoid arthritis, which are more common in women than men, the thoracic manifestations of rheumatoid arthritis are more common in men.

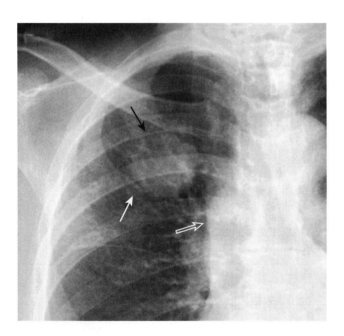

Figure 4-14. **Adenocarcinoma, right upper lobe.** *A mass is evident in the right upper lobe (closed white arrow). Its margin is slightly lobulated and is indistinct along the superolateral border (closed black arrow). Also, prominence of the soft tissues in the right paratracheal region (open white arrow) suggests associated adenopathy. CT scan of the chest confirmed the presence of the mass and demonstrated paratracheal and right hilar adenopathy. The mass was biopsied and was an adenocarcinoma, primary to the lung. Adenocarcinoma of the lung most commonly presents as a peripheral nodule.*

Box 4-9

Bronchogenic Carcinoma

There are four major cell types of bronchogenic carcinoma: adenocarcinoma, squamous cell carcinoma, small cell and large cell carcinoma.

Adenocarcinomas, in particular, can present as a solitary peripheral pulmonary nodule.

As a rule, on conventional chest radiographs, nodules or masses in the lung are more sharply marginated than airspace disease with a relatively clear demarcation between the nodule and the surrounding normal lung tissue.

CT scans may demonstrate spiculation or irregularity to the lung nodule that may not be apparent on conventional radiographs.

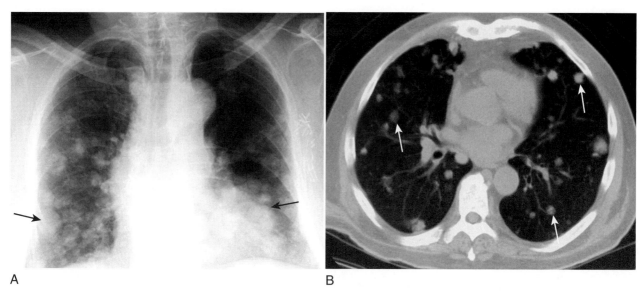

A   B

Figure 4-15. **Metastases to the lung.** *Frontal radiograph of the chest* **(A)** *demonstrates multiple nodules of varying size throughout both lungs (closed black arrows). The diagnosis of exclusion, whenever multiple nodules are found in the lungs, is metastatic disease. On a chest CT scan in another patient* **(B),** *there are multiple nodules of varying sizes with irregular margins seen in both lungs (closed white arrows). The patient in* **A** *had a breast carcinoma, and the patient in* **B** *had colorectal carcinoma. These nodules are sometimes called* **cannon-ball metastases** *seen with hematogenous spread of malignancy to the lungs.*

Box 4-10

Metastases to the Lung

Metastases to the lung can be divided into three categories, depending on the pattern of disease demonstrated in the lung: hematogenous metastases, lymphangitic spread, and direct extension.

Hematogenous metastases arrive via the bloodstream and usually produce two or more nodules in the lungs, sometimes called **cannonball metastases** because of their large, round appearance.

The pathogenesis of **lymphangitic spread to the lungs** is somewhat controversial but most likely involves blood-borne spread to the pulmonary capillaries and then invasion of adjacent lymphatics. An alternative means of lymphangitic spread is obstruction of central lymphatics usually in the hila with retrograde dissemination through the lymphatics in the lung.

Regardless of the mode of transmission, lymphangitic spread to the lung tends to resemble pulmonary interstitial edema except it tends to be localized to a segment or one lung. Findings include Kerley lines, fluid in the fissures, and pleural effusions.

Direct extension is the least common form of tumor spread to the lungs because the pleura is surprisingly resistant to the spread of malignancy through direct violation of its layers. Direct extension would most likely produce a localized pleural-based mass in the lung, frequently with adjacent rib destruction.

Primary tumors that classically produce nodular metastases to the lung include breast, colorectal, renal cell, bladder and testicular, head and neck carcinomas, soft tissue sarcomas, and malignant melanoma.

Primary tumors that classically produce the lymphangitic pattern of metastases to the lung include breast, lung, stomach, pancreatic, and infrequently, prostate carcinoma.

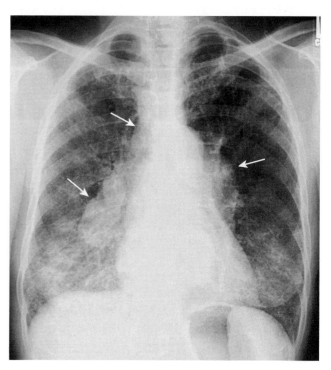

Figure 4-16. **Sarcoidosis.** *A frontal radiograph of the chest reveals bilateral hilar and right paratracheal adenopathy (closed white arrows), a classical distribution for the adenopathy in sarcoidosis. In addition, the patient has diffuse, bilateral interstitial lung disease that is reticulonodular in nature (see close-up view of this same patient in Fig. 4-8C). In some patients with this stage of disease, the adenopathy regresses while the interstitial disease remains. In the overwhelming majority of patients with sarcoid, the disease completely resolves.*

Box 4-11

Sarcoidosis

Besides the bilateral hilar and right paratracheal adenopathy characteristic of this disease, about half of patients with thoracic sarcoid also demonstrate interstitial lung disease.

The interstitial lung disease is frequently a mixture of both reticular and nodular components.

There is a progression of disease in sarcoid that tends to start with adenopathy, proceed to a combination of both interstitial lung disease and adenopathy, and then progress to a stage in which the adenopathy regresses while the interstitial lung disease remains.

Most patients with parenchymal lung disease will undergo complete resolution of the disease.

 ## TAKE-HOME POINTS: Recognizing Airspace versus Interstitial Lung Disease

Parenchymal lung disease can be divided into airspace (alveolar) and interstitial (infiltrative) patterns.

Recognizing the pattern of disease can help in reaching the correct diagnosis.

Characteristics of airspace disease include fluffy, confluent densities that are indistinctly marginated and may demonstrate air bronchograms.

Characteristics of interstitial lung disease include discrete "particles" or "packets" of disease with distinct margins that tend to occur in a pattern of lines (reticular), dots (nodular), or frequently a combination of the two (reticulonodular).

Examples of airspace disease include pulmonary alveolar edema, pneumonia, and aspiration.

Examples of interstitial lung disease include pulmonary interstitial edema, pulmonary fibrosis, metastases to the lung, bronchogenic carcinoma, sarcoidosis, and rheumatoid lung.

An *air bronchogram* is typically a sign of airspace disease and occurs when something other than air (such as inflammatory exudate or blood) surrounds the bronchus, allowing the air inside the bronchus to become visible.

When two objects of the same radiographic density are in contact with each other, their normal silhouette, which is formed by the edge or margin between them, will disappear. The disappearance of the margin between these two structures is called the silhouette sign and is useful throughout radiology in identifying either the location or the density of the abnormality in question.

5 Recognizing the Causes of an Opacified Hemithorax

- Mr. Jones presents to the emergency department very short of breath. His frontal chest radiograph is shown in Fig. 5-1.
- As you can see, Mr. Jones' left hemithorax is almost completely opaque.
  - To be able to treat him correctly, you have to know what is producing the opacification and the answer is on the radiograph if you know how to approach this problem.
- **There are three major causes of an opacified hemithorax** (plus one other that is less common):
  - **Atelectasis of the entire lung**
  - **A very large pleural effusion**
  - **Pneumonia of an entire lung**
  - And a fourth cause: **pneumonectomy**—removal of an entire lung
- Mr. Jones' treatment will vary greatly, depending on whether he has atelectasis (which may require emergent bronchoscopy), a large effusion (which may require emergent thoracentesis), or pneumonia (which would require starting antibiotics).

Table 5-1

PNEUMOTHORAX VERSUS OBSTRUCTIVE ATELECTASIS

Feature	Pneumothorax	Obstructive Atelectasis
Pleural space	Air in the pleural space separates the visceral from the parietal pleura.	The visceral and parietal pleurae do not separate from each other.
Density	The pneumothorax itself will appear "black" (air density). The hemithorax may appear more lucent than normal.	Atelectasis is the absence of air in the lung. The hemithorax will appear more opaque ("whiter") than normal.
Shift	There is never a shift of the heart or trachea *toward* the side of a pneumothorax.	There is *almost always a shift* of the heart and trachea *toward* the side of atelectasis.

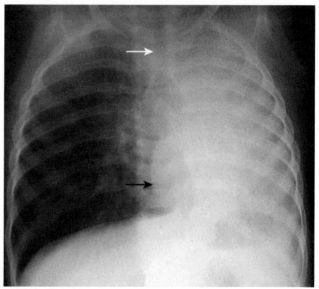

Figure 5-2. **Child with wheezing and shortness of breath.** *Frontal chest radiograph shows opacification of the entire left hemithorax. There is a shift of the heart toward the left such that the right heart border no longer projects to the right of the spine. The heart now overlies the spine (closed black arrow). The trachea (closed white arrow) has moved leftward from the midline toward the side of the opacification. These findings are characteristic of atelectasis of the entire lung, the left lung in this case. The child had asthma. Bronchoscopy was performed and a large mucus plug that was obstructing the left main bronchus was removed.*

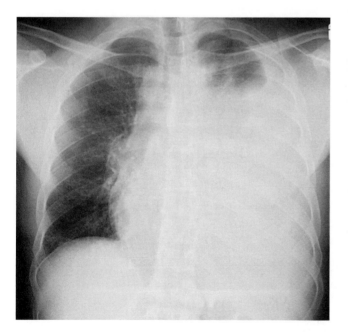

Figure 5-1. *Mr. Jones comes into the emergency department short of breath. This is his frontal chest radiograph. Would you recommend emergent bronchoscopy for atelectasis, emergent thoracentesis for a large pleural effusion, or a course of antibiotics for his large pneumonia? The answer is on the radiograph (and in this chapter).*

Atelectasis of the Entire Lung

- **Atelectasis of an entire lung** usually results from **complete obstruction of the right or left main bronchus.**
  - With bronchial obstruction, no air can enter the lung.
  - The remaining air in the lung is absorbed into the bloodstream through the pulmonary capillary system.
  - This leads to **loss of volume** of the affected lung.
- **In obstructive atelectasis,** even though there is volume loss within the affected lung, **the visceral and parietal pleura almost never separate from each other.**
  - That is an important fact about atelectasis and is sometimes confusing to beginners who try to picture atelectasis and a pneumothorax as both producing collapse of a lung without understanding why they look completely different (Table 5-1).
- Because the visceral and parietal pleura do not separate in atelectasis, mobile structures in the thorax are "pulled" toward the side of the atelectasis, producing a *shift* (movement) of those mobile structures **toward the side of opacification.**
- The most visible mobile structures in the thorax are the **heart, the trachea, and the hemidiaphragms.**
- **In obstructive atelectasis, one or all of these structures will shift toward the side of opacification (toward side of volume loss)** (Fig. 5-2).
- Table 5-2 summarizes the movement of the mobile structures in the thorax in patients with atelectasis.

Table 5-2

RECOGNIZING A "SHIFT" IN ATELECTASIS OR PNEUMONECTOMY

Structure	Normal Position	Right-Sided Atelectasis or Pneumonectomy	Left-Sided Atelectasis or Pneumonectomy
Heart	Midline	Heart moves rightward; left heart border may come to lie near left side of spine	Heart moves leftward; right heart border overlaps the spine
Trachea	Midline	Shifts toward right	Shifts toward left
Hemidiaphragm	Right slightly higher than left	Right hemidiaphragm moves upward and may disappear (silhouette sign)	Left hemidiaphragm moves upward and may disappear (silhouette sign)

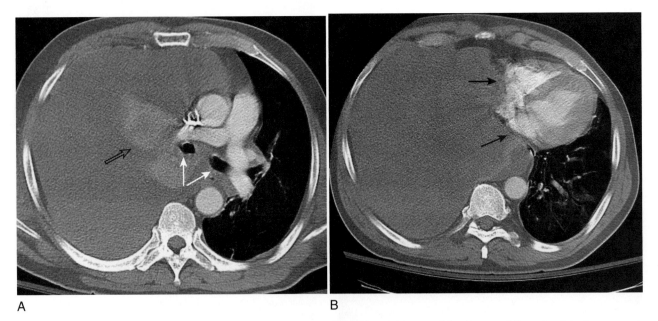

A   B

Figure 5-3. **CT scan of a large right pleural effusion.** *Two contrast-enhanced axial CT scans of the thorax at different levels in the same patient demonstrate complete opacification of the right hemithorax (remember, with CT scans, as with conventional radiographs, the patient's right is on your left and the patient's left is on your right). The right lung has been displaced from the lateral chest wall and is compressed centrally* **(A)** *(open black arrow). The right and left main bronchi (closed white arrows) are both displaced to the left. In* **B,** *which is a section at a lower level, the heart is displaced to the left (closed black arrows), away from the side of opacification. This is a large pleural effusion. Almost 2 L of serosanguineous fluid were removed at thoracentesis. The fluid contained malignant cells from a primary bronchogenic carcinoma.*

Table 5-3

RECOGNIZING A "SHIFT" IN PLEURAL EFFUSION

Structure	Normal Position	Right-Sided Effusion	Left-Sided Effusion
Heart	Midline	Heart moves leftward; apex may lie near chest wall	Heart moves rightward; more of heart protrudes to right of spine
Trachea	Midline	Shifts toward left	Shifts toward right
Hemidiaphragm	Right higher than left	Right hemidiaphragm disappears on chest radiograph (silhouette sign)	Left hemidiaphragm disappears on chest radiograph (silhouette sign)

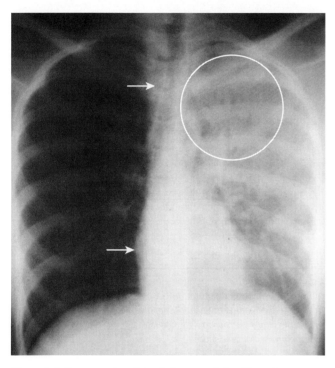

Figure 5-4. **Pneumonia of the left upper lobe.** *There is near-complete opacification of the left hemithorax with no shift of the heart and little shift of the trachea (closed white arrows). There are air bronchograms suggested within the upper area of opacification (circle). These findings suggest a pneumonia rather than atelectasis or pleural effusion. The patient had Streptococcus pneumoniae present in the sputum and improved quickly on antibiotics.*

Massive Pleural Effusion

- If fluid, whether blood, an exudate, or a transudate, fills the pleural space so as to opacify almost the entire hemithorax, then it will have predictable effects:
  - The **fluid acts like a mass** compressing the underlying lung tissue to some degree.
  - When enough pleural fluid accumulates, the **large effusion "pushes" mobile structures away** and there is a **shift of the heart and trachea away from the side of opacification** (Fig. 5-3).
- Table 5-3 summarizes the movement of the mobile structures in the thorax in patients with a large pleural effusion.

Pneumonia of an Entire Lung

- Inflammatory exudate fills the airspaces, causing consolidation and opacification of the lung.
- The hemithorax becomes opaque because the lung no longer contains air, but there is **neither a pull toward the side of the pneumonia by volume loss nor a push away** from the side of the pneumonia by a large effusion.
- There is **no shift of the heart or trachea.**
  - There **may be air bronchograms** present (Fig. 5-4).
- Table 5-4 summarizes the movement of the mobile structures in the thorax in patients with pneumonia of the entire lung.

Post-pneumonectomy

- Pneumonectomy means the removal of an entire lung.

Table 5-4

RECOGNIZING A "SHIFT" IN PNEUMONIA

Structure	Normal Position	Right-Sided Pneumonia	Left-Sided Pneumonia
Heart	Midline	There is usually no shift of the heart from its normal position	There is usually no shift of the heart from its normal position
Trachea	Midline	Midline	Midline
Hemidiaphragm	Right higher than left	Right hemidiaphragm may disappear on chest radiograph (silhouette sign)	Left hemidiaphragm may disappear on chest radiograph (silhouette sign)

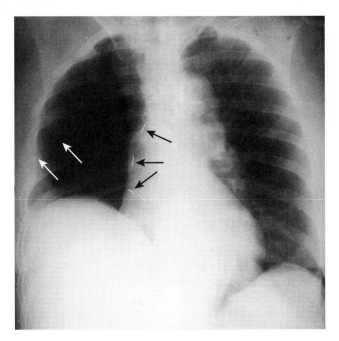

Figure 5-5. Post-pneumonectomy day 1, right lung.
A pneumonectomy is the removal of the entire lung. This postoperative radiograph was obtained less than 24 hours after this patient underwent a pneumonectomy on the right side for a bronchogenic carcinoma. There are surgical clips in the region of the right hilum (closed black arrows) and the right fifth rib has been surgically removed in order to perform the pneumonectomy (closed white arrows). Over the next several weeks, the right hemithorax will fill with fluid and there will be a gradual shift of the heart and mediastinal structures toward the side of the pneumonectomy (see Fig. 5-6).

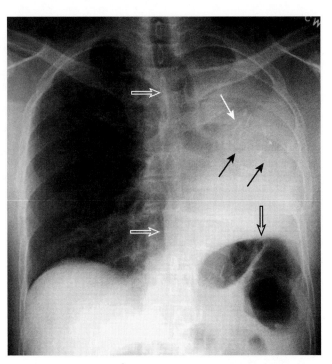

Figure 5-6. Post-pneumonectomy 2 years later, left lung. *This is a different patient than in Figure 5-5. There is complete opacification of the left hemithorax. The heart and trachea (open white arrows) are deviated toward the side of opacification and the splenic flexure of the colon is shifted upward indicating that the left hemidiaphragm is elevated (open black arrow). These signs are characteristic of volume loss. In addition, there are surgical clips surrounding the left hilum (closed white arrow) and the left sixth rib has been surgically removed (closed black arrows), both signs indicating that the patient has undergone a prior pneumonectomy on the left. The surgery had been performed 2 years earlier for a bronchogenic carcinoma. The fluid that gradually filled the left hemithorax immediately following the pneumonectomy has probably fibrosed and there is now a shift toward the pneumonectomized side.*

- In order to perform this procedure, **either the fifth or sixth rib on the affected side is almost always removed.**
- In most cases, **metallic surgical clips will be visible in the region of the hilum** on the pneumonectomized side.
- For about 24 hours following the surgery, only air occupies the hemithorax from which the lung has been removed (Fig. 5-5).
- Over the course of the next 2 weeks, the hemithorax gradually fills with fluid.
- By about 4 months after surgery, the pneumonectomized hemithorax should be completely opaque.
- The mobile mediastinal structures gradually shift toward the side of opacification.
- Eventually, **fibrous tissue forms in the pneumonectomized hemithorax** and in most patients **the entire hemithorax is opaque.**
  - The **heart and trachea shift toward the side of opacification.**
  - The chest study **looks identical to that of a patient with atelectasis of the entire lung.**
- **How to tell the difference between atelectasis of an entire lung versus post-pneumonectomy** if no history of prior surgery is available.

- Look for the missing fifth or sixth rib and look for the surgical clips in the hilum (Fig. 5-6).
- So let's return to the frontal radiograph of Mr. Jones with the opacified hemithorax, who has been waiting patiently in the emergency department while you read this chapter.
  - How would you treat his abnormality?
    - You'll notice there is a shift of the heart and trachea **away** from the side of opacification.
    - This is characteristic of a **very large pleural effusion** (Fig. 5-7).
    - Mr. Jones had a thoracentesis performed in which almost 2 L of serosanguineous fluid were removed.
  - The cytologic specimens showed malignant cells, and Mr. Jones was found to have a large left-sided bronchogenic carcinoma.

WebLink
More information on differentiating the causes of an opacified hemithorax is available to registered users on StudentConsult.com.

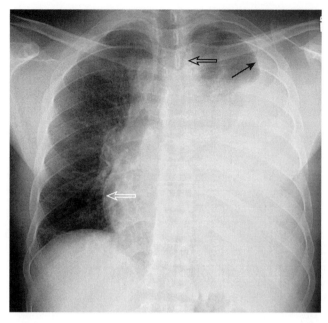

Figure 5-7. ***Mr. Jones' frontal chest radiograph.*** *There is opacification of almost the entire left hemithorax. There is also a shift of the trachea toward the right (open black arrow), and the heart is displaced toward the right as manifested by the amount of the right heart border extending into the right hemithorax (open white arrow). Both of these mobile structures have moved away from the side of opacification. There is also a* **meniscus sign** *present as fluid is seen to extend higher along the lateral margin of the pleural space (closed black arrow). These signs are characteristic of a large left pleural effusion. Thoracentesis revealed malignant cells from a left-sided bronchogenic carcinoma.*

TAKE-HOME POINTS: Recognizing the Causes of an Opacified Hemithorax

The differential possibilities for an opacified hemithorax should include atelectasis of the entire lung, a very large pleural effusion, pneumonia of the entire lung, or post-pneumonectomy.

The trachea, heart and hemidiaphragms are mobile structures that have the capability of moving **(shifting)** if there is either something pushing on them or something pulling them.

With atelectasis, there is a shift toward the side of the opacified hemithorax because of volume loss in the affected lung.

With a large pleural effusion, there is a shift away from the side of opacification because the large pleural effusion acts as if it were a mass.

With pneumonia of an entire lung, there is usually no shift, but air bronchograms may be present.

In the post-pneumonectomy patient, there is eventually volume loss on the side from which the lung has been removed, and the clues to such surgery may include surgical absence of the fifth or sixth rib on the affected side or metallic surgical clips in the hilum.

6 Recognizing Atelectasis

What Is Atelectasis?

- Common to all forms of atelectasis is a **loss of volume in some or all of the lung, usually leading to increased density of the lung involved.**
  - The lung normally appears "black" on a chest radiograph because it contains air.
  - When something of fluid or soft tissue density is substituted for that air or when the air in the lung is resorbed (as it can be in atelectasis), that part of the lung becomes whiter (more dense or more opaque).
- Unless mentioned otherwise, statements in this chapter that refer to "atelectasis" are referring to *obstructive atelectasis.*
- This might be a good time to review the chart from **Chapter 5, Recognizing the Causes of an Opacified Hemithorax** (see Table 5-1) highlighting the different appearances of the lung in a large pneumothorax and atelectasis of the entire lung (Fig. 6-1).

Signs of Atelectasis

- **Displacement (shift) of the interlobar fissures** (major and minor) toward the area of atelectasis (Fig. 6-2).
- **Increase in the density of the affected lung** (see Fig. 6-2)
- **Displacement (shift) of the mobile structures of the thorax**
  - The **mobile structures** are those capable of movement due to changes in lung volume:
    - **Trachea**
      - **Normally midline in location,** the trachea above the aortic knob is centered on the spinous processes of the vertebral bodies (also midline structures) on a nonrotated frontal chest x-ray.
      - There is **always a slight rightward deviation of the trachea at the site of the left-sided aortic knob.**
      - With atelectasis, especially of the upper lobes, the trachea may shift toward the side of the volume loss (Fig. 6-3).
  - **Heart**
    - **At least 1 cm of the right heart border normally projects to the right of the spine** on a nonrotated frontal radiograph.
    - With atelectasis, especially of the lower lobes, the heart may shift to one side or the other.
      - When the heart shifts toward the left, the right heart border will overlap the spine (Fig. 6-4).
      - When the heart shifts toward the right, the left heart border will approach the midline (Fig. 6-5).
  - **Hemidiaphragm**
    - The **right hemidiaphragm is almost always higher than the left** by about half the interspace distance between two adjacent ribs.
      - In about 10% of normal people, the left hemidiaphragm is higher than the right.
    - In the presence of atelectasis, especially of the lower lobes, the hemidiaphragm on the affected side will usually be displaced upward (Fig. 6-6).
- **Overinflation of the unaffected ipsilateral lobes or the contralateral lung**

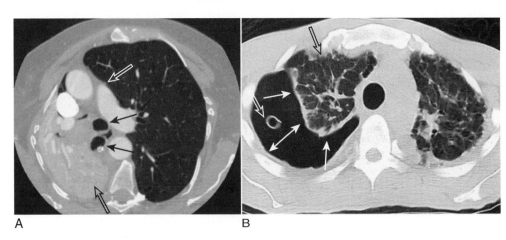

Figure 6-1. **Obstructive atelectasis versus a pneumothorax.** *Two different causes of lung collapse and the difference in their radiologic appearance. **A,** There is atelectasis of the entire right lung (open black arrow) from an obstructing endobronchial lesion. The visceral and parietal pleurae remain in contact with each other and other mobile structures in the mediastinum, such as the right and left main bronchi (closed black arrows), shift toward the atlectasis. The left lung overexpands and crosses the midline (open white arrow). **B,** This patient has a large right-sided pneumothorax. Air (double white arrow) interposes between the visceral (closed white arrows) and parietal pleurae, causing the lung to undergo passive atelectasis (open black arrow). There is a chest tube in the right hemithorax (open white arrow) that had been removed from suction.*

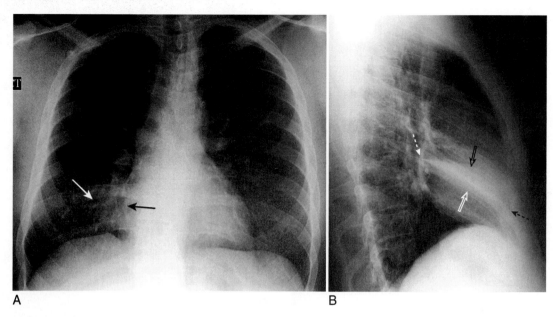

*Figure 6-2. **Right middle lobe atelectasis.** Frontal **(A)** and lateral **(B)** views of the chest show an area of increased density (closed white arrow), which is silhouetting the normal right heart border (closed black arrow) indicating its anterior location in the right middle lobe. On the lateral view **(B)**, the minor fissure is displaced downward (open black arrow) and the major fissure is displaced upward (open white arrow). Note the anterior location of the middle lobe and the fan-shaped appearance of the atelectatic lobe with its apex at the hilum (dotted white arrow) and its base adherent to the chest wall (dotted black arrow).*

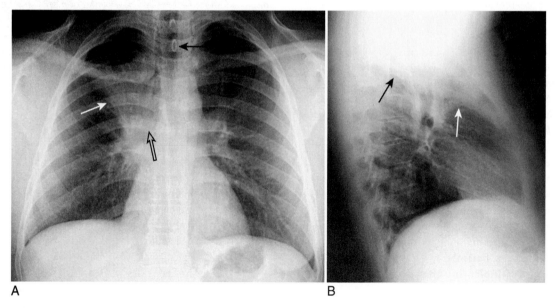

*Figure 6-3. **Right upper lobe atelectasis.** A fan-shaped area of increased density is seen on the frontal projection **(A)** representing the airless right upper lobe (open black arrow). The minor fissure is displaced upward (closed white arrow). The trachea is shifted to the right (closed black arrow). The lateral **(B)** demonstrates a similar wedge-shaped density near the apex of the lung. The minor fissure (closed white arrow) is pulled upward and the major fissure is pulled forward (closed black arrow). This is a child who had asthma leading to formation of a mucus plug, which obstructed the right upper lobe bronchus.*

- The greater the volume loss and the more chronic its presence, the more the lung on the side **opposite** the atelectasis or the **unaffected lobe(s) in the ipsilateral lung** will attempt to **overinflate** to compensate for the volume loss.

- This may be noticeable in the lateral projection by an **increase in the size of the retrosternal clear space** and on the frontal projection by **extension of the overinflated contralateral lung across the midline** (Fig. 6-7).

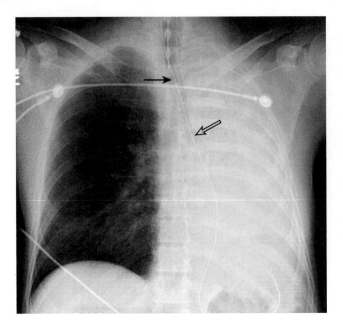

Figure 6-4. **Atelectasis of the left lung.** There is complete opacification of the left hemithorax with shift of the trachea (closed black arrow) and the esophagus (marked here by a nasogastric tube) (open black arrow) toward the side of the atelectasis. The right heart border, which should project about a centimeter to the right of the spine, has been pulled to the left side and is no longer visible. The patient had an obstructing bronchogenic carcinoma in the left main bronchus.

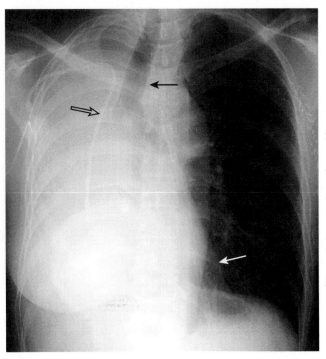

Figure 6-5. **Atelectasis of the right lung.** There is complete opacification of the right hemithorax with shift of the trachea (closed black arrow) toward the side of the atelectasis. The left heart border is displaced far to the right and now almost overlaps the spine (closed white arrow). This patient had an endobronchial metastasis in the right main bronchus from her left-sided breast cancer (did you notice the left breast was surgically absent?) and was already receiving chemotherapy through an indwelling central venous catheter (open black arrow).

* The signs of atelectasis are summarized in Box 6-1.

Types of Atelectasis

* **Subsegmental atelectasis** (also called *discoid atelectasis* or *plate-like atelectasis*) (Fig. 6-8)
    * **Linear densities of varying thickness usually parallel to the diaphragm**
        * Most commonly **seen at the lung bases**
        * Does not produce a sufficient amount of volume loss to cause a shift of the mobile thoracic structures
    * Occurs **mostly in patients who are "splinting,"** i.e., not taking a deep breath:
        * **Postoperative patients**
        * **Patients with pleuritic chest pain**
    * **Not due to bronchial obstruction**
        * Most likely related to **deactivation of surfactant** that leads to collapse of airspaces in a nonsegmental or nonlobar distribution.
    * On a single study, without prior examinations for comparison, subsegmental atelectasis and **chronic, linear scarring can look identical.**
        * Subsegmental atelectasis **typically disappears within a matter of days** with resumption of normal, deep breathing, whereas **scarring remains.**
* **Compressive atelectasis**
    * Loss of volume due to **passive compression of the lung** can be caused by:

* A poor inspiratory effort in which there is passive atelectasis of the lung at the bases (see Fig. 6-9A)
* A **large pleural effusion, large pneumothorax** or a **space-occupying lesion** (such as a large mass in the lung)
* When caused by a poor inspiratory effort, passive atelectasis may mimic airspace disease at the bases.
    * **Pitfall:** Be suspicious of compressive atelectasis if the patient has taken less than an 8-posterior-rib breath.
    * **Solution:** Check the lateral projection for confirmation of real airspace disease at the base.
* When caused by a large effusion or pneumothorax, the loss of volume associated with compressive atelectasis may balance the increased volume produced by either fluid (as in pleural effusion) or air (as in pneumothorax) (Fig. 6-9).
    * Consequently, **the combination of atelectasis and a large effusion** or atelectasis and a large **pneumothorax may not be associated with a shift** of the mobile chest structures.
* In an older patient with an **opacified hemithorax, no air bronchograms, and little or no shift of the**

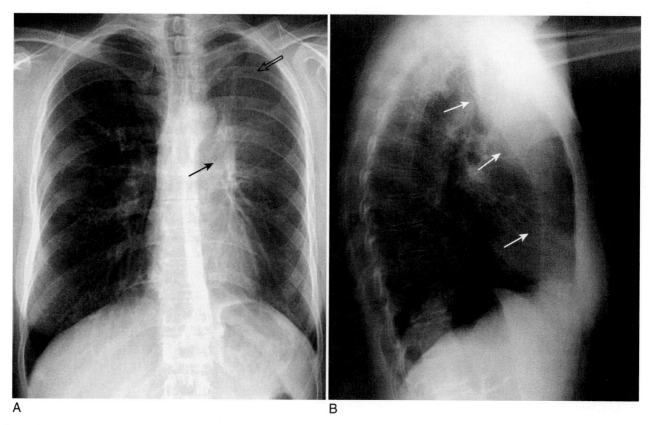

A   B

Figure 6-6. **Left upper lobe atelectasis.** *On the frontal projection* **(A),** *there is a hazy density surrounding the left hilum (open black arrow) and there is a soft tissue mass in the left hilum (closed black arrow). Notice how the left hemidiaphragm has been pulled up to the same level as the right. The lateral projection* **(B)** *shows a bandlike zone of increased density (closed white arrows) representing the atelectatic left upper lobe sharply demarcated by the major fissure, which has been pulled anteriorly. The patient had a squamous cell carcinoma of the left upper lobe bronchus that was producing complete obstruction of that bronchus.*

mobile thoracic structures, it is important to **suspect an obstructing bronchogenic carcinoma,** perhaps with metastases to the pleura (Fig. 6-10).

- **Round atelectasis**
  - This form of compressive atelectasis is **usually seen at the periphery of the lung base** and develops from a **combination of prior pleural disease** (such as from asbestos exposure or tuberculosis) **and the formation of a pleural effusion that produces adjacent compressive atelectasis.**
  - When the pleural effusion recedes, the underlying pleural disease leads to a portion of the **atelectatic lung becoming "trapped."**
  - This **produces a masslike lesion** that can be confused with a tumor.
  - On CT scan of the chest, the bronchovascular markings characteristically lead from the *round atelectasis* back to the hilum, producing a *comet-tail* appearance (Fig. 6-11).
- **Obstructive atelectasis** (see Fig. 6-4)
  - Obstructive atelectasis is associated with the **resorption of air from the alveoli,** through the pulmonary capillary

bed, **distal to an obstructing lesion** of the bronchial tree.
- The rate at which air is absorbed and the lung collapses depends on its gas content when occluded.
  - It takes about **18 to 24 hours for an entire lung to collapse** with the patient breathing room air but **less than an hour** with the patient breathing near 100% oxygen.
  - The **affected segment, lobe, or lung collapses** and becomes more opaque (whiter) because it contains no air.
  - The **collapse leads to volume loss** in the affected segment/lobe/lung.
  - Because the visceral and parietal pleurae invariably remain in contact with each other as the lung loses volume, there is a pull on **the mobile structures of the thorax toward the area of atelectasis.**
- The types of atelectasis are summarized in Table 6-1.

Patterns of Collapse in Lobar Atelectasis
- Obstructive atelectasis produces **consistently recognizable patterns of collapse** depending on the location of the atelectatic segment or lobe and the degree to which such

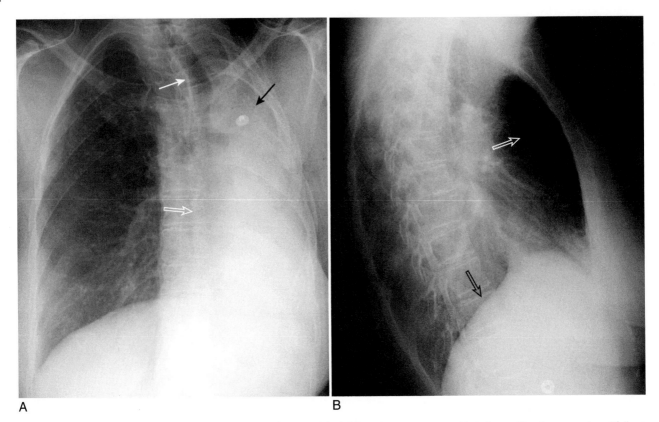

A   B

Figure 6-7. **Left-sided pneumonectomy.** *Complete opacification of the left hemithorax **(A)** is most likely from a fibrothorax produced following complete removal of the lung. There is associated marked volume loss with shift of the trachea to the left (closed white arrow). The left fifth rib was surgically removed during the pneumonectomy (closed black arrow). The right lung has herniated across the midline in an attempt to "fill-up" the left hemithorax, which is seen by the increased lucency extending across the midline in A (open white arrow) and the increased lucency behind the sternum in **B** (open white arrow). Notice that because only the right hemithorax has an aerated lung remaining, only the right hemidiaphragm is visible on the lateral projection (open black arrow). The left hemidiaphragm has been silhouetted by the airless hemithorax above it.*

Box 6-1

Signs of Atelectasis
Displacement* of the major or minor fissure
Increased density of the atelectatic portion of lung
Shift* of the mobile structures in the thorax, i.e., the heart, trachea, or hemidiaphragms
Compensatory overinflation of the unaffected segments, lobes, or lung

*Toward the atelectasis.

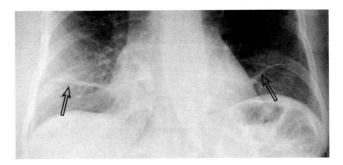

Figure 6-8. **Subsegmental atelectasis.** *Close-up view of the lung bases demonstrates several linear densities extending across all segments of the lower lobes, paralleling the diaphragm (open black arrows). This is a characteristic picture of subsegmental atelectasis, sometimes also called **discoid atelectasis** or **plate-like atelectasis**. The patient was postoperative from abdominal surgery and was unable to take a deep breath. The atelectasis disappeared within a few days after surgery.*

factors as collateral airflow between lobes and obstructive pneumonia allow the affected lobe to collapse.

- Lobes collapse in a fanlike configuration with the **base of the fan-shaped triangle anchored at the pleural surface and the apex of the triangle anchored at the hilum.**
- Other, unaffected lobes will undergo compensatory hyperinflation in an attempt to "fill" the affected

hemithorax, and this hyperinflation may limit the amount of shift of the mobile chest structures.

- **Pitfall:** The **more atelectatic a lobe or segment becomes** (that is, the smaller its volume), the **less visible it becomes on the chest radiograph.**

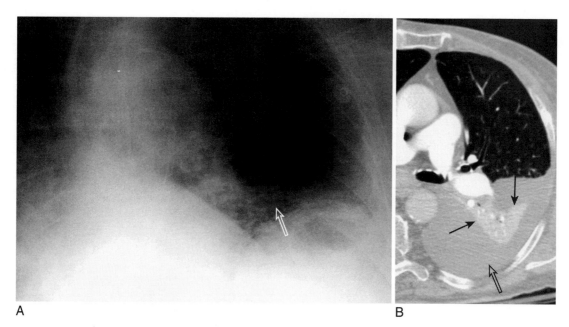

A   B

Figure 6-9. Compressive (passive) atelectasis. *Passive compression of the lung can occur either from a poor inspiratory effort* **(A),** *which is manifest as increased density at the lung bases (open white arrow) or secondary to a large pleural effusion or pneumothorax* **(B).** *Axial CT scan of the chest showing only the left hemithorax* **(B)** *demonstrates a large left pleural effusion (open black arrow). The left lower lobe (closed black arrows) is atelectatic, having been compressed by the pleural fluid surrounding it.*

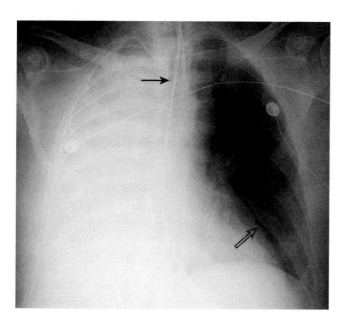

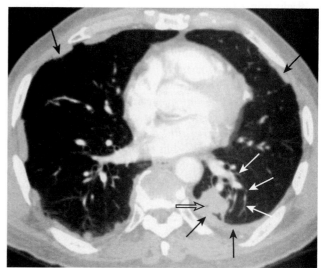

Figure 6-10. Atelectasis and effusion in balance, an ominous combination. *There is complete opacification of the right hemithorax. There are neither air bronchograms to suggest pneumonia nor any shift of the trachea (closed black arrow) or heart (open black arrow). The absence of any shift suggests the possibility of atelectasis and pleural effusion in balance, a combination that should raise suspicion for a central bronchogenic carcinoma (producing obstructive atelectasis) with metastases (producing a large pleural effusion).*

Figure 6-11. Round atelectasis, left lower lobe. *There is a masslike density in the left lower lobe (open black arrow). The patient has underlying pleural disease in the form of pleural plaques from asbestos exposure (closed black arrows). There are* **comet-tail-** *shaped bronchovascular markings that emanate from the "mass" and extend back to the hilum (closed white arrows). This combination of findings is characteristic of round atelectasis and should not be mistaken for a tumor.*

Table 6-1

TYPES OF ATELECTASIS

Type	Cause	Remarks
Subsegmental atelectasis	Splinting, especially in postoperative patients and those with pleuritic chest pain	May be related to deactivation of surfactant; does not usually lead to volume loss; disappears in days
Compressive atelectasis	Passive external compression of the lung from poor inspiration, large pneumothorax, or large pleural effusion	Volume loss of compressive atelectasis can balance volume increase from effusion or pneumothorax, resulting in no shift
Obstructive atelectasis	Obstruction of a bronchus from malignancy or mucus plugging	Visceral and parietal pleurae maintain contact; mobile structures in the thorax shift toward the atelectasis

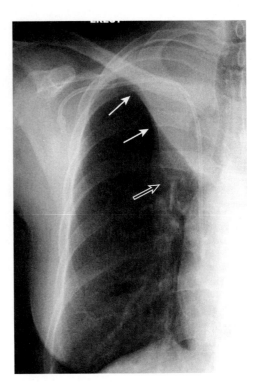

Figure 6-12. ***Right upper lobe atelectasis and hilar mass: S sign of Golden.*** *There is a soft tissue mass in the right hilum (open white arrow). There is opacification of the right upper lobe from atelectasis. The minor fissure is displaced upward toward the area of increased density (closed white arrows)* indicating right upper lobe volume loss. *The curved edge formed by the mass and the elevated minor fissure is called the S sign of Golden. The patient had a large squamous cell carcinoma obstructing the right upper lobe bronchus.*

- This can lead to the false assumption of improvement when, in fact, the atelectasis is worsening.
- **Solution:** This can usually be resolved with a careful analysis of the study to check for the degree of displacement of the interlobar fissures or with a CT scan of the chest.
- **Right upper lobe atelectasis** (see Fig. 6-3)
  - On the frontal radiograph
    - There is an upward shift of the minor fissure.
    - There is a rightward shift of the trachea.
  - On the lateral radiograph
    - There is a upward shift of the minor fissure and forward shift of the major fissure.
  - If there is a mass in the right hilum producing right upper lobe atelectasis, the combination of the hilar mass and the upward shift of the minor fissure produces a characteristic appearance on the frontal radiograph named the ***S sign of Golden*** (Fig. 6-12).
- **Left upper lobe atelectasis** (see Fig. 6-6)
  - On the frontal radiograph
    - There is a hazy area of increased density around the left hilum.
    - There is a leftward shift of the trachea.
    - There may be elevation of the left hemidiaphragm.
    - Compensatory overinflation of the lower lobe may cause the superior segment of the left lower lobe to extend to the apex of the thorax on the affected side.
  - On the lateral radiograph
    - There is forward displacement of the major fissure and the opacified upper lobe forms a band of increased density running roughly parallel to the sternum.

- **Lower lobe atelectasis** (Fig. 6-13)
  - On the frontal radiograph
    - Both the right and left lower lobes collapse to form a triangular density that extends from its apex at the hilum to its base at the medial portion of the affected hemidiaphragm.
    - There is elevation of the hemidiaphragm on the affected side.
    - The heart may shift toward the side of the volume loss.
    - On the right (only), there is a downward shift of the minor fissure (see Fig. 6-13C).
  - On the lateral radiograph
    - There is both downward and posterior displacement of the major fissure until the completely collapsed lower lobe forms a small triangular density posteriorly at the costophrenic angle (see Fig. 6-13B).
- **In the critically ill patient, atelectasis occurs most frequently in the left lower lobe.**
  - **Always check that the left hemidiaphragm is seen in its entire extent** through the heart as **left lower lobe atelectasis will manifest by disappearance (silhouetting) of all or part of the left hemidiaphragm** (see Fig. 6-13A).

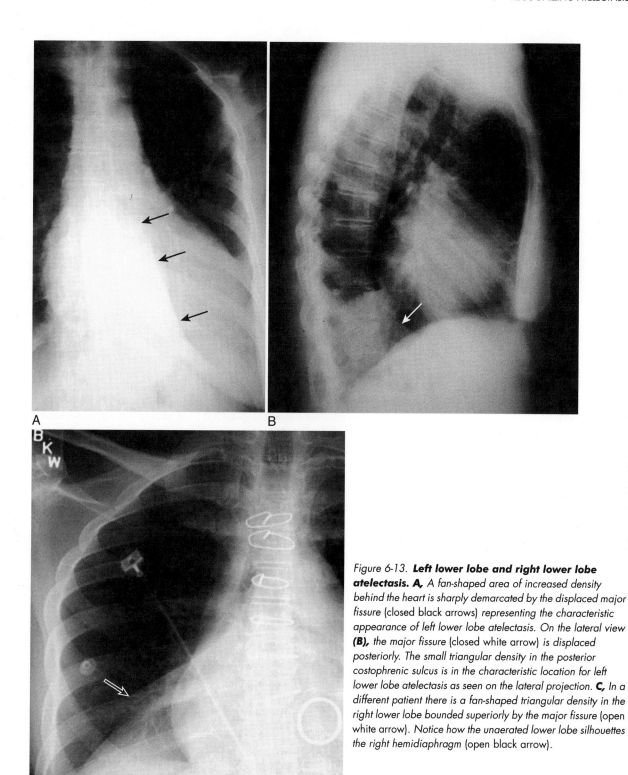

Figure 6-13. **Left lower lobe and right lower lobe atelectasis. A,** *A fan-shaped area of increased density behind the heart is sharply demarcated by the displaced major fissure (closed black arrows) representing the characteristic appearance of left lower lobe atelectasis. On the lateral view* **(B),** *the major fissure (closed white arrow) is displaced posteriorly. The small triangular density in the posterior costophrenic sulcus is in the characteristic location for left lower lobe atelectasis as seen on the lateral projection.* **C,** *In a different patient there is a fan-shaped triangular density in the right lower lobe bounded superiorly by the major fissure (open white arrow). Notice how the unaerated lower lobe silhouettes the right hemidiaphragm (open black arrow).*

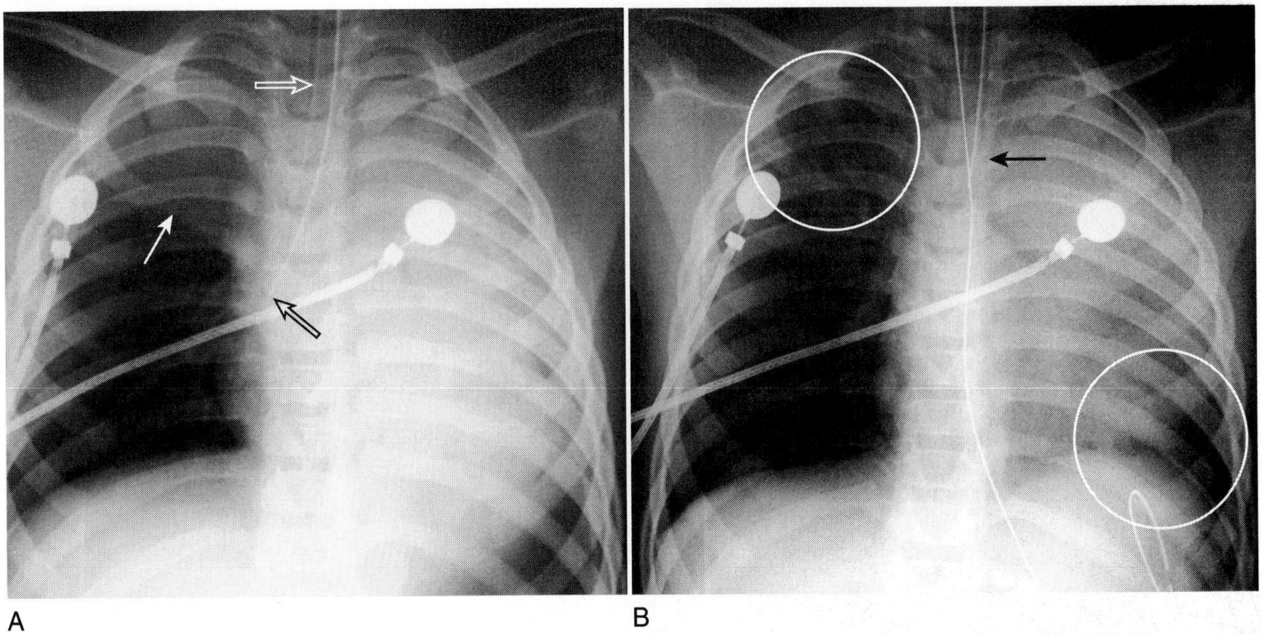

A   B

Figure 6-14. ***Right upper lobe and left lung atelectasis from an endotracheal tube.*** *The tip of the endotracheal tube extends beyond the carina into the bronchus intermedius (open black arrow), which aerates only the right middle and lower lobes* **(A)**. *The right upper lobe and entire left lung are opaque from atelectasis. The minor fissure is elevated (closed white arrow) and the trachea (as marked by the endotracheal tube) is displaced to the left (open white arrow).* **B,** *One hour later, the tip of the endotracheal tube has been retracted (closed black arrow) and the right upper lobe and a portion of the left lower lobe are again aerated (white circles).*

- **Right middle lobe atelectasis** (see Fig. 6-2)
  - On the frontal radiograph
    - There is a triangular density silhouetting the right heart border with its base pointing toward the hilum.
    - The minor fissure is displaced downward.
  - On the lateral radiograph
    - There is a triangular density with its base directed anteriorly and its apex at the hilum.
    - The minor fissure may be displaced inferiorly and the major fissure superiorly.
- **Endotracheal tube too low** (Fig. 6-14)
  - If the tip of an endotracheal tube enters the right lower lobe bronchus, only the right lower lobe tends to be aerated and remain expanded.
  - Within a short time, atelectasis of the entire left lung and the right upper lobe will develop.
  - Once the tip of the endotracheal tube is withdrawn above the carina, the atelectasis usually clears quite rapidly.
- **Atelectasis of the entire lung** (see Figs. 6-4 and 6-5)
  - On the frontal radiograph
    - There is **opacification of the atelectatic lung** due to loss of air.
    - There is a **shift of all the mobile structures** of the thorax **toward the side of the atelectatic lung.**
  - On the lateral radiograph
    - The **hemidiaphragm on the side of the atelectasis will be silhouetted by the nonaerated lung above it.**
    - Look closely on the lateral exposure, and you'll see **only one hemidiaphragm** instead of two.

How Atelectasis Resolves
- Depending in part on the rapidity with which the segment, lobe, or lung became atelectatic, atelectasis has the capacity to **resolve within hours or last for many days even after the obstruction has been removed.**
- Slowly resolving lobar or whole-lung atelectasis may manifest patchy areas of airspace disease surrounded by progressively increasing areas of aerated lung until the atelectasis has completely cleared.
- The most common causes of obstructive atelectasis are summarized in Table 6-2.

WebLink
More information on recognizing atelectasis is available to registered users on StudentConsult.com.

Table 6-2

MOST COMMON CAUSES OF OBSTRUCTIVE ATELECTASIS

Cause	Remarks
Tumors	Includes bronchogenic carcinoma (especially squamous cell), endobronchial metastases, carcinoid
Mucus plug	Especially in bedridden individuals; postoperative patients; those with asthma, cystic fibrosis
Foreign body aspiration	Especially peanuts; toys; following a traumatic intubation
Inflammation	As in scarring caused by tuberculosis

TAKE-HOME POINTS: Recognizing Atelectasis

Common to all forms of atelectasis is volume loss, but the radiographic appearance of atelectasis will differ depending on the type of atelectasis.

The three most commonly observed types of atelectasis are subsegmental atelectasis (also known as discoid or plate-like atelectasis), compressive or passive atelectasis, and obstructive atelectasis.

Subsegmental atelectasis usually occurs in patients who are not taking a deep breath (splinting) and produces linear densities usually at the lung bases most commonly parallel to the diaphragm.

Compressive atelectasis occurs passively when the lung is collapsed by a poor inspiration (at the bases), or from a large adjacent pleural effusion or pneumothorax. When the underlying abnormality is removed, the lung usually expands.

Round atelectasis is a type of passive atelectasis in which the lung does not re-expand when a pleural effusion recedes, usually due to pre-existing pleural disease. Round atelectasis may produce a masslike lesion on chest radiographs and can mimic a tumor.

Obstructive atelectasis occurs distal to an occluding lesion of the bronchial tree because of reabsorption of the air in the distal airspaces via the pulmonary capillary bed.

Obstructive atelectasis produces consistently recognizable patterns of collapse based on the assumptions that the visceral and parietal pleura invariably remain in contact with each other and every lobe of the lung is anchored at or near the hilum.

Signs of obstructive atelectasis include displacement of the fissures, increased density of the affected lung, shift of the mobile structures of the thorax toward the atelectasis, and compensatory overinflation of the unaffected ipsilateral or contralateral lung.

Atelectasis tends to resolve quickly if it occurs acutely; the more chronic the process, the longer it takes to resolve.

7 Recognizing a Pleural Effusion

Normal Anatomy and Physiology of the Pleural Space
- **Normal anatomy**
  - The **parietal pleura lines the inside of the thoracic cage** and the **visceral pleura adheres to the surface of the lung** parenchyma including its interface with the mediastinum and diaphragm.
  - The **enfolds of the visceral pleura form the interlobar fissures,** the major (oblique) and minor (horizontal) on the right, only the major on the left.
  - The space between the visceral and parietal pleura, i.e., the *pleural space,* **is a potential space normally containing only about 2 to 5 mL of pleural fluid.**
- **Normal physiology**
  - Normally, several hundred milliliters of fluid are produced and reabsorbed each day.
  - **Fluid is produced primarily at the parietal pleura** from the pulmonary capillary bed and is **resorbed at the visceral pleura and by lymphatic drainage through the parietal pleura.**

Causes of Pleural Effusions
- Fluid accumulates in the pleural space when the rate at which the fluid forms exceeds the rate by which it is cleared.
  - **The rate of formation may be increased** by
    - **Increasing hydrostatic pressure,** as in left-sided heart failure
    - **Decreasing colloid osmotic pressure,** as in hypoproteinemia
    - **Increasing capillary permeability,** as can occur in toxic disruption of the membrane in pneumonia or hypersensitivity reactions
  - **The rate of resorption may be decreased** by
    - **Decreased absorption** of fluid **by lymphatics either from lymphangitic blockade by tumor or from increased venous pressure,** which decreases the rate of fluid transport via the thoracic duct.
    - **Decreased pressure in pleural space,** as in atelectasis of the lung due to bronchial obstruction
- Pleural **effusions can also form when there is transport of peritoneal fluid from the abdominal cavity** through the diaphragm or via lymphatics from a subdiaphragmatic process.

Types of Pleural Effusions
- Pleural effusions are **divided into exudates** or **transudates** depending on their **protein content** and their **LDH (lactate dehydrogenase) concentrations.**
- **Transudates** tend to form when there is
  - **Increased capillary hydrostatic pressure** or **decreased osmostic pressure,** such as occurs in

- **Congestive heart failure,** primarily left-sided heart failure, which is the most common cause of a transudative pleural effusion
  - **Hypoalbuminemia**
  - **Cirrhosis**
  - **Nephrotic syndrome**
- Exudates
  - **Most common cause of exudative pleural effusion is malignancy.**
  - **Empyema**—an exudate containing pus
  - **Hemothorax**—fluid hematocrit > 50% blood hematocrit
  - **Chylothorax**—contains increased triglycerides or cholesterol

Recognizing the Different Appearances of Pleural Effusions
- Forces that influence the appearance of pleural fluid on a chest radiograph depend on the position of the patient, the force of gravity, the amount of fluid, and the degree of elastic recoil of the lung.
- The descriptions that follow, unless otherwise indicated, assume the patient is in the upright position.

SUBPULMONIC EFFUSION
- It is believed that **almost all pleural effusions first collect beneath the lung** between the parietal pleura lining the diaphragm and the visceral pleura of the lower lobe.
- If the effusion remains entirely subpulmonic in location, it can be difficult to detect on conventional radiographs except for contour alterations in what appears to be the hemidiaphragm but is actually the fluid-lung interface beneath the lung.
- The different appearances of subpulmonic effusions are summarized in Table 7-1 and Figures 7-1 and 7-2.
- *Subpulmonic* does **not** mean *loculated.*
  - **Most subpulmonic effusions flow freely** as the patient changes position.

BLUNTING OF THE COSTOPHRENIC ANGLES
- As the subpulmonic effusion grows in size, it first fills and *blunts* the **posterior costophrenic sulcus,** visible on the lateral view of the chest (Fig. 7-3).
  - This occurs with approximately **75 mL of fluid.**
- **When the effusion reaches about 300 mL in volume, it blunts the lateral costophrenic angle,** visible on the frontal chest radiograph (Fig. 7-4).
- **Pitfall:** Pleural thickening caused by fibrosis can also produce blunting of the costophrenic angle.
  - **Solutions:** Scarring sometimes produces a characteristic *ski-slope appearance* of blunting, unlike the meniscoid appearance of a pleural effusion (Fig. 7-5).

Table 7-1

RECOGNIZING A SUBPULMONIC EFFUSION

View	Right-Sided Findings (Fig. 7-1)	Left-Sided Findings (Fig. 7-2)
Frontal view	The highest point of the apparent hemidiaphragm* is displaced more laterally than the highest point of a normal hemidiaphragm would be. These are more difficult to recognize than left-sided subpulmonic effusions because the liver is the same density as the pleural fluid above it.	The distance between the stomach bubble and the apparent left hemidiaphragm is increased (should normally be only about 1 cm from top of stomach bubble to bottom of aerated left lower lobe). The highest point of the apparent hemidiaphragm* is displaced more laterally than the highest point of a normal hemidiaphragm.
Lateral view	Posteriorly, the apparent hemidiaphragm has a curved arc, but as it meets the junction with the major fissure, the apparent hemidiaphragm* assumes a flat edge that drops sharply to the anterior chest wall.	Posteriorly, the apparent hemidiaphragm has a curved arc but as it meets the junction with the major fissure, the apparent hemidiaphragm* assumes a flat edge that drops sharply to the anterior chest wall.

*__Apparent hemidiaphragm__ is the term used because the shadow being cast is actually from the subpulmonic fluid interfacing with the lung. The actual hemidiaphragm is invisible, silhouetted by the soft tissue in the abdomen below it and the pleural fluid above it.

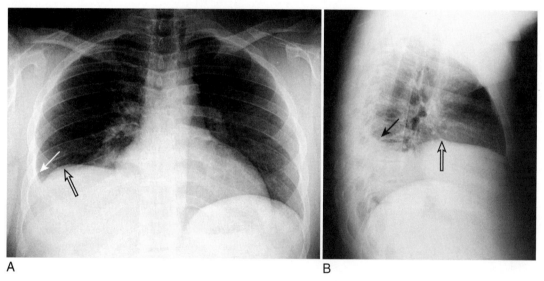

A   B

Figure 7-1. __Right-sided subpulmonic effusion.__ *In the frontal projection* __(A),__ *the highest point of the apparent hemidiaphragm (open black arrow) is more lateral than normal. This edge does not represent the actual right hemidiaphragm, which has been rendered invisible by the pleural fluid that has accumulated above it, but the interface between the effusion and the base of the lung (thus the term "apparent hemidiaphragm"). There is blunting of the right costophrenic sulcus (closed white arrow). On the lateral projection* __(B),__ *there is blunting of the posterior costophrenic sulcus (closed black arrow). The apparent hemidiaphragm is rounded posteriorly but then changes its contour as the effusion interfaces with the major fissure on the left side (open black arrow).*

- **Pleural thickening will not change in location** with a change in patient position, as most effusions will.

THE MENISCUS SIGN

- Because of the natural elastic recoil of the lungs, **pleural fluid appears to rise higher along the lateral margin of the thorax than it does medially** in the frontal projection.
  - This produces a characteristic *meniscus* shape to the effusion in the upright position.
- In the lateral projection, the fluid assumes a U-shape ascending equally high both anteriorly and posteriorly (Fig. 7-6).

- Identifying an abnormal lung density that demonstrates a meniscoid-shape is strongly suggestive of a pleural effusion.
- Effect of patient positioning on the appearance of pleural fluid:
  - In the **upright position,** pleural fluid falls to the base of the thoracic cavity owing to the force of gravity.
  - In the **supine position,** the same free-flowing effusion will layer along the posterior pleural space and produce a homogeneous "haze" over the entire hemithorax when viewed *en face* (Fig. 7-7).

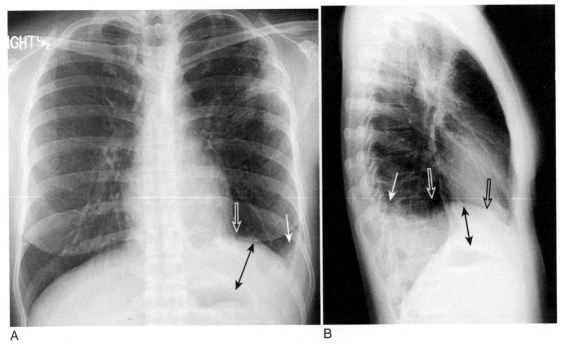

A   B

Figure 7-2. **Left-sided subpulmonic effusion.** *In both the frontal* **(A)** *and lateral* **(B)** *projections, there is more than 1 cm distance between the air in the stomach and the apparent left hemidiaphragm (double black arrows). The edge between the aerated lung and the open white arrows does not represent the actual left hemidiaphragm, which has been rendered invisible by the pleural fluid that has accumulated above it, but the interface between the effusion and the base of the lung. There is blunting of the left costophrenic sulcus (closed white arrows) on both projections. On the lateral projection* **(B),** *the apparent hemidiaphragm is rounded posteriorly (open white arrow) but then changes its contour as the effusion interfaces with the major fissure (open black arrow).*

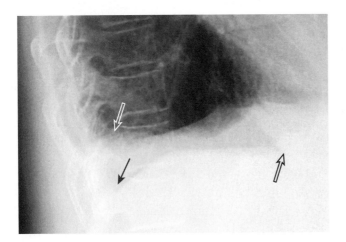

Figure 7-3. **Blunting of the right posterior costophrenic sulcus on the lateral projection.** *When approximately 75 mL of fluid has accumulated in the pleural space, the fluid will typically ascend in the thorax and blunt the posterior costophrenic sulcus (angle) first (open white arrow). This can be visualized only on the lateral projection. The normal, sharp posterior costophrenic angle is seen on the opposite side (closed black arrow). Notice how the normal hemidiaphragm is silhouetted by the heart anteriorly (open black arrow) indicating this is the left hemidiaphragm that is in contact with the heart. The pleural effusion is on the right side.*

- When the patient is **semirecumbent,** pleural fluid will form a triangular density of varying thickness at the lung base with the apex, or thinnest part, of the triangle ascending to varying heights in the hemithorax, depending on how recumbent the patient is and how much fluid is present.
- **Pitfall:** Depending on the patient's degree of recumbence, the lower lung fields may appear denser if the patient is upright and the fluid settles to the base of the thorax or more lucent as the patient becomes more recumbent and the effusion begins to layer posteriorly.
- **Solution:** In the best of all worlds, each portable chest radiograph should be exposed with the patient in the same position.
- **The lateral decubitus view of the chest**
  - The effect of positioning on the appearance of pleural fluid can be used for diagnostic advantage by having the patient lie on the side containing the effusion while taking a chest exposure using an x-ray beam directed horizontally.
  - If the patient lies on the right side, it is called a *right lateral decubitus* and if he lies on the left side, it is called a *left lateral decubitus* view of the chest.

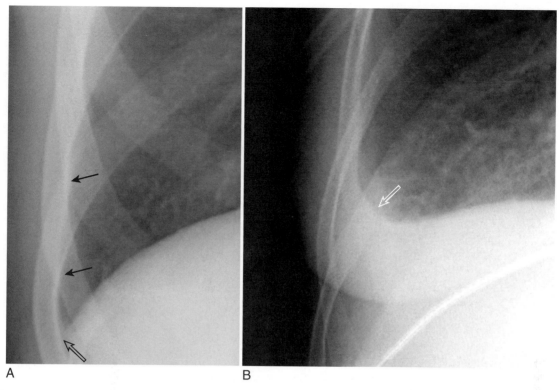

Figure 7-4. Normal and blunted right lateral costophrenic angle. *The hemidiaphragm usually makes a sharp and acute angle as it meets the lateral chest wall on the frontal projection* **(A)** *to produce the lateral costophrenic sulcus (open black arrow). Notice how normally aerated lung extends to the inner margin of each of the ribs (closed black arrows). When an effusion reaches about 300 mL in volume* **(B),** *the lateral costophrenic sulcus loses its acute angulation and becomes blunted (open white arrow).*

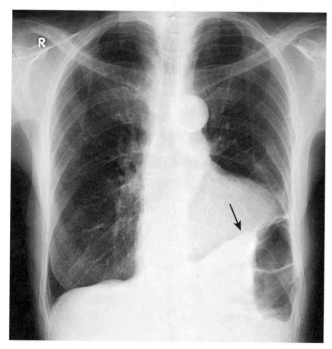

Figure 7-5. Scarring producing blunting of the left costophrenic angle. *Scarring from such things as previous infection, surgery, or blood in the pleural space sometimes produces a characteristic* **ski-slope appearance** *of blunting (closed black arrow), unlike the meniscoid appearance of a pleural effusion. This fibrosis would not change in appearance or location with change in the patient's position as free-flowing pleural fluid would.*

- **Decubitus views can be used to**
  - **Confirm the presence of a pleural effusion.**
  - **Determine whether a pleural effusion flows freely** in the pleural space or not, **an important factor to know before attempting to drain** pleural fluid.
  - **"Uncover" a portion of the underlying lung** hidden by the effusion.
- If a pleural effusion can flow freely in the pleural space, the fluid will produce a characteristic **bandlike area of increased density along the inner margin of the chest cage on the dependent side of the body.**
  - With a **right lateral decubitus view of the chest,** the patient's right side will be dependent and a **right pleural effusion will layer** along the dependent surface (Fig. 7-8A).
  - With a **left lateral decubitus view of the chest,** the patient's left side will be dependent and a **left pleural effusion will layer** along the dependent surface (Fig. 7-8B).
- **Fluid** may be present but **may not flow freely** in the pleural space **if there are adhesions present** which impede the flow of the fluid (see "Loculated Effusions").
- **Decubitus views** of the chest **can demonstrate effusions as small as 15 to 20 mL.**

OPACIFIED HEMITHORAX

- When the **hemithorax in an adult contains about 2 L** of fluid, the **entire hemithorax will be opacified** (Fig. 7-9).

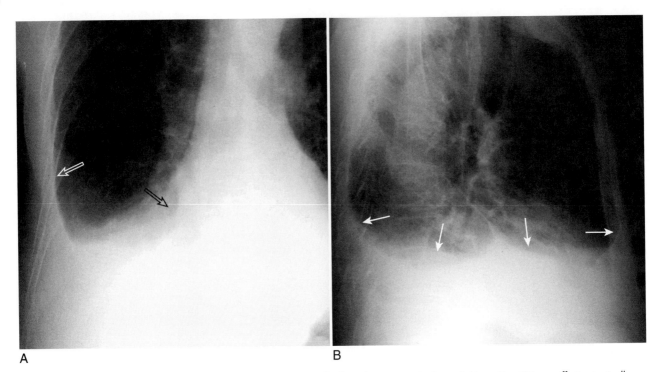

A   B

Figure 7-6. **Right pleural effusion, meniscoid appearance.** *On the frontal projection in the upright position* **(A),** *an effusion typically ascends more laterally (open white arrow) than it does medially (open black arrow) because of factors affecting the natural elastic recoil of the lung. On the lateral projection* **(B)** *the fluid ascends about the same amount anteriorly and posteriorly, forming a U-shaped density (closed white arrows).*

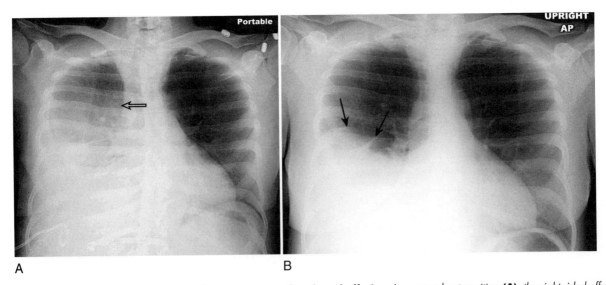

A   B

Figure 7-7. **Effect of patient positioning on the appearance of a pleural effusion.** *In a recumbent position* **(A),** *the right-sided effusion layers along the posterior pleural surface and produces a "haze" over the entire hemithorax that is densest at the base and less dense toward the apex of the lung (open black arrow). In the same patient x-rayed a few minutes later in a more upright position* **(B),** *pleural fluid falls to the base of the thoracic cavity due to the force of gravity (closed black arrows). This simple change in position can produce the mistaken impression that an effusion has improved (or worsened if the supine study follows the erect examination) when there has actually been no change in the amount of pleural fluid. Ideally, the patient should be x-rayed in the same position each time for a meaningful comparison.*

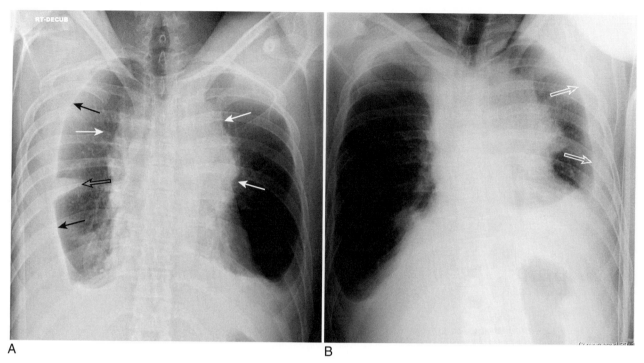

A   B

Figure 7-8. **Decubitus views of the chest. A,** A **right lateral decubitus view** *of the chest. The film is exposed with the patient lying on their right side on the examining table while a horizontal x-ray beam is directed posteroanteriorly (PA). Because the patient's right side is dependent, any free-flowing pleural fluid will layer along the right side (closed black arrows), forming a bandlike density. Notice how the fluid flows into the minor fissure (open black arrow).* **B,** A **left lateral decubitus view** *of the chest. When the same patient lies on the table with their left side down, free fluid on the left side layers along the left lateral chest wall (open white arrows). This patient has pleural effusions and bulky mediastinal adenopathy (closed white arrows in A) from lymphoma.*

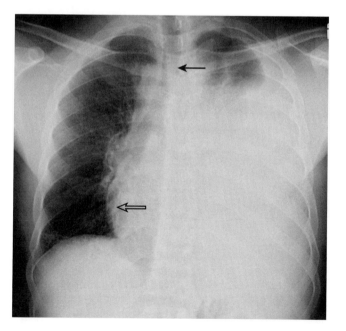

Figure 7-9. **Large left pleural effusion.** *The left hemithorax is almost completely opacified and there is a shift of the mobile mediastinal structures such as the trachea (closed black arrow) and the heart (open black arrow) away from the side of opacification. This is characteristic of a large pleural effusion, which acts like a mass. In most adults, it requires about 2 L of fluid to fill or almost fill the entire hemithorax such as this.*

- As fluid fills the pleural space, the lung tends to undergo passive collapse (atelectasis) (see Chapter 6).
- **Large effusions are sufficiently opaque** on conventional chest radiographs **so as to mask whatever disease may be present in the lung** enveloped by them.
  - **CT is the modality usually employed** to visualize the underlying lung that is rendered impenetrable by a large effusion.
- **Large effusions** act like a mass and **displace the heart and trachea away** from the **side of opacification** (see Fig. 5-3).
- **Pitfall:** Don't order a lateral decubitus view of the chest if the entire hemithorax is opacified because there can be no change in the position of the fluid and the underlying lung will be no more visible in the decubitus position than it was with the patient upright.
  - **Solution:** CT scan of the chest is a better means of evaluating the underlying lung if the hemithorax is opacified.
- For more on the opacified hemithorax, go to Chapter 5, Recognizing the Causes of an Opacified Hemithorax.

LOCULATED EFFUSIONS

- **Adhesions in the pleural space,** caused most often by old empyema or hemothorax, **may limit the normal mobility of a pleural effusion** so that it remains in the same location no matter what position the patient assumes.
- Imaging findings

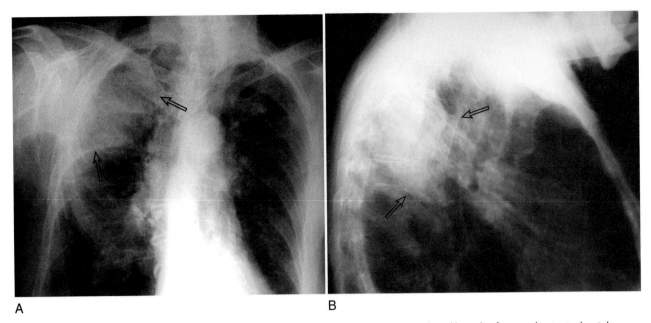

A   B

Figure 7-10. **Loculated pleural effusion in frontal (A) and lateral (B) projections.** *A pleural-based soft tissue density in the right upper lung field represents a loculated pleural effusion (open black arrows). Loculated effusions can be suspected when an effusion has an unusual shape or location in the thorax; for example, the effusion defies gravity by remaining at the apex of the lung even though the patient is upright. Loculation occurs because of pleural adhesions that prevent the fluid from flowing freely in the pleural space. Adhesions can result from such diseases as prior infection or prior hemothorax.*

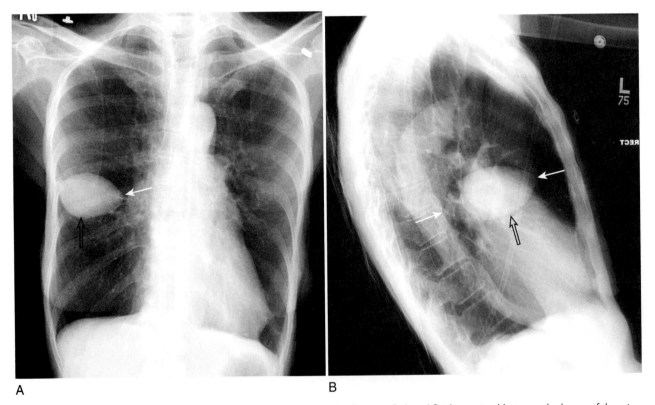

A   B

Figure 7-11. **Pseudotumor in the minor fissure.** *A sharply marginated collection of pleural fluid contained between the layers of the minor fissure produces a characteristic lenticular shape (open black arrows) that frequently has pointed ends on each side where they insinuate into the fissure so that pseudotumors look like a lemon on frontal **(A)** or lateral **(B)** chest radiographs (closed white arrows). Pseudotumors almost always occur in patients with congestive heart failure and, although they disappear when the underlying condition is treated, they frequently return each time the patient's failure recurs.*

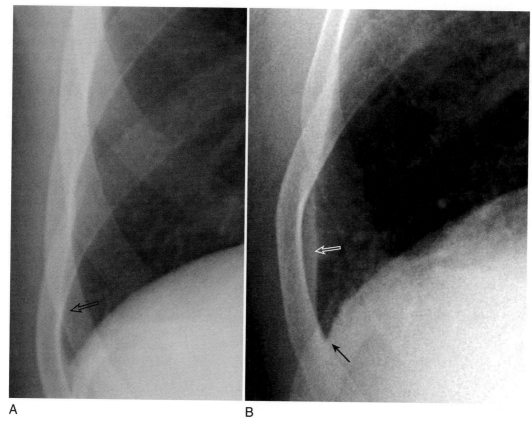

Figure 7-12. Normal versus laminar pleural effusion. In **A**, notice how normally aerated lung extends to the inner margin of each of the ribs (open black arrow). In **B**, there is a thin band of increased density that extends superiorly from the lung base (open white arrow) but does not appear to cause blunting of the costophrenic angle (closed black arrow). This is the appearance of a laminar pleural effusion that is most often associated with either congestive heart failure or lymphangitic spread of malignancy in the lung. This patient was in congestive heart failure.

- Loculated effusions **can be suspected when an effusion has an unusual shape or location in the thorax,** e.g., the effusion defies gravity by remaining at the apex of the lung even though the patient is upright (Fig. 7-10).
- **Loculation of pleural fluid has therapeutic importance** because such collections tend to be traversed by multiple adhesions, which make it difficult to drain the noncommunicating pockets of fluid with a single pleural drainage tube in the same way free-flowing effusions can be drained.

FISSURAL PSEUDOTUMORS

- *Pseudotumors* (also called *vanishing tumors*) are sharply marginated collections of pleural fluid contained either between the layers of an **interlobar pulmonary fissure** or in a subpleural location just beneath the fissure.
- They are **transudates** that **almost always occur in patients with congestive heart failure (CHF).**
- The imaging findings of a pseudotumor are characteristic, so they should not be mistaken for an actual tumor (from which they derive their name).

- They are **lenticular in shape,** most often occur in the **minor fissure (75%),** and frequently have **pointed ends on each side** where they insinuate into the fissure, much like the shape of a lemon.
- They **do not tend to flow freely** with a change in patient positioning.
- They **disappear when the underlying condition (usually CHF) is treated** but they **tend to recur in the same location** each time the patient's failure recurs (Fig. 7-11).

LAMINAR EFFUSIONS

- A laminar effusion is a form of pleural effusion in which the fluid assumes a **thin, bandlike density along the lateral chest wall, especially near the costophrenic angle.**
  - The lateral costophrenic angle appears to maintain its sharpness.
- Laminar effusions are **almost always the result of** elevated left atrial pressure, as in **congestive heart failure** or secondary to **lymphangitic spread of malignancy.**
- They **are usually not free-flowing.**
- They can be recognized by the band of increased density that separates the air-filled lung from the inside margin of

the contiguous ribs at the lung base on the frontal chest radiograph.
- In normal subjects, aerated lung should extend to the inside of each contiguous rib (Fig. 7-12).

HYDROPNEUMOTHORAX

- The presence of *both* air in the pleural space (pneumothorax) *and* abnormal amounts of fluid in the pleural space (pleural effusion or hydrothorax) is called a *hydropneumothorax.*
- Some of the more common causes of a hydropneumothorax are **trauma, surgery,** or a **recent pleural tap to remove fluid** in which air enters the pleural apace.
  - *Bronchopleural fistula,* an abnormal and relatively uncommon connection between the bronchial tree and the pleural space most often due to tumor, surgery, or infection, can also produce both air and fluid in the pleural space.
- Unlike pleural effusion alone, whose mensicoid shape is governed by the elastic recoil of the lung, a **hydropneumothorax produces an air-fluid level in the hemithorax** marked by a straight edge and a sharp air-over-fluid interface when the exposure is made with a horizontal x-ray beam (Fig. 7-13).
- CT is frequently necessary to distinguish between some presentations of hydropneumothorax and a **lung abscess,** both of which may have a similar appearance on conventional chest radiographs.

Side Specificity of Pleural Effusions

- **Diseases that usually produce bilateral effusions.**
  - **Congestive heart failure**
    - Usually about the same amount of fluid in each hemithorax
    - **If there are markedly different amounts** in each hemithorax, **suspect a parapneumonic effusion or malignancy** on the side with the greater volume of fluid.
  - **Lupus erythematosus**—usually bilateral, but when unilateral, the effusions are usually left-sided.
- **Diseases that can produce effusions on either side.**
  - **Tuberculosis** and other exudative effusions associated with infectious agents, including viruses
  - **Pulmonary thromboembolic disease**
  - **Trauma**
- **Diseases that usually produce left-sided effusions.**
  - **Pancreatitis**
  - **Dressler's syndrome** (Box 7-1; Fig. 7-14)
  - **Distal thoracic duct obstruction**
- **Diseases that usually produce right-sided effusions.**
  - **Abdominal disease related to liver or ovary**—some ovarian tumors can be associated with a right pleural effusion and ascites *(Meigs' syndrome).*
  - **Rheumatoid arthritis**—the effusion can remain unchanged for years.
  - **Proximal thoracic duct obstruction**

WebLink
More information on recognizing pleural effusions is available to registered users on StudentConsult.com.

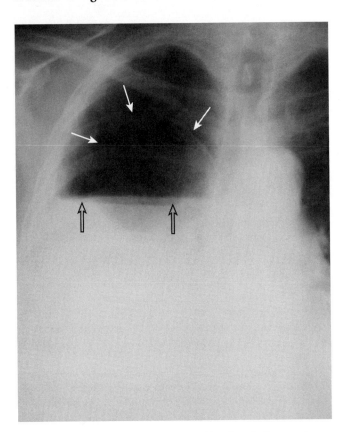

Figure 7-13. **Hydropneumothorax.** *Unlike pleural effusions alone, whose mensicoid shape is governed by the elastic recoil of the lung, hydropneumothorax produces an air-fluid level in the hemithorax (open black arrows) marked by a straight edge and a sharp air over fluid interface when the exposure is made with a horizontal x-ray beam. The visceral pleural line is seen as well (closed white arrows). Surgery, trauma, a recent thoracentesis to remove pleural fluid, and bronchopleural fistulae are among the causes of a hydropneumothorax. This person was stabbed in the right side and this actually represents a hemopneumothorax, but conventional radiography is unable to distinguish between blood and any other fluid. A CT scan of the chest or a pleural tap would be necessary to better define the pleural fluid.*

Box 7-1

Dressler's Syndrome
Postpericardiotomy/postmyocardial infarction syndrome
Typically occurs 2–3 weeks after a transmural myocardial infarct, producing a left pleural effusion, pericardial effusion and patchy airspace disease at the left lung base
Associated with chest pain and fever; usually responds to high-dose aspirin or steroids

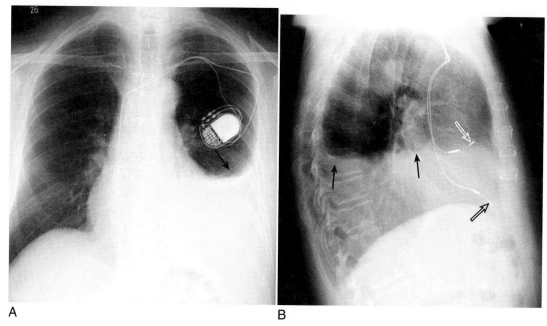

Figure 7-14. **Dressler's syndrome (postpericardiotomy/postmyocardial infarction syndome).** *This syndrome typically occurs 2 to 3 weeks after a transmural myocardial infarct. It also can occur following pericardiotomy such as occurs in patients undergoing coronary artery bypass surgery, as in this case. The combination of chest pain and fever, left pleural effusion (closed black arrows), patchy left lower lobe airspace disease, and pericardial effusion several weeks following a myocardial infarction or open-heart surgery should suggest the syndrome. It usually responds to high-dose aspirin or steroids. This patient has a dual lead pacemaker in place and, on the lateral projection* **(B),** *the leads are seen in the region of the right atrium (open white arrow) and right ventricle (open black arrow).*

⊞ TAKE-HOME POINTS: Recognizing a Pleural Effusion

Pleural effusions collect in the potential space between the visceral and parietal pleurae and are either transudates or exudates depending on their protein content and LDH concentration.

There are normally a few milliliters of fluid in the pleural space; about 75 mL are required to blunt the posterior costophrenic sulcus (seen on the lateral view) and about 200–300 mL to blunt the lateral costophrenic sulcus (seen on the frontal view); approximately 2 L of fluid will cause opacification of the entire hemithorax in an adult.

Most pleural effusions begin by collecting in the pleural space between the hemidiaphragm and the base of the lung; these are called **subpulmonic effusions.**

As the amount of fluid increases, it forms a **meniscus** shape on the upright frontal chest radiograph due to the natural elastic recoil properties of the lung.

Large pleural effusions act like a mass and characteristically produce a shift of the mobile mediastinal structures (e.g., the heart) away from the side of the effusion.

In the absence of pleural adhesions, effusions will flow freely and change location with a change in the patient's position; with pleural adhesions (usually from old infection or hemothorax) the fluid may assume unusual appearances or occur in atypical locations; such effusions are said to be **loculated.**

A **pseudotumor** is a type of loculated effusion that occurs in the fissures of the lung (mostly the minor fissure) and is most frequently secondary to congestive heart failure; it clears when the underlying failure is treated.

Laminar effusions are best recognized at the lung base just above the costophrenic angles on the frontal projection and, when seen, most often occur as a result of either congestive heart failure or lymphangitic spread of malignancy.

A **hydropneumothorax** is both air and abnormal amounts of fluid in the pleural space and is recognizable on an upright view of the chest by a straight, air-fluid interface rather than the typical meniscus shape of pleural fluid alone.

Whether an effusion is unilateral or bilateral, mostly right-sided or mostly left-sided, can be an important clue to its cause.

8 Recognizing Pneumonia

General Considerations

- Pneumonia can be generally defined as **consolidation of lung produced by inflammatory exudate, usually as a result of an infectious agent.**
- **Most pneumonias produce airspace disease, either lobar or segmental.**
- **Other pneumonias demonstrate interstitial disease,** and others produce findings in both the airspaces and the interstitium.
- Most microorganisms that produce pneumonia are **spread to the lungs via the tracheobronchial tree, either through inhalation or aspiration** of the organisms.
  - In some instances, microorganisms are spread via the bloodstream and, in even fewer cases, by direct extension.
- Because many different microorganisms can produce similar imaging findings in the lungs, it is **difficult to identify with certainty the causative organism from the roentgenographic presentation alone.**
  - However, **certain patterns** of disease **are very suggestive** of a particular causative organism (Table 8-1).
- Some use the term "infiltrate" to be synonymous with pneumonia, although many diseases, from amyloid to pulmonary fibrosis, can infiltrate the lung.

General Characteristics of Pneumonia

- Because **pneumonia** fills the involved airspaces or interstitial tissues with some form of fluid or inflammatory exudate, it **will appear denser (whiter) than the surrounding normally aerated lung.**
- **Pneumonia may contain air bronchograms** if the bronchi themselves are not filled with inflammatory exudate or fluid (see Chapter 4, "Characteristics of Airspace Disease") (Fig. 8-1).
  - When the bronchi are filled with fluid, as in bronchopneumonia, there will be no air bronchograms present.
  - Air bronchograms are **much more likely to be visible when the pneumonia involves the central portion** of the lung near the hilum.
    - Near the periphery of the lung, air bronchograms are usually too small to be visible.
  - Remember that anything of fluid or soft tissue density that replaces the normal gas in the airspaces may also produce this sign, so **an air bronchogram is not specific for pneumonia** (see Chapter 4, Recognizing Airspace versus Interstitial Lung Disease).
- **Airspace pneumonias appear fluffy** and their **margins are indistinct.**
  - **Where pneumonia abuts a pleural surface,** such as an interlobar fissure or the chest wall, **it will be sharply marginated.**

- Interstitial pneumonia, on the other hand, may produce prominence of the interstitial markings in the affected part of the lung or may spread to adjacent airways and resemble airspace disease.
- Except for the presence of air bronchograms, airspace **pneumonia is usually homogeneous in density** (Fig. 8-2).
- In some types of pneumonia (i.e., bronchopneumonia), **the bronchi as well as the airspaces contain inflammatory exudate.**
  - This can lead to **atelectasis associated with the pneumonia.**
- Box 8-1 summarizes the keys to recognizing pneumonia.

Patterns of Pneumonia

- Pneumonias may be distributed in the lung in several patterns described as *lobar, segmental, interstitial, round,* and *cavitary* (Table 8-2).

Table 8-1

PATTERNS THAT MIGHT SUGGEST A CAUSATIVE ORGANISM

Pattern of Disease	Likely Causative Organism
Upper lobe cavitary pneumonia with spread to the opposite lower lobe	*Mycobacterium tuberculosis* (TB)
Upper lobe lobar pneumonia with bulging interlobar fissure	*Klebsiella pneumoniae*
Lower lobe cavitary pneumonia	*Pseudomonas aeruginosa* or anaerobic organisms (*Bacteroides*)
Perihilar interstitial disease or perihilar airspace disease	*Pneumocystis carinii (jiroveci)*
Thin-walled upper lobe cavity	*Coccidioides* (coccidioidomycosis, TB)
Airspace disease with effusion	Streptococci, staphylococci (TB)
Diffuse nodules	*Histoplasma, Coccidioides* (TB, histoplasmosis, coccidiomycosis)
Soft-tissue, fingerlike shadows in upper lobes	*Aspergillus* (allergic bronchopulmonary aspergillosis)
Solitary pulmonary nodule	*Cryptococcus*
Spherical soft tissue mass in a thin-walled upper lobe cavity	*Aspergillus* (aspergilloma)

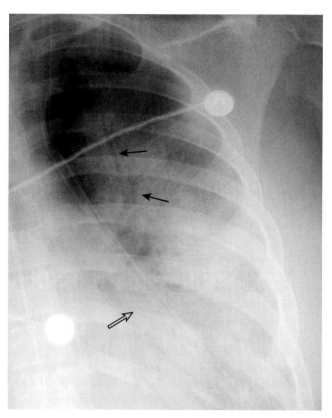

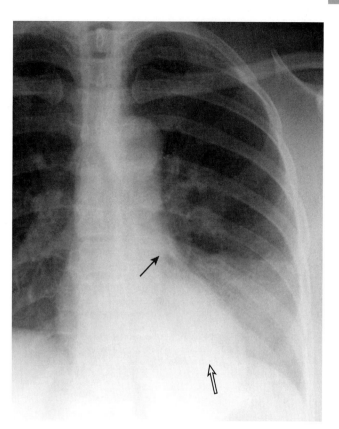

Figure 8-1. **Lingular pneumonia.** *There are several black, branching structures* (closed black arrows) *that represent typical air bronchograms seen centrally in airspace disease in this patient with pneumococcal pneumonia. The disease is homogeneous in density, except for the presence of the air bronchograms. The disease can be localized to the lingula because the pneumonia is obscuring the left heart border* (open black arrow), *an example of the* **silhouette sign.** *The consolidated lingula, being an anterior structure, is in contact with the left heart border, also an anterior structure, and because they are now of the same radiographic density (fluid or soft tissue), the edge between them disappears.*

Figure 8-2. **Left lower lobe pneumococcal pneumonia.** *Airspace disease in the left lower lobe contains an air bronchogram centrally* (closed black arrow). *The disease is of homogeneous density except for the presence of the air bronchogram. The disease is in contact with the medial portion of the left hemidiaphragm, which is ''silhouetted'' by the fluid density of the consolidated lower lobe in contact with the soft tissue density of the diaphragm* (open black arrow).

Box 8-1

Recognizing a Pneumonia—Key Signs
Pneumonia is more opaque than surrounding normal lung.
In airspace disease, the margins may be fluffy and indistinct except where they abut a pleural surface such as the interlobar fissures where the margin will be sharp.
Interstitial pneumonias will cause a prominence of the interstitial tissues of the lung in the affected area; in some cases, the disease can spread to the alveoli and resemble airspace disease.
Affected area tends to be homogeneous in density.
Lobar pneumonias may contain air bronchograms.
Segmental pneumonias may be associated with atelectasis in the affected portion of the lung.

- Remember, these terms simply describe the distribution of the disease in the lungs; they aren't diagnostic of pneumonia because many other diseases can produce the same patterns of disease distribution in the lung.

LOBAR PNEUMONIA
- The **prototypical lobar pneumonia is pneumococcal pneumonia** caused by *Streptococcus pneumoniae* (Fig. 8-3).
- Although we are calling it lobar pneumonia, the patient may present with the disease before the entire lobe is involved.
  - In its most classical form, the disease fills most or all of a lobe of the lung.
- Because lobes are bound by interlobar fissures, **one or more of the margins of a lobar pneumonia may be sharply marginated.**

- Where the disease is not bound by a fissure, it will have an **indistinct and irregular margin.**
- Lobar pneumonias almost always produce a ***silhouette sign*** where they come in contact with the heart, aorta, or diaphragm, and they almost always contain ***air***

Table 8-2

PATTERNS OF APPEARANCE OF PNEUMONIAS

Pattern	Characteristics
Lobar	Homogeneous consolidation of affected lobe with air bronchogram
Segmental (bronchopneumonia)	Patchy airspace disease frequently involving several segments simultaneously; no air bronchogram; atelectasis may be associated
Interstitial	Reticular interstitial disease usually diffusely spread throughout lungs early in a disease process; frequently progresses to airspace disease
Round	Spherical pneumonia usually seen in the lower lobes of children; may resemble a mass
Cavitary	Produced by numerous microorganisms, chief among them being *Mycobacterium tuberculosis*

bronchograms if they involve the central portions of the lung.

SEGMENTAL PNEUMONIA (BRONCHOPNEUMONIA)

- The **prototypical bronchopneumonia is caused by *Staphylococcus aureus.***
  - Many gram-negative bacteria, such as *Pseudomonas aeruginosa*, produce the same picture.
- The disease is spread centrifugally via the tracheobronchial tree to **many foci at the same time.**
- Therefore, **it frequently involves several segments** of the lung.
- Because lung segments are not bound by fissures, all of the **margins of segmental pneumonias tend to be fluffy and indistinct** (Fig. 8-4).
- Unlike lobar pneumonia, **segmental bronchopneumonias produce exudate that fills the bronchi.**
  - **Air bronchograms are usually not present.**
  - **Frequently, some volume loss (atelectasis) is associated with bronchopneumonia.**

INTERSTITIAL PNEUMONIA

- The **prototypes for interstitial pneumonia are viral pneumonia and *Mycoplasma pneumoniae*** as well as ***Pneumocystis*** pneumonia in patients with AIDS.
- Interstitial pneumonias **tend to involve the airway walls and alveolar septa** and may produce, especially early in their course, a **fine, reticular pattern in the lungs.**

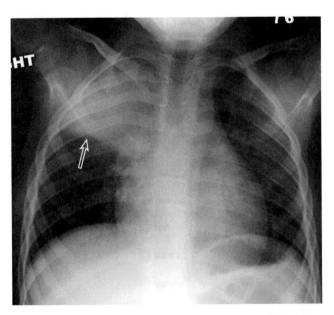

Figure 8-3. ***Right upper lobe pneumococcal pneumonia.*** *There is airspace disease in the right upper lobe that occupies all of that lobe (open white arrow). Because lobes are bound by interlobar fissures (in this case the minor or horizontal fissure is located at the open white arrow), the inferior margin of the pneumonia is sharply marginated. There is some volume loss associated with this particular pneumonia, as evidenced by the superior displacement of the minor fissure. The disease is homogeneous and there are faint air bronchograms centrally.*

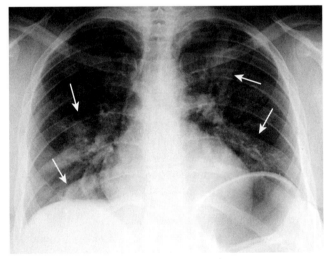

Figure 8-4. ***Staphylococcal bronchopneumonia.*** *There are multiple irregularly marginated patches of airspace disease in both lungs (closed white arrows). This is a characteristic distribution and appearance of bronchopneumonia. The disease is spread centrifugally via the tracheobronchial tree to many foci at the same time so it frequently involves several segments of the lung. Lung segments are not bound by fissures, so all the margins of segmental pneumonias tend to be fluffy and indistinct. No air bronchograms are present, in part because inflammatory exudate fills the bronchi as well as the airspaces around them.*

- Most **interstitial pneumonia eventually spreads to the adjacent alveoli** and produces patchy or confluent airspace disease, **making the original interstitial nature of the pneumonia impossible to recognize** radiographically.
- *Pneumocystis carinii (jiroveci)* **pneumonia (PCP)**
  - PCP is the **most common clinically recognized infection** in patients with acquired immunodeficiency syndrome (AIDS).
    - Classically presents as a **perihilar, reticular interstitial pneumonia,** or
    - **Airspace disease that may mimic the central distribution of pulmonary edema** (Fig. 8-5)
    - Other presentations such as unilateral airspace disease or widespread, patchy airspace disease can occur but are less common.
    - There are usually **no pleural effusions and no hilar adenopathy.**
    - Opportunistic infections **usually occur with CD4 cell counts under 200** per cubic mL of blood.

ROUND PNEUMONIA

- Some pneumonias, mostly in children, can assume a **spherical shape** on chest radiographs.
- These *round pneumonias* are almost always **posterior** in the lungs, usually **in the lower lobes.**
- Causative agents are frequently *Haemophilus influenzae, Streptococcus,* and *Pneumococcus.*

- A round pneumonia could be confused with a tumor mass except that symptoms associated with infection usually accompany the lung findings and tumors are uncommon in children (Fig. 8-6).

CAVITARY PNEUMONIA

- The prototypical organism is *Mycobacterium tuberculosis.*
- **Primary tuberculosis (primary TB)**
  - **Cavitation is rare** in primary TB.
  - Primary TB **affects the upper lobes slightly more than the lower,** produces airspace disease that **may be associated with ipsilateral hilar adenopathy** (especially in children) and **large, often unilateral, pleural effusions** (especially in adults) (Fig. 8-7).
- **Postprimary tuberculosis (reactivation tuberculosis)**
  - **Cavitation is common.**
    - The cavity is usually **thin-walled.**
    - It has a **smooth inner margin.**
    - **There is usually no air-fluid level** (Fig. 8-8).
  - Postprimary tuberculosis almost always **affects the apical or posterior segments of the upper lobes or the superior segments of the lower lobes.**
  - **Bilateral upper lobe disease is very common.**
  - **Transbronchial spread** (from one upper lobe to the opposite lower lobe, or to another lobe in the lung) **should make you think of *Mycobacterium tuberculosis*** as the causative organism.
  - **Healing occurs with fibrosis and retraction.**
- **Miliary tuberculosis**
  - Considered to be a manifestation of primary TB, although clinical appearance of miliary TB may not occur for many years after initial infection.

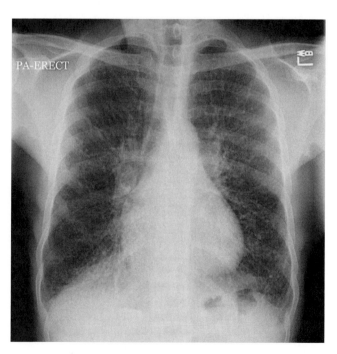

Figure 8-5. Pneumocystis carinii (jiroveci) pneumonia (PCP). *There is diffuse interstitial lung disease that is primarily reticular in nature. Without the additional history that this patient had acquired immunodeficiency syndrome (AIDS), this could be mistaken for pulmonary interstitial edema or for a chronic, fibrotic process such as sarcoidosis. No pleural effusions are present, as might be expected with pulmonary interstitial edema, and there is no evidence of hilar adenopathy, as might occur in sarcoid.*

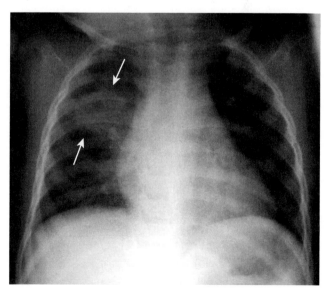

Figure 8-6. Round pneumonia. *A soft tissue density in the right upper lobe of this 1-year-old child has a rounded appearance (closed white arrows). The child had a cough and fever. This is a characteristic appearance of a round pneumonia, most common in children and frequently due to either Haemophilus, streptococcal, or pneumococcal infection.*

Figure 8-7. **Primary tuberculosis.** *Prominence of the left hilum is caused by left hilar adenopathy (closed white arrows). Unilateral hilar adenopathy may be the only manifestation of primary infection with Mycobacterium tuberculosis, especially in children. When it produces pneumonia, primary TB affects the upper lobes slightly more than the lower. It produces airspace disease that may be associated with ipsilateral hilar adenopathy (especially in children) and large, often unilateral, pleural effusions (especially in adults).*

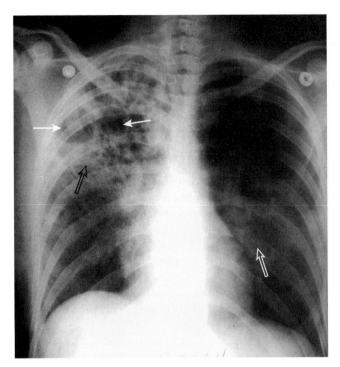

Figure 8-8. **Postprimary tuberculosis (reactivation tuberculosis).** *A cavitary pneumonia is in the right upper lobe (open black arrow). Numerous thin-walled cystic lesions (cavities) are seen throughout the airspace disease (closed white arrows). A cavitary upper lobe pneumonia is presumptively TB, until proved otherwise. In addition, airspace disease is seen in the left lower lobe (open white arrow), another finding suggestive of TB that can spread via a transbronchial route to the opposite lower lobe or another lobe in the same lung. (The apparent absence of lung markings in the left upper lung field is an artifact of the reproduction.)*

- When first visible, the **small nodules measure only about 1 mm;** they can grow to 2 to 3 mm if left untreated (Fig. 8-9).
- **When miliary TB is treated, clearing is usually rapid.**
- **Miliary TB seldom,** if ever, **heals with calcification.**
- **Other infectious agents** may produce cavitary disease:
- **Staphylococcal pneumonia** can cavitate and produce thin-walled *pneumatoceles.*
- **Streptococcal pneumonia,** *Klebsiella* **pneumonia, and coccidioidomycosis** are among some of the other pneumonias that can cavitate.

Aspiration Pneumonia

- Aspiration pneumonia almost always occurs in the **most dependent portions of the lung.**
- When the person is **upright,** the most dependent portions of the lung will usually be the **lower lobes.**
  - The **right side is more often affected than the left** because of the straighter and wider nature of the right main bronchus.
- When a person is recumbent, aspiration usually occurs into the superior segments of the lower lobes or the posterior portion of the upper lobes.

- **Acute aspiration** will produce radiographic findings of **airspace disease.**
  - Its location, the rapidity with which it appears, and the group of patients predisposed to aspirate are clues to its diagnosis (Fig. 8-10).
- **Recognizing the different types of aspiration** (Table 8-3)
  - The clinical and radiologic course of aspiration depends on what was aspirated.
    - **Aspiration of bland (neutralized) gastric juices or water**
      - This is technically **not a pneumonia,** is handled by the lung as if it were pulmonary edema fluid, and **classically remains for only a day or two before clearing** through resorption (see Fig. 4-7).
    - **Aspiration that produces pneumonia due to microorganisms in the lung**
      - Although **we all constantly aspirate numerous microorganisms present in the normal oropharyngeal flora,** there are some patients in whom these microorganisms can develop into pneumonia including those who are immunocompromised, elderly, or debilitated or who have underlying lung disease.

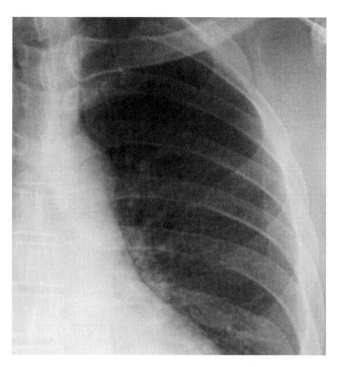

Figure 8-9. **Miliary tuberculosis.** *Innumerable small round nodules are present in this close-up view of the left upper lobe in a patient with miliary tuberculosis. At the start of the disease, the nodules are so small they are frequently difficult to detect on conventional radiographs. When they reach about 1 mm or larger, they become visible. Miliary tuberculosis clears relatively rapidly with appropriate treatment and does not heal with calcification.*

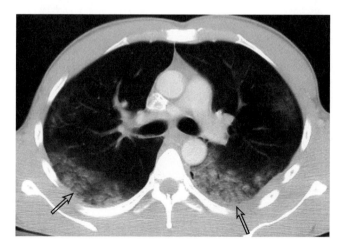

Figure 8-10. **Aspiration, both lower lobes.** *Single, axial CT image of the chest demonstrates bilateral lower lobe airspace disease in a patient who had aspirated (open black arrows). Aspiration usually affects the most dependent portions of the lung. In the upright position, the lower lobes are affected; in the recumbent position, aspiration affects the superior segments of the lower lobes and the posterior portions of the upper lobes. Aspiration of water or neutralized gastric acid will usually clear in 24 to 48 hours, depending on the volume aspirated.*

Table 8-3

THREE PATTERNS OF ACUTE ASPIRATION

Aspirate	Characteristics
Bland gastric acid or water	Rapidly appearing and rapidly clearing airspace disease in dependent lobe(s); not a pneumonia
Infected aspirate	Usually lower lobe; frequently cavitates and may take months to clear
Unneutralized stomach acid	Immediate appearance of dependent airspace disease that frequently becomes secondarily infected

- Usually caused by **anaerobic organisms,** such as *Bacteroides*
- Produce **lower lobe airspace disease** that **frequently cavitates**
- May take **months** to resolve
- **Aspiration of unneutralized stomach acid** (*Mendelson's syndrome*)
  - **Chemical pneumonitis develops,** producing dependent lobe airspace disease or **pulmonary edema.**
  - May appear within **hours** of the aspiration
  - Takes **days or longer to clear** and may become **secondarily infected**

Localizing Pneumonia

- Although it is true that an antibiotic will travel to every lobe of the lung without regard for which actually harbors the pneumonia, determining the location of a pneumonia may provide clues to the causative organism (e.g., upper lobes, think of TB) and the presence of associated pathology (e.g., lower lobes, think of recurrent aspiration).
- It is always **best to localize disease on conventional radiographs using two views taken at 90° to each other** (*orthogonal views*), such as frontal and lateral chest radiographs.
- Sometimes, only a frontal radiograph may be available, as with critically ill or debilitated patients who require a portable bedside examination.
- Nevertheless, it is still frequently **possible to localize the pneumonia using only the frontal radiograph** by analyzing which structure's edges are obscured by the disease (i.e., the silhouette sign).
- **Silhouette sign** (see also Chapter 4, "Characteristics of Airspace Disease")
  - If two objects of the **same** radiographic density **touch** each other, then the **edge between them disappears** (see Fig. 4-4).
    - The silhouette sign is valuable in localizing and identifying tissue types throughout the body, not just the chest.

Table 8-4

USING THE SILHOUETTE SIGN ON THE FRONTAL CHEST RADIOGRAPH

Structure That Is No Longer Visible	Disease Location
Ascending aorta	Right upper lobe
Right heart border	Right middle lobe
Right hemidiaphragm	Right lower lobe
Descending aorta	Left upper or lower lobe
Left heart border	Lingula of left upper lobe
Left hemidiaphragm	Left lower lobe

- You can utilize the silhouette sign to localize a pneumonia, even if only a frontal projection is available (Table 8-4).
- The *spine sign* (Fig. 8-11)
  - Normally on the lateral chest x-ray, the **thoracic spine appears to get darker (blacker) as you survey it from the shoulder girdle to the diaphragm.**
    - This is because the x-ray beam normally needs to penetrate more tissue (more bones, more muscle) around the shoulders than it does just above the diaphragm (just the aerated lungs).
- **When disease** of soft tissue or fluid density **involves the posterior portion of the lower lobe,** more of the x-ray beam will be absorbed by the new, added density and **the spine will appear to become "whiter" (more opaque) just above the posterior costophrenic sulcus.**
  - This is called the *spine sign* and it provides another way to localize disease in the lungs.
- This **lower lobe disease may not be apparent on the frontal projection** if it falls below the plane of the highest point of the affected hemidiaphragm.
- Therefore, the *spine sign* may indicate the presence of lower lobe **disease,** like lower lobe pneumonia, **which may be otherwise invisible on the frontal projection.**

How Pneumonia Resolves

- Pneumonia can resolve in 2 to 3 days if the organism is sensitive to the antibiotic administered, especially pneumococcal pneumonia.
- **Most pneumonias typically resolve from within** (vacuolize), gradually disappearing in a patchy fashion over days or weeks (Fig. 8-12).
- If a pneumonia **does not** resolve in weeks, **consider an underlying** obstructing lesion, such as a **neoplasm,** that is preventing adequate drainage from that portion of the lung.

WebLink

More information on recognizing pneumonia is available to registered users on StudentConsult.com.

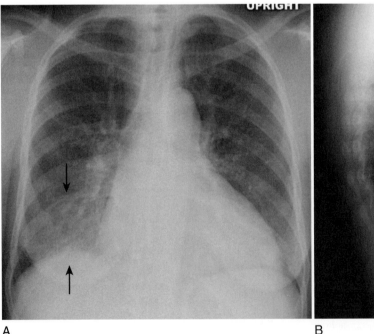
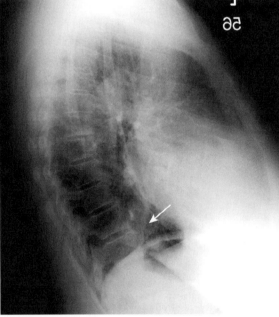

A
B

Figure 8-11. **The spine sign.** *Frontal and lateral views of the chest demonstrate airspace disease on the lateral film* **(B)** *in the right lower lobe that may not be immediately apparent on the frontal film (you can see the pneumonia in the right lower lobe in* **A** *[closed black arrows]). Normally, the thoracic spine appears to get "blacker" as you view it from the neck to the diaphragm because there is less tissue for the x-ray beam to traverse just above the diaphragm than in the region of the shoulder girdle (see also Fig. 2-12). In this case, a right lower lobe pneumonia superimposed on the lower spine in the lateral view (closed white arrow) makes the spine appear "whiter" (more dense) just above the diaphragm. This is called the* **spine sign.**

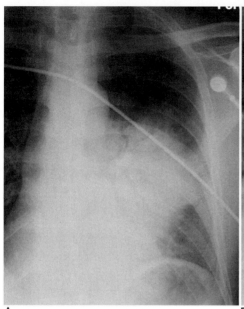
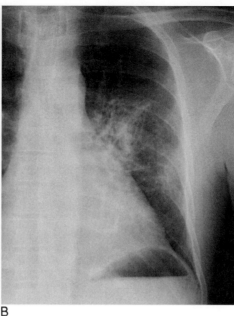

A   B

Figure 8-12. **Resolving pneumonia.** *Pneumonia can resolve in days if the organism is sensitive to the antibiotic administered, especially pneumococcal pneumonia. Most pneumonias, like that in the left upper lobe on radiographs taken 7 days apart shown in* **A** *and* **B,** *typically resolve from within (vacuolize), gradually disappearing in a patchy fashion over days or weeks. If a pneumonia does not resolve in weeks, you should consider the presence of an underlying obstructing lesion, such as a neoplasm, that is preventing adequate drainage from that portion of the lung.*

TAKE-HOME POINTS: Recognizing a Pneumonia

Pneumonia is more opaque than the surrounding normal lung, and its margins may be fluffy and indistinct except for where it abuts a pleural margin; it tends to appear homogeneous in density; it may contain air bronchograms; it may be associated with atelectasis.

Although there is considerable overlap in the patterns of pneumonia different organisms produce, some appearances are highly suggestive of particular etiologic agents.

Lobar pneumonia (prototype: pneumococcal pneumonia) tends to be homogeneous, occupy most or all of a lobe, have air bronchograms centrally, and produce the silhouette sign.

Segmental pneumonia (prototype: staphylococcal pneumonia) tends to be multifocal, does not have air bronchograms, and can be associated with volume loss because bronchi are also filled with inflammatory exudate.

Interstitial pneumonia (prototype: viral pneumonia or PCP) tends to involve the airway walls and alveolar septa and may produce, especially early in the course, a fine, reticular pattern in the lungs; later in the course, it can produce airspace disease.

Round pneumonia (prototype: *Haemophilus*) usually occurs in children in the lower lobes posteriorly and can resemble a mass, although masses in children are uncommon.

Cavitary pneumonia (prototype: tuberculosis) has cavities produced by lung necrosis as its hallmark; postprimary tuberculosis usually involves the upper lobes; it can spread via a transbronchial route that can infect the opposite lower lobe or another lobe in the same lung.

Aspiration occurs in the most dependent portion of the lung at the time of the aspiration, usually the lower lobes or the posterior segments of the upper lobes; aspiration can be bland and clear quickly, can be infected and take months to clear, or may be from a chemical pneumonitis, which can take weeks to clear.

Pneumonia can be localized with just a frontal radiograph by using the silhouette sign as an aid.

Pneumonias frequently resolve by "breaking up" so that they contain patchy areas of newly aerated lung within the confines of the previous area of consolidation (vacuolization).

9 Recognizing Pneumothorax, Pneumomediastinum, Pneumopericardium, and Subcutaneous Emphysema

Normal Anatomy
- The **pleura is composed of two layers, the outer parietal and inner visceral.**
  - The pleural space lies between them.
- Normally there are **several milliliters of fluid but no air in the pleural space.**
- The visceral pleura is adherent to the lung.
- **Neither the parietal pleura nor the visceral pleura is normally visible** on a conventional chest radiograph, except where two layers of visceral pleura enfold to form the major and minor fissures.

Recognizing a Pneumothorax
- A **pneumothorax occurs when air enters the pleural space.**
  - The negative pressure normally present in the pleural space rises higher than the intralveolar pressure and the lung collapses.
  - The parietal pleura remains on the inner surface of the chest wall, but the visceral pleura advances toward the hilum with the collapsing lung.
  - The **visceral pleura becomes visible as a thin, white line** outlined by air on both sides, marking the outer border of the lung and indicating the presence of a pneumothorax.
- The visible visceral pleura is called the *visceral pleural white line* or simply the *visceral pleural line.*
- **You must be able to identify the visceral pleural line (Fig. 9-1) to make the definitive diagnosis of a pneumothorax!**
- Even as the lung collapses, it tends to maintain its usual lunglike shape so that the curvature of **the visceral pleural line parallels the curvature of the chest wall;** that is, the visceral pleural line is **convex outward toward the chest wall** (Fig. 9-2).
  - Most other processes that mimic a pneumothorax do not demonstrate this spatial relationship with the chest wall.
- There is usually, but not always, an **absence of lung markings peripheral to the visceral pleural line.**
- **Pitfall:** Pleural adhesions may keep part, but not all, of the visceral pleura adherent to the parietal pleura.
  - On conventional radiographs, it may be possible to visualize lung markings in front or in back of the visceral pleural line and to overlook the presence of a pneumothorax because lung markings appear to extend to the chest wall (Fig. 9-3).

- **Absence of lung markings alone is not sufficient for the diagnosis of pneumothorax.**
- **The presence of lung markings distal to the visceral pleural line is not sufficient to eliminate the possibility of a pneumothorax.**

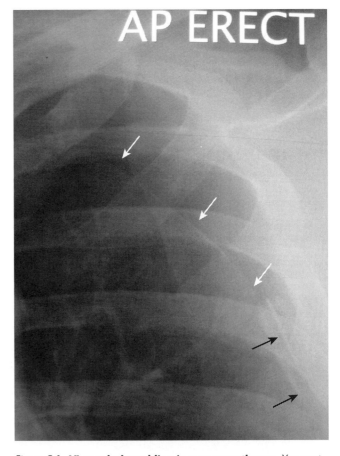

Figure 9-1. *Visceral pleural line in a pneumothorax.* You must see the visceral pleural line to make the definitive diagnosis of a pneumothorax (closed white arrows). The visceral and parietal pleura are normally not visible, both normally lying adjacent to the lateral chest wall. When air enters the pleural space, the visceral pleura advances toward the hilum with the collapsing lung and becomes visible as a very thin, white line with air outlining it on either side. Notice how the contour of the pneumothorax parallels the curvature of the adjacent chest wall. This patient already has a chest tube inserted (closed black arrows).

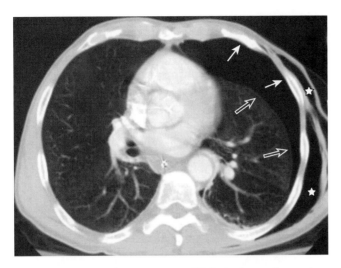

Figure 9-2. ***Pneumothorax seen on CT.*** *As the lung collapses, it tends to maintain its usual shape so that the curve of the visceral pleural line (open white arrows) parallels the curve of the chest wall (closed white arrows); that is, the visceral pleural line is convex outward toward the chest wall. This is important in differentiating a pneumothorax from artifacts or other diseases that can mimic a pneumothorax. As it collapses, the lung on the side of the pneumothorax also tends to remain lucent until the lung loses almost all of its normal volume, at which point it appears opaque. This patient also has subcutaneous emphysema—air in the soft tissues—of the left lateral chest wall (white stars). The patient had been stabbed by a friend.*

- The **presence of an air-fluid interface in the pleural space** is proof that there is a pneumothorax (see Fig. 7-13).
  - For more about recognizing a hydropneumothorax, see **Chapter 7, Recognizing a Pleural Effusion.**
- In the supine position, air in a relatively large pneumothorax may collect anteriorly and inferiorly in the thorax and manifest itself by **displacing the costophrenic sulcus inferiorly** while, at the same time, producing **increased lucency of that costophrenic sulcus.**
  - This is called the ***deep sulcus sign*** and it is presumptive evidence for the presence of a pneumothorax on a supine chest radiograph (Fig. 9-4).
    - The key signs for recognizing a pneumothorax are summarized in Box 9-1.

Recognizing the Pitfalls in Overdiagnosing a Pneumothorax

- Several pitfalls can lead to the mistaken diagnosis of a pneumothorax.
- **Pitfall 1: Absence of lung markings mistaken for a pneumothorax**
  - The simple absence of lung markings is not sufficient to warrant the diagnosis of a pneumothorax because there are other diseases that produce such a finding in part or all of a hemithorax.
  - These other diseases include
    - **Bullous disease of the lung** (Fig. 9-5)
    - **Large cysts in the lung**

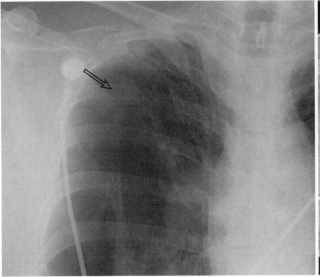

A

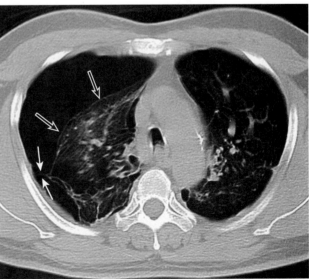

B

Figure 9-3. ***Pneumothorax with pleural adhesions.*** *There may be lung markings (open black arrow) visible on a conventional radiograph of the chest* ***(A) distal*** *to the visceral pleural line if there are pleural adhesions. This can be confusing on conventional radiographs, and a CT scan of the chest is frequently obtained to make the definitive diagnosis. On a CT scan of the same patient* ***(B),*** *the pleural adhesion (closed white arrows) prevents the lung from fully collapsing. Adhesions most frequently result from prior infection or blood in the pleural space. The visceral pleural line parallels the chest wall (open white arrows). Remember, it is not the absence of lung markings but the visualization of the visceral pleural line that is needed to make the diagnosis of pneumothorax.*

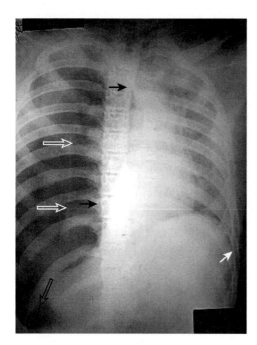

Figure 9-4. **Deep sulcus sign, tension pneumothorax.** *In the supine position, air in a relatively large pneumothorax may collect anteriorly and inferiorly in the thorax and manifest itself by displacing the costophrenic sulcus inferiorly while, at the same time, producing increased lucency of that sulcus (open black arrow). This is called the* **deep sulcus sign** *and is an indication of a pneumothorax on a supine radiograph. Notice how much lower the right costophrenic sulcus appears than the left sulcus (closed white arrow). The visceral pleural line is also visible in this patient (open white arrows) and there is a shift of the heart and trachea toward the opposite side (closed black arrows), indicating the likelihood of a tension pneumothorax. This patient was also stabbed by a friend.*

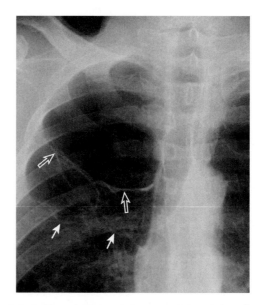

Figure 9-5. **Bullous disease, right upper lobe.** *A thin white line is visible on this close-up of the right upper lobe (open white arrows), and there are no lung markings peripheral to it. But unlike the visceral pleural line of a pneumothorax, this white line is convex* **away** *from the chest wall and does not parallel the curve of the chest wall. This is the classic appearance of a bulla in a patient with emphysema. It is important to differentiate between a pneumothorax and a bulla because inadvertently placing a chest tube into a bulla will almost always* **produce** *a pneumothorax, which may be difficult to re-expand. The walls of several bullae are visible in this patient (closed white arrows). On rare occasions, the bullae can grow so large as to render the hemithorax seemingly devoid of visible lung tissue* **(vanishing lung syndrome)**. *(See also Chapter 14.)*

Box 9-1

Recognizing a Pneumothorax—Signs to Look For
Visualization of the visceral pleural line—a must for the diagnosis
Convex curve of the visceral pleural line paralleling the contour of the chest wall
Absence of lung markings distal to the visceral pleural line (most times)
The **deep sulcus sign** of an inferiorly displaced costophrenic angle seen on a supine view
The presence of an air-fluid interface in the pleural space

- **Pulmonary embolism,** which can lead to a lack of perfusion and hence a decrease in the number of vessels visible in a particular part of the lung (*Westermark's sign of oligemia*) (see Chapter 14).
- In none of these diseases would the treatment ordinarily include the insertion of a chest tube and, in fact,

introduction of a chest tube into a bulla might actually **produce** an intractable pneumothorax.
  - **Solution:** Look at the contour of the structure you believe is the visceral pleural line.
    - Unlike the margin of a bulla, the **visceral pleural line** will be **convex outward** toward the chest wall and will **parallel the curve of the chest wall** (Fig. 9-6).
- **Pitfall 2: Mistaking a skin fold for a pneumothorax**
  - When the patient lies directly on the radiographic cassette (as for a portable supine radiograph), a fold of the patient's skin may become trapped between the patient's back and the surface of the cassette.
  - This can produce an *edge* in the expected position of the visceral pleural line which **may, in fact, parallel the chest wall** just as you would expect the pleural line in a pneumothorax (Fig. 9-7).
  - **Solution:** Unlike the thin, white line of the visceral pleura, **skin folds produce a relatively thick, white band of density.**
- **Pitfall 3: Mistaking the medial border of the scapula for a pneumothorax**

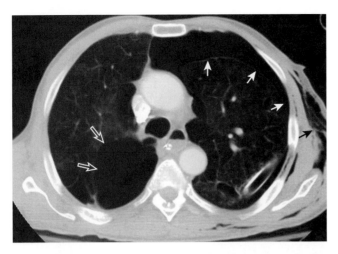

Figure 9-6. *Bullous disease on right; pneumothorax on left.* This section from a chest CT demonstrates the different appearances of bullous disease, seen on the right with its border convex **away** from the posterior chest wall (open white arrows), and a pneumothorax seen here on the left with its border convex **toward** and paralleling the anterior chest wall (closed white arrows). This patient also has subcutaneous emphysema on the left (closed black arrow).

- Ordinarily, the patient is positioned for an erect frontal chest radiograph in such a way that the scapulae are retracted lateral to the outer margin of the rib cage, thus eliminating the medial border of the scapula from overlapping the lung fields.

- With supine radiographs, **the medial border of the scapula may superimpose on the upper lobe and mimic the visceral pleural line** of a pneumothorax (Fig. 9-8).
- **Solution:** Before you diagnose a pneumothorax because you think you see the visceral pleural line, make sure you can **trace the outlines of the scapula** on the side in question and identify its medial border as being separate from the suspected pneumothorax.

Types of Pneumothoraces

- Pneumothoraces can be categorized as *primary*, i.e., occurring in what appears to have been normal lung (*spontaneous pneumothorax* being an example), or *secondary*, i.e., those that occur in diseased lung (as in emphysema).
- They have also been classified based on the presence or absence of a "shift" of the mobile mediastinal structures, such as the heart and trachea.
- **Simple**—there is usually **no shift of the mediastinal structures** (Fig. 9-9).
- **Tension**—there is **frequently a shift of the mediastinal structures away from the side of the pneumothorax** associated with cardiopulmonary compromise (Fig. 9-10).
  - Progressive loss of air into pleural space through a one-way, check-valve mechanism may cause a shift of the heart and mediastinal structures **away** from side of pneumothorax.

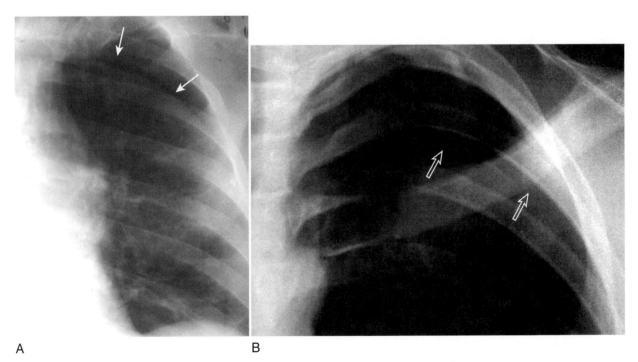

A   B

Figure 9-7. *Skin fold mimicking a pneumothorax.* When patients lay directly on the radiographic cassette as they might for a portable, supine radiograph, a fold of the patient's skin may become trapped between the patient's back and the surface of the cassette. This can produce an **edge** (closed white arrows) in the expected position of a pneumothorax and that edge may, in fact, parallel the chest wall just as you would expect a pneumothorax to do **(A)**. Unlike the thin, white line of the visceral pleura (open white arrows), as seen in a different patient with a pneumothorax in **(B)**, skin folds produce relatively thick, white bands of density. A skin fold is an **edge;** the visceral pleura produces a **line.**

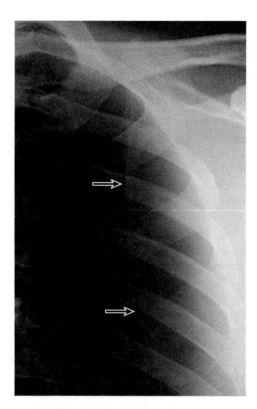

Figure 9-8. *Scapular edge mimicking a pneumothorax.* *The patient is usually positioned for an erect frontal chest radiograph in such a way that the medial edges of the scapulae are retracted lateral to the outer edge of the rib cage, thus reducing the risk that the scapulae will produce superimposed densities on the frontal chest radiograph. In supine radiographs, the medial border of the scapula (open white arrows) will frequently superimpose on the upper lung field and may mimic the visceral pleural line of a pneumothorax. Before you diagnose a pneumothorax, make sure you can identify the medial border of the scapula as being separate from the suspected pneumothorax.*

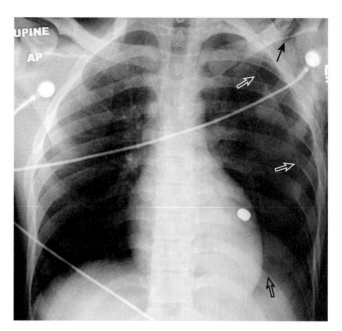

Figure 9-9. *Pneumothorax with no shift.* *There is a large left-sided pneumothorax (open white arrows) with no shift of the heart or trachea to the right. There is also a hemothorax (open black arrow) obscuring the left hemidiaphragm, but not forming an air-fluid interface because this radiograph was obtained with the patient supine. Subcutaneous emphysema is seen in the region of the left shoulder (closed black arrow). Can you detect why the patient had all of these findings? Yes, that's a bullet superimposed on the heart (but on CT it was posterior to the heart in the left lower lobe). He was not shot by a friend.*

- The air may be entering through a rent in the parietal pleura, visceral pleura, or from the tracheobronchial tree.
- The continuously **increasing intrathoracic pressure may lead to cardiopulmonary compromise by impairing venous return to the heart.**
- Besides a shift of the mobile mediastinal structures away from the side of the pneumothorax, there may be **inversion of the hemidiaphragm** (especially on the left) and there may be **flattening of the heart contour on the side under tension.**
- The question **"How large is the pneumothorax?"** is common and oft-repeated but the actual issue is "Does this patient require a chest tube to drain the pneumothorax?" Box 9-2 summarizes the answer.
- **Mediastinal shifts with a pneumothorax**
  - In most pneumothoraces, there is **usually no shift of the heart or trachea** (see Fig. 9-9).
  - In a **tension pneumothorax, there is a shift of the heart or trachea away** from the side of pneumothorax

associated with cardiopulmonary compromise (see Fig. 9-10).
- There is **never a shift** of the mobile mediastinal structures **toward the side of a pneumothorax.**

Causes of a Pneumothorax
- **Spontaneous**
  - Often from **rupture of an apical, subpleural bleb** or bulla and **characteristically occurring in tall, thin males between 20 and 40 years of age.**
  - Most common cause of a pneumothorax
- **Traumatic**
  - **May be either accidental or iatrogenic**
    - Through chest wall, e.g., stab wound
    - Internal, e.g., rupture of a bronchus from a motor vehicle collision
    - Iatrogenic, e.g., following transbronchial biopsy
- **Diseases that decrease lung compliance**
  - Chronic fibrotic diseases, e.g., eosinophilic granuloma
  - **Diseases that stiffen the lung,** e.g., hyaline membrane disease in infants
  - **Rupture of an alveolus or bronchiole,** e.g., asthma (Fig. 9-11)

Other Ways to Diagnose a Pneumothorax
- **Expiratory chest x-rays**
  - Based on the theory that the **volume of air in the lung will normally decrease** on expiration, but the **size of a pneumothorax will not,** small pneumothoraces not

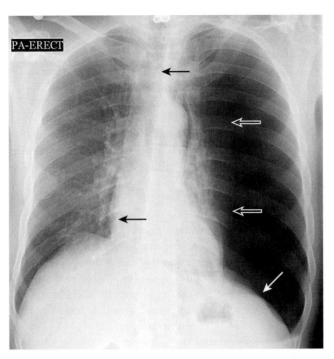

Figure 9-10. **Large left-sided tension pneumothorax.**
*Progressive loss of air into pleural space through a one-way
check-valve mechanism may cause a shift of the heart and mediastinal
structures away from side of pneumothorax and lead to
cardiopulmonary compromise by impairing venous return to the heart.
In this patient with a spontaneous pneumothorax, the left lung is almost
totally collapsed (open white arrows) and there is a shift of the trachea
and heart to the right (closed black arrows). The left hemidiaphragm is
depressed because of the elevated left intrathoracic pressure (closed
white arrow).*

Box 9-2

How Large Is the Pneumothorax?

Size measurements of pneumothoraces on conventional radiographs correlate poorly with CT scans of their actual size.

There is poor correlation between the size of the pneumothorax and the degree of clinical impairment.

The 2 cm rule: if the distance between the lung margin and the chest wall at the apex is < 2 cm, a chest tube is usually not needed; a distance > 2 cm usually requires chest tube drainage.

Assessment of the patient's clinical status is the most important determinant in deciding whether chest tube drainage is required.

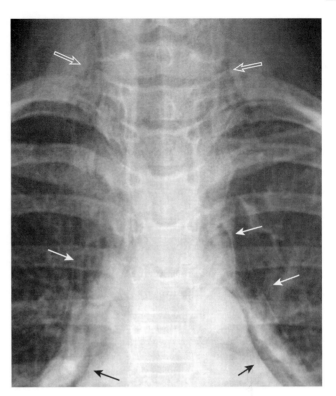

Figure 9-11. **Pneumomediastinum, pneumopericardium, and
subcutaneous emphysema.** *This patient with asthma developed
spontaneous pneumomediastinum most likely from rupture of an
alveolus followed by formation of pulmonary interstitial emphysema.
The air tracked back to the hila, then into the mediastinum where it
produced streaky black linear densities (closed white arrows)
extending to the neck. In the neck, there is subcutaneous emphysema
(open white arrows). In adults, air does not usually enter the
pericardium except by direct penetration, so it is somewhat unusual
that this patient also developed pneumopericardium (closed black
arrows). Notice how the air in the pericardial space does not extend
above the reflections of the aorta and pulmonary artery.*

visible on an inspiratory radiograph may become visible on a radiograph exposed in **full expiration.**

- Routine expiratory views are no longer recommended for the detection of pneumothoraces.
- **Decubitus chest x-rays**
  - Because air rises to the highest point, lateral decubitus films of the chest with the affected side "up" and the x-ray beam directed horizontally (parallel to the floor) may detect a small pneumothorax not seen in the supine position.
- **Delayed films** are sometimes obtained about **6 hours after a penetrating injury** to the chest in patients in whom no pneumothorax is visible on the initial examination because of the occasional appearance of a delayed traumatic pneumothorax.
- **CT of the chest**
  - Today, CT of the chest has essentially replaced expiratory and decubitus views if there is a strong clinical suspicion of a pneumothorax that is not demonstrated on conventional radiographs (Fig. 9-12).
  - **CT is able to detect extremely small amounts of air in the pleural space.**

Pulmonary Interstitial Emphysema (PIE*)

---

*Don't become confused by how many "PIES" there are at the imaging bakery. "PIE" is used as an abbreviation for: *pulmonary interstitial edema* (most common usage), *pulmonary interstitial emphysema,* and *pulmonary infiltrates with eosinophilia.*

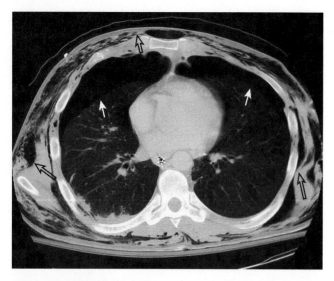

*Figure 9-12. **Bilateral pneumothoraces.** Conventional radiography is the initial modality used for detecting pneumothorax but smaller pneumothoraces may be visible only on CT scans of the chest. This patient has bilateral pneumothoraces (closed white arrows). Air will rise to the highest point (the patient is supine in the CT scanner). There is also extensive subcutaneous emphysema present (open black arrows), which developed because of an "air leak" from a chest tube that had been inserted earlier.*

- When the pressure or volume in the alveolus becomes sufficiently elevated, the **alveolus may rupture.**
- This extra-alveolar air may take one of two paths:
  - If the alveolus is close to a pleural surface, the **air may burst outward into the pleural space and create a pneumothorax.**
  - Alternatively, the **air can track backward along the bronchovascular bundles in the lung to the mediastinum,** then into the neck and out to the subcutaneous tissues of the chest and abdominal wall.
  - The air can eventually track downward into the abdomen as well as retroperitoneum.
- The air that tracks backward toward the hilum does so along the **perivascular connective tissue of the lung** forming **small, cystic collections** of extra-alveolar air which **dissect retrograde through the bronchovascular sheaths** to the hila.
  - While it is confined to the interstitial network of the lung, this air is called *pulmonary interstitial emphysema* or *perivascular interstitial emphysema (PIE).*
- Presumably because of the looser connective tissue in the lungs of children and young adults, **pulmonary interstitial emphysema is more likely to occur in those under the age of 40.**
  - **Assisted, mechanical ventilation increases the risk of developing pulmonary interstitial emphysema** and its formation **heralds a significant risk for the imminent appearance of a pneumothorax,** frequently within a matter of a few hours or days.

- Other causes of increased intra-alveolar pressure and rupture include asthma and barotrauma.
- **Pulmonary interstitial emphysema is usually not recognizable** because the air collections are so small and because there is usually a **considerable amount of coexisting disease** in the lung that obscures it.
- **Pitfall:** In infants with hyaline membrane disease (respiratory distress syndrome), pulmonary interstitial emphysema may lead to the appearance of *pseudo-clearing* of the lungs (which can appear less dense overall from the formation of the innumerable small air pockets) but its presence actually portends more serious complications.

Recognizing Pneumomediastinum

- When intra-alveolar pressure rises sufficiently to rupture the alveolus, air can **track backward along the bronchovascular bundles in the lung** to the mediastinum.
- **About 1 in 3 patients with pulmonary interstitial emphysema will develop pneumomediastinum** (more than 3 in 4 develop pneumothorax).
- **Pneumomediastinum may also develop when there is perforation of an air-containing mediastinal viscus,** such as the esophagus or tracheobronchial tree.
  - **Rupture of the distal esophagus** can occur with increased intra-esophageal pressure from retching or vomiting in *Boerhavve's syndrome.*
  - **Rupture of the tracheobronchial tree** is most often **secondary to significant trauma,** either **iatrogenic,** such as during a traumatic **intubation,** or **accidental,** such as from a penetrating wound or severe blunt trauma.
- **Radiographic findings of pneumomediastinum:**
  - **Linear streak-like lucency associated with a thin white line paralleling the left heart border**
  - **Streaky air outlining the great vessels** (aorta, superior vena cava, carotid arteries)
  - Linear streaks of **air parallel to the spine in the upper thorax extending into the neck** and surrounding the esophagus and trachea (Fig. 9-13)
  - *Continuous diaphragm sign*
    - With pneumomediastinum, **air can outline the central portion of the diaphragm** beneath the heart, producing an unbroken superior surface of the diaphragm that extends from one lateral chest wall to the other (Fig. 9-14).

Recognizing Pneumopericardium

- **Pneumopericardium is usually due to direct penetrating injuries** to the pericardium **either caused iatrogenically** (during cardiac surgery) **or accidentally** (from penetrating trauma).
  - Pneumopericardium is **more common in pediatric patients** than adults and may develop in neonates with hyaline membrane disease.
- It is **rare for air in the pleural space to enter the pericardium,** except in those who have had a surgical "window" incised in the pericardium to allow free exchange between the pleural and pericardial spaces.

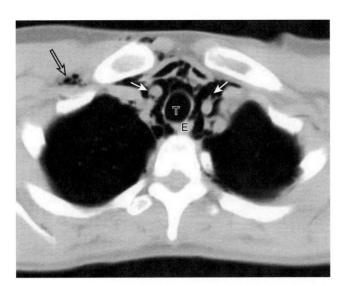

Figure 9-13. **Pneumomediastinum seen on CT.** *CT scan through the upper thorax demonstrates air in the mediastinum outlining the outside of the trachea (T) as well as the esophagus (E) and the major vessels leading to the neck (closed white arrows). There is a small amount of subcutaneous emphysema (open black arrow).*

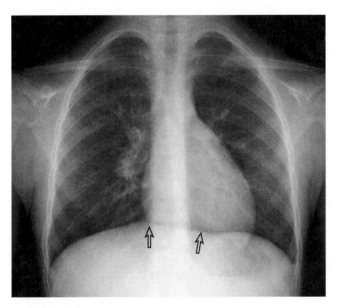

Figure 9-14. **Continuous diaphragm sign of pneumomediastinum.** *With pneumomediastinum, air can outline the central portion of the diaphragm beneath the heart producing an unbroken diaphragmatic contour that extends from one lateral chest wall to the other (open black arrows). This is called the* **continuous diaphragm sign.** *Normally, the diaphragm is not visible in the center of the chest because there is no air in the mediastinum and the soft tissue density of the heart rests upon and silhouettes the soft tissue density of the diaphragm in its central portion.*

- Pneumopericardium produces a **continuous** band of **lucency that encircles the heart but extends no higher than the root of the great vessels** (which corresponds to the height of the main pulmonary artery) (Fig. 9-15).

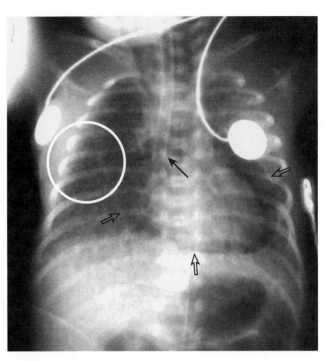

Figure 9-15. **Pneumopericardium, pulmonary interstitial emphysema.** *This is a premature infant with underlying* **hyaline membrane disease** *(respiratory distress syndrome) who is on a ventilator. A lucency surrounds the heart (open black arrows), representing air in the pericardial space. Notice how the air does not extend above the reflection of the aorta and main pulmonary artery.* **Pneumopericardium** *usually occurs from direct violation of the pericardium by trauma. In infants, it can occur from air that dissects along the bronchovascular bundles of the lungs (pulmonary interstitial emphysema). The lungs have a "bubbly" appearance (white circle) suggesting small pockets of air, a finding of* **pulmonary interstitial emphysema.** *The tip of the endotracheal tube extends too far and is in the right main bronchus (closed black arrow).*

- Pneumomediastinum, in contrast, will extend above the root of the great vessels into the uppermost thorax.
- **CT is usually necessary to make the diagnosis of pneumopericardium.**

Recognizing Subcutaneous Emphysema

- **Air can extend into the soft tissues of the neck, chest, and abdominal walls** from the mediastinum, or it can dissect in the subcutaneous tissues from a thoracotomy drainage tube or a penetrating injury to the chest wall.
- **Air dissecting along muscle bundles** produces a **characteristic comblike, striated appearance** that superimposes on the underlying lung, often making it difficult to evaluate the lungs by conventional radiography (Fig. 9-16).
- Although dramatic radiographically, **subcutaneous emphysema usually produces no serious clinical effects by itself.**

WebLink

More information on recognizing a pneumothorax, pneumomediastinum, pneumopericardium and subcutaneous emphysema is available to registered users on StudentConsult.com.

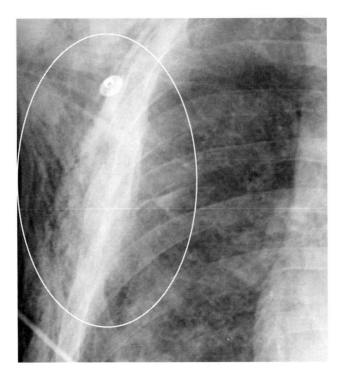

Figure 9-16. Subcutaneous emphysema. *Air can extend into the subcutaneous tissues of the neck, chest, and abdominal walls from the mediastinum, or it can dissect in the soft tissues from a thoracotomy drainage tube or a penetrating injury to the chest wall. Air dissecting along muscle bundles produces a characteristic comblike, striated appearance that overlies the lung (white oval). Although dramatic radiographically, subcutaneous emphysema usually produces no serious clinical effects by itself.*

 TAKE-HOME POINTS: Recognizing Pneumothorax, Pneumomediastinum, Pneumopericardium, and Subcutaneous Emphysema

There is normally no air in the pleural space; air in the pleural space is called a pneumothorax.

You must see the visceral pleural white line to diagnose a pneumothorax.

Beware of the pitfalls that resemble pneumothoraces: bullae, skin folds, and the medial border of the scapula.

Simple pneumothoraces are those with no shift of the heart or mobile mediastinal structures; most pneumothoraces are simple.

Tension pneumothoraces (usually associated with cardiorespiratory compromise) produce a shift of the heart and mediastinal structures away from the side of the pneumothorax by virtue of a check-valve mechanism that allows air to enter the pleural space but not leave.

Most pneumothoraces are spontaneous, either primary or secondary.

Conventional chest radiographs are poor at estimating the size of a pneumothorax; CT is better; the most important assessment is the clinical status of the patient.

Besides the conventional erect chest radiograph, other ways to diagnose a pneumothorax include expiratory exposures, decubitus views, delayed images, and CT scans.

Spontaneous pneumothoraces often occur as a result of rupture of a small apical, subpleural bleb; they most often occur in younger men; spontaneous (nontraumatic) pneumothoraces can also be secondary to such diseases as emphysema or asthma.

Pulmonary interstitial emphysema results from an increase in the intraalveolar pressure that leads to rupture of an alveolus and dissection of air back toward the hila along the bronchovascular bundles; it is frequently difficult to visualize.

Pneumomediastinum can occur when air tracks back to the mediastinum from a ruptured alveolus or from perforation of an air-containing viscus such as the esophagus or trachea; it can produce the continuous diaphragm sign on a frontal radiograph.

Pneumopericardium usually is due to direct penetration of the pericardium rather than dissection of air from a pneumomediastinum; it can be difficult to differentiate from a pneumomediastinum.

Air dissecting into the neck and chest wall can produce subcutaneous emphysema which, because of its superimposition on the lungs, can make evaluation of the underlying lung more difficult.

10 The ABCs of Heart Disease: Recognizing Adult Heart Disease from the Frontal Chest Radiograph

- This chapter presents a system for diagnosing cardiac disease in adults by asking a **series of questions** in a **set fashion,** the answers to which are certain **fundamental observations** made from the **frontal chest radiograph** alone.
  - This system is PG-13; that is, for adolescents and adults. Infant hearts do not display many of the recognizable contours discussed here, so cardiovascular evaluation in infants depends much more on parameters such as the pulmonary vasculature, the location of the great vessels, and the clinical findings.
- In a moment, we'll get to the questions; first, we'll review the "answers."
- The answers are a set of fundamental observations, described here, all based on the frontal chest radiograph alone.

Heart Size
- The **cardiothoracic ratio** is the **maximum transverse diameter of the heart** divided by the **greatest internal diameter of the thoracic cage** (from inside of rib to inside of rib) (see Fig. 3-1).
  - The maximum internal diameter of the rib cage usually occurs at the level of the diaphragm.
  - **In normal people, the cardiothoracic ratio is usually less than 50%.**
  - The cardiothoracic ratio is a handy way of separating most normal hearts from most abnormal hearts.
    - Unfortunately, it has its pitfalls.

- **Pitfall 1: The heart may appear to be enlarged** (i.e., be greater than 50% of the cardiothoracic ratio), **but still be a normal heart.**
  - This may be due to an *extracardiac cause* for the apparent cardiac enlargement from:
    - **The patient's inability to take a deep breath** because of
      - **Obesity**
      - **Pregnancy**
      - **Ascites**
    - **Abnormalities of the chest cage that compress the heart,** such as
      - Pectus excavatum deformity (see Fig. 3–2)
  - **Solution:** Look at the patient. The factors named above that will truly limit a patient's ability to take a deep breath will not be subtle findings.

- **Pitfall 2: Sometimes the heart can appear normal in size** (i.e., measure less than 50% of the cardiothoracic ratio), **but still be an abnormal heart.**
  - This can occur **when there is obstruction to the outflow of blood from the ventricles** and the **ventricles respond, at first, by undergoing hypertrophy, which does not produce recognizable cardiac enlargement.**
  - **Solution:** Because not all abnormal hearts are enlarged, **recognition of cardiac abnormalities in these individuals depends on an assessment of the contours of the heart** (Fig. 10-1).

Cardiac Contours
- There are seven identifiable cardiac contours on the frontal chest radiograph.

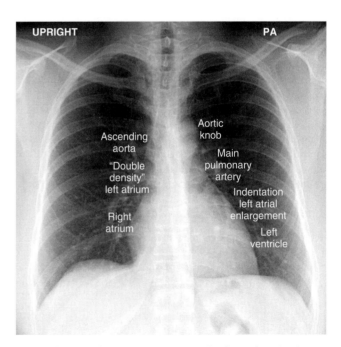

*Figure 10-1. **Cardiac contours seen in the frontal projection.** There are seven identifiable cardiac contours on the frontal chest radiograph. On the right side of the heart, from top to bottom, are the ascending aorta, the indentation between the ascending aorta and the right atrium (where an enlarged left atrium may appear), and the right atrium itself. On the left, from top to bottom, are the aortic knob, the main pulmonary artery, an indentation (where an enlarged left atrium may appear), and the left ventricle.*

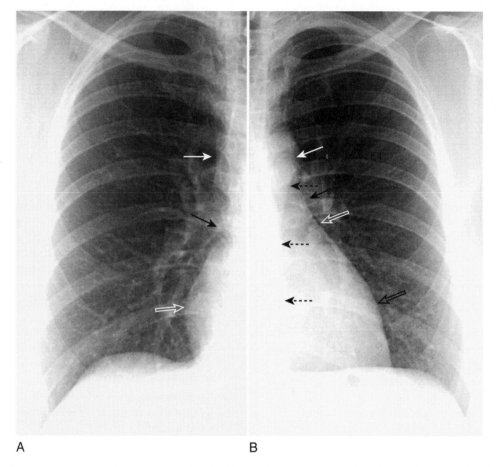

A   B

Figure 10-2. **Cardiac contours. A,** *Cardiac contours, right side of heart. The first contour is a low-density, almost straight edge visible just to the right of the trachea reflecting the size of the ascending aorta (closed white arrow). Where the contour of the ascending aorta meets the contour of the right atrium, there is usually a slight indentation (closed black arrow). The right heart border is formed by the right atrium (open white arrow). In an adult, the right atrium will almost never enlarge without concomitant enlargement of the right ventricle.* **B,** *Cardiac contours, left side of heart. The first contour on the left side of the heart is the aortic knob (closed white arrow). The aortic knob is a radiographic structure formed by the foreshortened aortic arch superimposed on a portion of the proximal descending aorta. The next contour below the aortic knob is the main pulmonary artery (closed black arrow). This is the shadow of the pulmonary artery before it divides into a right and left pulmonary artery. Just below the main pulmonary artery segment there is normally a slight indentation (open white arrow). The last contour of the heart on the left is formed by the left ventricle (open black arrow). The descending aorta almost disappears with the shadow of the spine (dotted black arrows).*

 ASCENDING AORTA

- The first contour on the right is the **ascending aorta.**
- It is a **low-density, almost straight edge** visible just to the right of the trachea reflecting the size of the ascending aorta (Fig. 10-2A).
  - Anatomically, this contour really represents the superior vena cava and brachiocephalic vessels, but for all practical purposes, it reflects the size of the more medially placed ascending aorta.
- The **ascending aorta can be small** as it is in atrial septal defect (ASD), or it can be **prominent** as it is in diseases that **increase the pressure or flow** in the aorta or affect its elasticity such as **aortic stenosis, aortic regurgitation, and arteriosclerotic cardiovascular disease.**

- **The normal ascending aorta should not project farther to the right than the right heart border on a nonrotated frontal radiograph** (Fig. 10-3).

"DOUBLE DENSITY" OF LEFT ATRIAL ENLARGEMENT
- Where the contour of the ascending aorta meets the contour of the right atrium, there is usually a slight indentation (see Fig. 10-2A).
- In patients with an **enlarged left atrium,** the right lateral wall of the enlarged left atrium may produce one of **two overlapping densities** in the region of this indentation.
  - One of the densities is normal: it's the contour of the **normal right atrium.**
  - The other overlapping density is abnormal: it's the contour of the **enlarged left atrium** (Fig. 10-4).

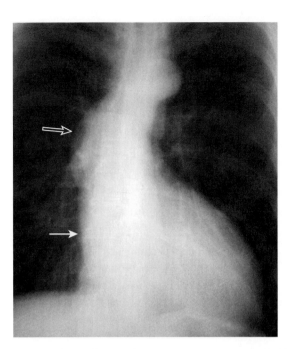

Figure 10-3. **Enlarged ascending aorta in aortic stenosis.** *The normal ascending aorta should never project farther to the right than the right heart border (closed white arrow) on a nonrotated frontal radiograph. In this patient, the ascending aorta (open white arrow) does project farther to the right than it should (the patient also has a scoliosis, which accentuates the prominence slightly). This patient had aortic stenosis. The prominence of the ascending aorta is due to* **poststenotic dilatation,** *characteristically seen just distal to hemodynamically significant stenoses in major arteries.*

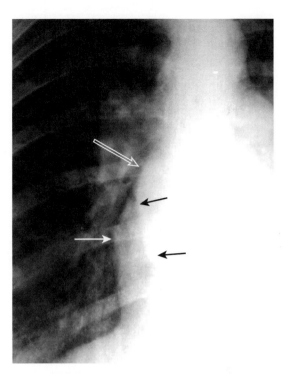

Figure 10-4. **"Double density" of left atrial enlargement.** *In patients with an enlarged left atrium, the right lateral wall of the enlarged left atrium may produce one of two overlapping densities at the junction between the ascending aorta and the right atrium (open white arrow). One of the densities is the normal right atrium (closed white arrow). The other overlapping density is abnormal and represents the enlarged left atrium (closed black arrows).*

- These two overlapping edges are called the **double density** of left atrial enlargement.

 RIGHT ATRIUM

- The **right heart border is formed by the right atrium** (see Fig. 10-2A).
- In an adult, **the right atrium will almost never enlarge without concomitant enlargement of the right ventricle.**
- Therefore, we'll consider the **right atrium and ventricle together as a single functional unit in adults,** and we will estimate right-sided cardiac enlargement in another way described later, but not by the size of the right atrium.
- For the purposes of this system, the right atrium is not an important contour.

 AORTIC KNOB

- The first contour on the left side of the heart is the aortic knob.
- The **aortic knob is a radiographic, not an anatomic, structure** seen on the frontal chest radiograph and formed by the foreshortened aortic arch together with a portion of the proximal descending aorta (see Fig. 10-2B).
- We can **measure the size of the aortic knob:**
  - In normal subjects, the aortic knob **measures less than 35 mm** when measured from the **lateral border of the air in the trachea to the lateral border of the aortic knob** (Fig. 10-5).

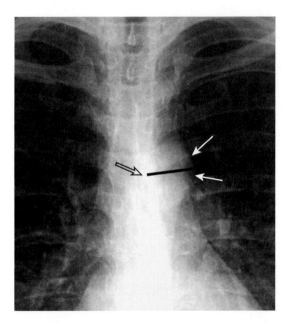

Figure 10-5. **Measuring the size of the aortic knob.** *In normal subjects, the aortic knob measures less than 35 mm (black line) from the lateral border of the air in the trachea (open black arrow) to the lateral border of the aortic knob (closed white arrows). The knob can be greater than 35 mm when there is increased pressure, increased flow, or changes in the elasticity of the aortic wall such as might occur in cystic medial necrosis or atherosclerosis.*

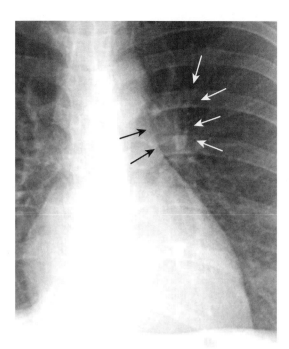

*Figure 10-6. **Locating the main pulmonary artery.*** *An assessment of the size of the main pulmonary artery is the keystone of this system, so it is very important for you to know how to find it, no matter what the shape of the heart. You can find the main pulmonary artery (closed black arrows) by finding the adjacent "squiggly" vessels that represent branches of the left pulmonary artery (closed white arrows). These branches of the left pulmonary artery are always immediate next door neighbors to the main pulmonary artery.*

- The knob can be **greater than 35 mm due to increased pressure, flow, or changes in the elasticity of the wall of the aorta** such as in systemic hypertension, cystic medial necrosis, or aortic dissection.

 MAIN PULMONARY ARTERY

- The next contour below the aortic knob is the main pulmonary artery (see Fig. 10-2B).
- **The main pulmonary artery is the keystone of this entire system.**
- First, **you must be able to find the main pulmonary artery** segment. Then, you can measure it.
  - You can find the main pulmonary artery by finding the adjacent "squiggly" vessels that represent branches of the **left pulmonary artery.**
  - These **branches of the left pulmonary artery** are always **immediately adjacent** to the **main pulmonary artery** (Fig. 10-6).
- We can **measure the main pulmonary artery** by drawing a **tangent line from the apex of the left ventricle to the aortic knob** and then measuring along a perpendicular to that tangent line, the distance between the tangent and the main pulmonary artery (Fig. 10-7).
  - In normal subjects, **the distance between the tangent line and the main pulmonary artery lies within a range of values between 0 mm (the main pulmonary is touching the tangent line) to as far away from the tangent line (medially) as 15 mm.**

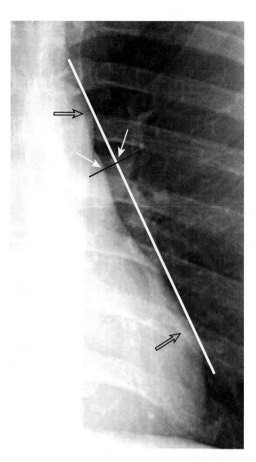

*Figure 10-7. **The tangent line.*** *You can measure the main pulmonary artery by drawing a real or imaginary tangent line (white line) from the apex of the left ventricle to the aortic knob (open black arrows) and then measuring along a perpendicular (black line) to that tangent, the distance between the tangent and the main pulmonary artery (distance between the two closed white arrows). In normal subjects, the distance between the tangent line and the main pulmonary artery lies within a range of values from 0 mm (meaning the main pulmonary is touching the tangent line) to as far away from the tangent line (medially or to the patient's right) as 15 mm.*

- This sounds complicated, but it isn't.
- This range of normal values establishes two major categories of abnormality in this system:
  - First, the **main pulmonary artery may project beyond the tangent line** (greater than 0 mm).
    - This can occur if there is **increased pressure** or **increased flow** in the pulmonary circulation (Fig. 10-8).
  - Second, the **main pulmonary artery may project more than 15 mm to the right of the tangent line (medially)** (Fig. 10-9).
    - This can occur for **two main reasons:**
      - One, there is something **intrinsically abnormal with the pulmonary artery** such as **absence or hypoplasia** of the pulmonary artery, which occurs in tetralogy of Fallot or truncus arteriosus.

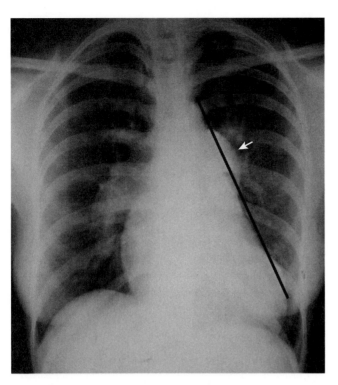

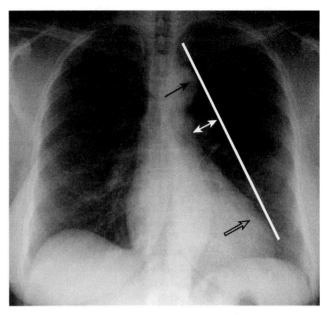

Figure 10-8. *Main pulmonary artery projects beyond the tangent line.* *If the main pulmonary artery (closed white arrow) projects beyond the tangent line (greater than 0 mm) (black line), this is almost always abnormal. This can occur if there is increased pressure or increased flow in the pulmonary circulation. In this patient, there was increased flow from a left-to-right shunt secondary to an atrial septal defect. Younger females may have main pulmonary artery segments that are normally prominent, but the main pulmonary artery, even though prominent, still does not usually project beyond the tangent line.*

Figure 10-9. *"Concave" main pulmonary artery segment.* *The main pulmonary artery may project more than 15 mm to the right of the tangent line (distance between white tangent line and main pulmonary artery is indicated by double white arrow). This can occur for two reasons: (1) there is something intrinsically abnormal with the pulmonary artery making it small or absent or (2) either the left ventricle (open black arrow) or the aortic knob (closed black arrow) is enlarged and pushes the tangent line away from the pulmonary artery. This patient has systemic hypertension and both the left ventricle and aortic knob are prominent.*

- These are uncommon diseases in adults.
  - Two, the main pulmonary artery may be more than 15 mm from the tangent line because either the **left ventricle** or **aortic knob** may **enlarge** and **push** the tangent line away from the pulmonary artery, which occurs with atherosclerosis and systemic hypertension.
- These are common diseases in adults.
  - **Pitfall:** Young females may have normal prominence of the main pulmonary artery, but it rarely projects beyond the tangent line.

CONCAVITY FOR LEFT ATRIUM
- The third contour on the left side of the heart is the indentation for the left atrium.
- Just below the main pulmonary artery segment (the concavity between the main pulmonary artery and the left ventricle) there is normally a slight indentation (see Fig. 10-2B).
- **Filling in of this concavity** by an enlarged left atrium produces **straightening** of **the left heart border.**
- Sometimes, the **left atrial appendage** may enlarge as well and produce a **convexity** in this region.

- This is almost always seen with markedly elevated left atrial pressure such as occurs in mitral valvular disease, usually **mitral stenosis** (Fig. 10-10).
- Box 10-1 summarizes the key findings relative to left atrial enlargement.

LEFT VENTRICLE
- The last cardiac contour on the left is formed by the left ventricle (see Fig. 10-2B).
- But we're going to identify which ventricle is producing cardiac enlargement by evaluating each ventricle's corresponding outflow tract rather than the shape or appearance of the left ventricle.
- **The easiest way to evaluate which ventricle (right or left) is enlarged is to examine the corresponding outflow tract for each ventricle.**
  - If the heart is enlarged (i.e., the **cardiothoracic ratio is greater than 50%**) and the **main pulmonary artery is large** (i.e., projects beyond the tangent line), then the cardiomegaly is made up of at least **right ventricular enlargement** (Fig. 10-11).
  - If the heart is enlarged (i.e., the **cardiothoracic ratio is greater than 50%**) and the **aorta is prominent** (ascending aorta, aortic knob, and descending aorta), then the cardiomegaly is made up of at least **left ventricular enlargement** (Fig. 10-12).

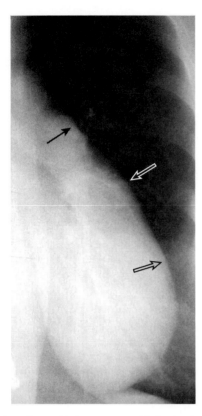

Figure 10-10. **Enlarged left atrium and left atrial appendage.** *Filling-in of the normal concavity between the main pulmonary artery (closed black arrow) and the left ventricle (open black arrow) can occur when the left atrium enlarges. This is called* **straightening** *of the left heart border. Sometimes, not only the left atrium but the left atrial appendage as well may enlarge and if this occurs, there will be a convexity in this region (open white arrow). This is usually seen in mitral valvular disease, in particular mitral stenosis. This patient had rheumatic heart disease leading to mitral stenosis.*

Box 10-1

Facts About the Left Atrium

Normally, the left atrium forms no border of the heart in the frontal projection.

When the left atrium enlarges, it may produce abnormal contours on both the left and right sides of the heart.

On the left side of the heart, it can fill in the concavity normally present below the main pulmonary artery. This is called **straightening of the left heart border.**

On the right side, it can produce one of two overlapping edges where the normal indentation between the ascending aorta and right atrium occurs. This is called the **double density of left atrial enlargement** and is less common than straightening of the left heart border.

The double density may occasionally be seen in normal individuals; always check the left heart border for straightening when you think you see a "double density."

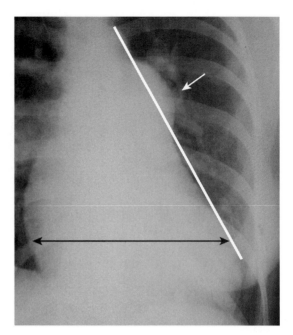

Figure 10-11. **Determining which ventricle is enlarged.** *The easiest way to evaluate which ventricle is enlarged (right or left) is to look at the corresponding outflow tract for each ventricle. If the heart is enlarged (i.e., the cardiothoracic ratio is greater than 50%) (black double arrow) and the main pulmonary artery is large (white arrow), i.e., projects beyond the tangent line (white line), then the cardiomegaly is made up of at least right ventricular enlargement because the pulmonary artery is the corresponding outflow tract for the right ventricle.*

- Once one ventricle is determined to be enlarged, it is usually not possible to assess if the other ventricle is also enlarged on a conventional chest radiograph.

DESCENDING AORTA

- The descending thoracic aorta produces a contour that is seen through the heart just to the left of the thoracic spine on a well-exposed frontal chest radiograph.
- Normally, the **descending aorta parallels the spine** and is **barely visible** on the frontal radiograph of the chest (see Fig. 10-2B).
- It may become *tortuous* or *uncoiled* or *enlarged* and swing farther away from the spine, such as in atherosclerosis or systemic hypertension.
- Box 10-2 summarizes the five most important cardiac contours visible on the frontal chest radiograph.

THE PULMONARY VASCULATURE

- Using just the information we've already discussed and the cardiac contours alone, you can arrive at a set of differential diagnoses for cardiac disease, but to make the actual diagnosis you unfortunately have to evaluate the pulmonary vasculature.
  - It is "unfortunate" because everyone, including those with a great deal of experience, has difficulty accurately evaluating the pulmonary vasculature.
- The **pulmonary vasculature can be classified into the following five categories:**

- **Normal flow**
- **Pulmonary venous hypertension**
- **Pulmonary arterial hypertension**
- **Increased flow**
- **Decreased flow** to the lungs (this fifth category is usually so difficult to assess accurately that we'll not concern ourselves with it here).
- To evaluate the pulmonary vasculature, **we shall look at the following three parameters:**

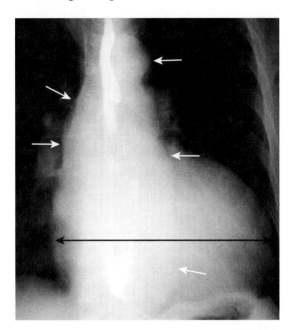

Figure 10-12. ***Determining which ventricle is enlarged.*** *If the heart is enlarged, i.e., the cardiothoracic ratio is greater than 50% (double black arrow), and the aorta is prominent (ascending aorta, aortic knob, and descending aorta) (closed white arrows), then the cardiomegaly is made up of at least left ventricular enlargement. Once one ventricle is determined to be enlarged, it is usually not possible to determine if the other ventricle is also enlarged on a conventional chest radiograph.*

Box 10-2

Five Most Important Cardiac Contours

Ascending aorta—should not project beyond right heart border.

Indentation on right side of heart where "double density" of left atrial enlargement will appear—overlapping of left and right atrial walls.

Aortic knob—should be less than 35 mm from the edge of the trachea.

Main pulmonary artery segment—should fall between 0 and 15 mm from tangent line.

Concavity where the left atrium, when it enlarges, will appear on the left side of the heart.

The right atrium and left ventricle are less important contours because we evaluate ventricular enlargement by looking at the outflow tracts for each ventricle.

- **The right descending pulmonary artery**
- **The distribution of flow in the lung from apex to base.**
- **The distribution of flow in the lungs from central to peripheral.**

NORMAL

- **The right descending pulmonary artery (RDPA)**
  - The RDPA is visible on almost all frontal chest radiographs as a large vessel just lateral to the right heart border (Fig. 10-13).
  - We will measure its diameter (before it branches).
    - Normally, the **right descending pulmonary artery measures less than 17 mm in diameter.**
    - So, right from the start, we have a handy way of separating most normal from abnormal pulmonary vasculature.
- Evaluate the **distribution of flow in the lungs from apex to base.**
  - Normally, in the upright position, **the blood flow to the bases is greater than the blood flow to the apices.**
    - This is due to the effect of **gravity.**
  - In normal subjects, the **size** (not the number) of the vessels at the base will therefore be greater than the **size** (not the number) of the vessels at the apex.
- **Evaluate the size of the pulmonary vessels in two imaginary circles about the size of a silver dollar,** one drawn at the **apex** of either lung and another at the right lung **base.**

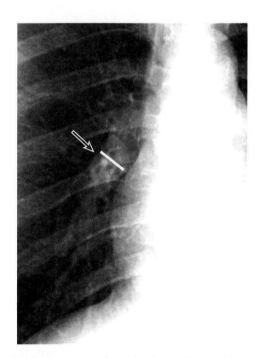

Figure 10-13. ***Measuring the right descending pulmonary artery.*** *The right descending pulmonary artery is visible on almost all frontal chest radiographs as a large vessel just lateral to the right heart border (open white arrow). It serves the right lower and right middle lobes. You can measure its diameter before it branches (white line) to make a more objective assessment of the pulmonary vasculature. In normal subjects, the right descending pulmonary artery measures less than 17 mm in diameter. This is a handy way to separate normal from most abnormal types of pulmonary vasculature.*

- You can't evaluate the vessels at the left base very easily because the heart obscures them.
- Normally, the **size of the vessels at the base will be greater than the size of the vessels at the apex, so long as the study is done with the patient upright** (Fig. 10-14).
- Please note that the difference in size of the upper and lower lobe vessels is due to the force of gravity in the upright position so that if a patient is lying supine when the image is exposed, the upper and lower lobe vessels will normally be the same size.
- Evaluate the **distribution of flow from central to peripheral**
  - Normally, the **pulmonary vessels,** whether they are arteries or veins, **taper gradually from central to peripheral.**

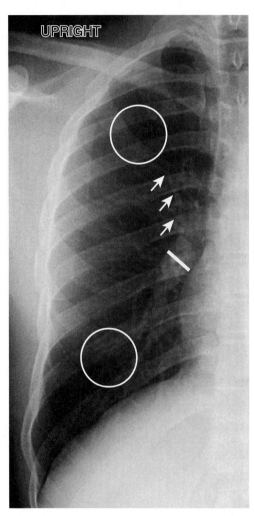

*Figure 10-14. **Three parameters used to assess the pulmonary vasculature.*** *Normally, in the upright position the right descending pulmonary artery should be less than 17 mm in diameter (white line). The distribution of flow from apex to base can be assessed by examining the size (not the number) of vessels in two imaginary circles at the right base and either apex (white circles). The vessels should be larger at the base in the upright position. The last assessment of the distribution of flow is made by examining the gradual and progressive tapering of vessels as they travel from the hilum to the periphery of the lung (closed white arrows).*

- In the lungs, there should be a gradual diminution in the size of the vessels as you examine them from the hila to the periphery of the lung (see Fig. 10-14).
- This gradual tapering defines the normal distribution of flow in the lungs from central to peripheral.

PULMONARY VENOUS HYPERTENSION

- Now, let's examine the abnormal states of the pulmonary vasculature and discuss how to recognize them.
- In **pulmonary venous hypertension,** there is a redistribution of flow in the lungs such that **the blood flow to the apex becomes equal to or greater than the blood flow to the base.**
  - As fluid leaks from lower lobe vessels under increasing venous pressure, there is an associated increase in the resistance to lower lobe flow and there is a redistribution of pulmonary flow to the upper lobes.
- Therefore, with pulmonary venous hypertension, the **size of the vessels at the apex becomes equal to or greater than the size of the vessels at the bases**—a reversal of the normal flow pattern (Fig. 10-15).
- This redistribution of flow in a cephalad direction from base to apex is known as **cephalization.**
  - **Cephalization is a sign of pulmonary venous hypertension.**

PULMONARY ARTERIAL HYPERTENSION

- In **pulmonary arterial hypertension** (usually referred to simply as *pulmonary hypertension* with the "arterial" understood), there is also a **redistribution of flow in the lungs,** but in this case the redistribution is **from central to peripheral.**
- Instead of the gradual tapering of blood vessels that normally occurs from the hila outward, **in pulmonary hypertension the peripheral vessels appear too small for the size of the central vessels from which they come.**
  - Another way to think of pulmonary hypertension is that the central vessels (i.e., the main pulmonary artery and the right descending pulmonary artery) appear too large for the size of the vessels that emanate from them.
- This **discrepancy in size between the central pulmonary vessels** (which are large) **and the peripheral pulmonary vasculature** (which is not enlarged and may be indistinguishable from normal) is called *pruning* (Fig. 10-16).
  - **Pruning is a sign of pulmonary arterial hypertension.**

INCREASED FLOW TO THE LUNGS

- With **increased flow to the lungs, all of the blood vessels are carrying more blood** than they normally would.
- Because they are carrying more blood, you would expect them to become larger than normal, and you would be correct.
- With increased flow to the lungs, **all the blood vessels everywhere in the lung are larger** than they would be in a normal person.
- The **key feature that differentiates increased flow to the lungs** from pulmonary arterial and pulmonary venous hypertension is that with increased flow the **distribution of flow** in the lungs is as it would be in a **normal** person.

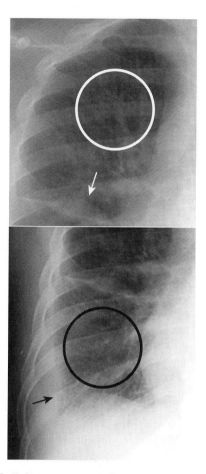

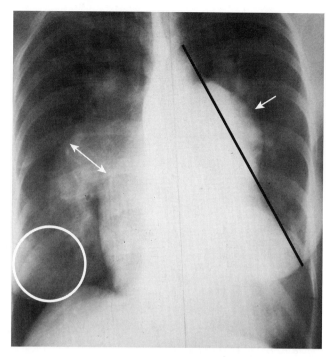

Figure 10-15. **Pulmonary venous hypertension.** *In pulmonary venous hypertension, there is a redistribution of flow in the lungs such that the blood flow to the apex becomes equal to or greater than the blood flow to the base. This is reflected in an increase in the size of the vessels at the apex (white circle), which become equal to or greater than the size of the vessels at the base (black circle). This is a reversal of the normal flow pattern. This redistribution of flow from apex to base in pulmonary venous hypertension is known as* **cephalization.** *Other signs of pulmonary venous hypertension in this patient with congestive heart failure are a laminar pleural effusion (closed black arrow) and fluid in the form of a pseudotumor in the minor fissure (closed white arrow).*

Figure 10-16. **Pulmonary arterial hypertension.** *In pulmonary arterial hypertension, there is a redistribution of flow in the lungs from central to peripheral. Instead of the gradual tapering of blood vessels that normally occurs from the hila outward, the peripheral vessels appear too small for the size of the central vessels from which they come. Another way to think of pulmonary hypertension is that the central vessels, i.e., the main pulmonary artery (closed white arrow) and the right descending pulmonary artery (double white arrow), appear too large for the size of the vessels that emanate from them (white circle). Notice how the main pulmonary artery projects beyond the tangent line (black line). This discrepancy in size between the central and peripheral vessels is called* **pruning.** *This patient had a long-standing left-to-right shunt that led to pulmonary arterial hypertension.*

- So, the lower lobe vessels are larger than the upper lobe vessels and there is a gradual tapering as vessels extend from central to peripheral, but all the blood vessels, everywhere in the lung, are larger than they should be.
- **How do you recognize that vessels are "larger than they should be"?** That takes some experience.
  - Part of it comes from **looking at a lot of pulmonary vessels** on chest radiographs.
  - The rest comes by developing an ability to recognize that there seem to be more blood vessels visible in the lungs than you are accustomed to seeing (Fig. 10-17).

DECREASED FLOW TO THE LUNGS
- **Decreased flow to the lungs is very difficult to recognize.**
- It may be manifest by small hila or by fewer than normal vessels in the lung.

- **In summary,** using the size of the RDPA and the distribution of flow in the lungs—apex to base and central to peripheral—you can define the four states of the pulmonary vasculature.
- Table 10-1 summarizes the key findings relative to the pulmonary vasculature and Figure 10-18 shows a side-by-side photographic comparison of the four important types.
- That completes all the observations you need to answer the fixed set of questions that actually constitute the system of "The ABCs of Heart Disease."
  - You have just learned the answers. Now, here are the questions.

The ABCs of Heart Disease System*

- The system depends for its success on the questions being asked in a set order with "A" being the first question, then "B" and so on.

*Grateful acknowledgment is made to Bernard J. Ostrum, MD, who along with his father Joseph Ostrum, MD, both radiologists and both teachers, pioneered the development of this approach to the diagnosis of heart disease by chest x-ray.

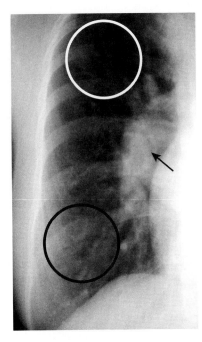

Figure 10-17. **Increased flow to the lungs.** *With increased flow to the lungs, all the blood vessels everywhere in the lung are larger than they would be in a normal person. This includes the right descending pulmonary artery (closed black arrow), the upper lobe vessels (white circle), and the lower lobe vessels (black circle). This is usually first recognized by realizing that there seem to be more blood vessels visible than one would expect normally. In increased flow to the lungs, the distribution of flow is as it would be in a normal person. So, even though there appear to be more blood vessels throughout the lung, the lower lobe vessels remain larger than the upper lobe vessels and there is still a gradual tapering as the vessels extend from central to peripheral. This patient had increased flow from a ventricular septal defect.*

- Your **assessment** of the heart **begins with** an evaluation of **cardiac size** using the **cardiothoracic ratio** and a determination that the heart is enlarged.
- Even if the heart is not enlarged, you should still **examine the cardiac contours** in the suggested systematic fashion below because some lesions can produce an abnormal cardiac contour without producing cardiomegaly.
- Evaluate the heart by asking the following four questions in this order:

A—Is the Left Atrium Enlarged?

- The first question is "A—**Is the left atrium enlarged?**" (A for atrium)
- To answer that question, look at the two places on the frontal chest radiograph where you might detect left atrial enlargement. Is there straightening of the left heart border or is there a double density on the right heart border? (See Figs. 10-4 and 10-10.)
- It is **more common** for **straightening to be present** with an enlarged left atrium **than for the double density** to be apparent.
- If there is either straightening or a double density, then the answer to question A is "yes."
- If the answer to question A is yes, then look at the pulmonary vasculature (Fig. 10-19).
- Your evaluation of the pulmonary vasculature should also be systematic, starting with assessment of the **size of the right descending pulmonary artery** and proceeding to an evaluation of the **distribution of flow in the lungs from apex to base** and then from **hilum to periphery.**
- If the answer to question A is "no," and the left atrium is not enlarged, then move to question B.
- Table 10-2 summarizes the causes and key findings associated with an enlarged left atrium.

Table 10-1

STATES OF THE PULMONARY VASCULATURE

Description of State	Size of Right Descending Pulmonary Artery	Distribution of Flow from Apex to Base	Distribution of Flow from Central to Peripheral	Remarks
Normal (Fig. 10-18A)	< 17 mm	Lower lobe larger than upper lobe	Gradual tapering from central to peripheral	These relationships require an upright chest to hold true
Venous hypertension (Fig. 10-18B)	> 17 mm	Upper lobe equal to or greater than size of lower lobe *(cephalization)*	Gradual tapering from central to peripheral	Diagnosis of cephalization requires upright chest
Arterial hypertension (Fig. 10-18C)	> 17 mm	Lower lobe larger than upper lobe	Rapid attenuation is size between central and peripheral vessels *(pruning)*	Can be difficult to recognize
Increased flow (Fig. 10-18D)	> 17 mm	Lower lobe larger than upper lobe	Gradual tapering from central to peripheral	All the vessels—everywhere in the lung—are larger than normal

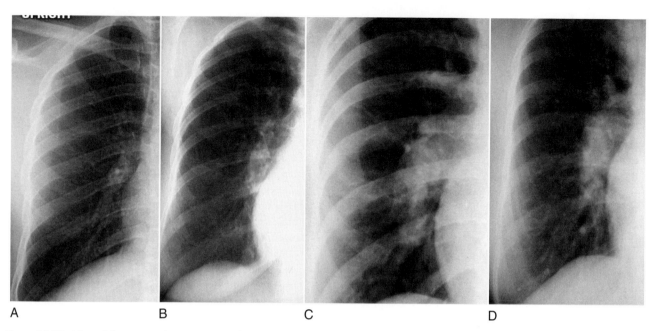

A   B   C   D

*Figure 10-18. Normal flow **(A)**, pulmonary venous hypertension **(B)**, pulmonary arterial hypertension **(C)**, and increased flow **(D)** to the lungs compared side by side. See Table 10-1.*

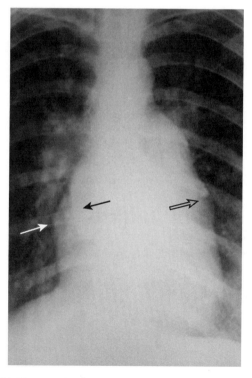

*Figure 10-19. **Mitral stenosis.** Question A is "Is the left atrium enlarged?" The answer to that question would be "yes" in this case. There is a convexity rather than a concavity on the left heart border due to an enlarged left atrium and enlarged left atrial appendage (open black arrow) and there is a double density on the right heart border caused by the enlarged left atrium (closed black arrow) superimposed on the normal right atrium (closed white arrow). This patient had mitral stenosis. Note that the heart is not enlarged and the underlying abnormality is diagnosable only by recognizing the abnormal contours of the heart.*

Table 10-2

"A" HEART

Type	Remarks
Normal	
Mitral regurgitation	Enlarged heart
Pulmonary venous hypertension	
Mitral stenosis	Normal or slightly enlarged heart
Left atrial myxoma	Rare
Papillary muscle dysfunction	Look for pulmonary edema, effusions
Left-sided heart failure	Common
Increased flow	
Ventricular septal defect	Normal-sized aorta
Patent ductus arteriosus	Enlarged aorta
Pulmonary arterial hypertension	
Mitral stenosis	Will also have pulmonary venous hypertension
Ventricular septal defect, patent ductus arteriosus	Will also have increased flow

B—Is the Main Pulmonary Artery Big or Bulbous?

- If the answer to question A is "no," then you ask question B, **"Is the main pulmonary artery segment big or bulbous?"** (B for big or bulbous).
- To answer question B, you draw the imaginary tangent line from the apex of the left ventricle to the aortic knob to determine if the main pulmonary artery protrudes beyond the tangent line.
- If the main pulmonary artery projects beyond the tangent line, then the answer to question B is "yes" (Fig. 10-20).
- If the answer to question B is yes, the next step is to examine the pulmonary vasculature.
- Once again, your evaluation of the pulmonary vasculature should be systematic, starting with assessment of the size of the right descending pulmonary artery and proceeding to an evaluation of the distribution of flow in the lungs.
  - You can't have pulmonary venous hypertension in a "B" heart because pulmonary venous hypertension presupposes elevation of left atrial pressure for its existence and, if the left atrial pressure were elevated, the left atrium would be enlarged, and it would have been an "A" heart, not a "B" heart.

- If the answer to question B is "no," then move to question C.
- Table 10-3 summarizes the causes and findings associated with a prominent main pulmonary artery.

C—Is the Main Pulmonary Artery Segment Concave?

- If the answer to question B was no, then you ask question C, **"Is the main pulmonary artery segment concave?"** (C is for concave).
- To answer question C, you will use the same tangent line from the apex of the left ventricle to the aortic knob as you did previously, measure along the same perpendicular to the tangent, but this time you will be determining if the main pulmonary artery is more than 15 mm medial to the tangent line (see Fig. 10-9).
  - "Away from the tangent line" means more than 15 mm **medial** to it or more than 15 mm to the **patient's right of the tangent line.**
- If the main pulmonary artery is more than 15 mm away from the tangent line, then the answer to question C is "yes."

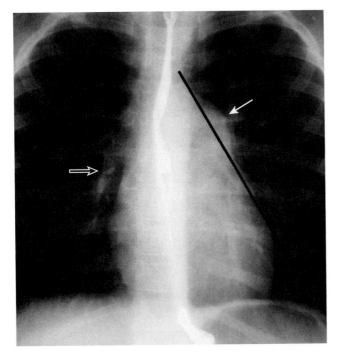

Figure 10-20. **Pulmonary stenosis.** *To answer question B, you should draw the tangent line from the apex of the left ventricle to the aortic knob (black line) to see if the main pulmonary artery protrudes beyond the tangent line. In this case, it does (closed white arrow). The right descending pulmonary artery is normal in size (open white arrow). The pulmonary vasculature is normal. This patient had valvular pulmonary stenosis since birth. The barium in the esophagus in this case, and others in this chapter, was part of an older method to assess cardiac chamber enlargement by having the patient swallow barium to mark the position of the esophagus.*

Table 10-3

"B" HEART

Type	Remarks
Normal	
Pulmonary stenosis	Left pulmonary artery sometimes asymmetrically enlarged
Idiopathic pulmonary artery dilatation	Only the main pulmonary artery is enlarged
Hyperdynamic states (e.g., anemia, hyperthyroid)	Vasculature usually normal
Pulmonary venous hypertension	Presupposes elevated left atrial pressure, which produces an "A" heart
Increased flow	
Atrial septal defect	Left atrium not often enlarged
Ventricular septal defect	Left atrium frequently enlarged
Patent ductus arteriosus	Left atrium frequently enlarged
Anomalous pulmonary venous return	Heart may have *snowman* shape
Pulmonary arterial hypertension	
Primary (idiopathic)	Normal lungs; disease of arteries themselves
Secondary	Multiple pulmonary emboli, arteritis, chronic obstructive pulmonary disease, schistosomiasis (lungs will be abnormal)

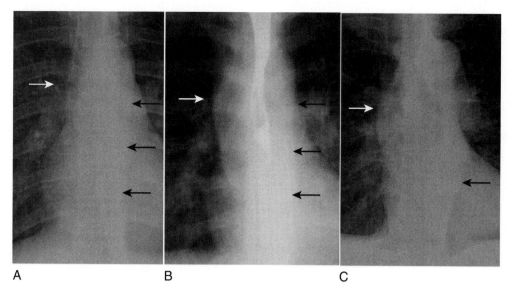

A   B   C

Figure 10-21. **Appearances of the aorta.** In **A,** which is normal, the ascending aorta is a low-density, almost straight edge—not convex outward (closed white arrow)—and the descending aorta almost disappears with the shadow of the thoracic spine (closed black arrows). In **B,** the ascending aorta is abnormal as it projects convex outward (closed white arrow) but the descending aorta remains normal (closed black arrows). In **C,** both the ascending and descending aorta are abnormal with the ascending aorta projecting convex outward (closed white arrow) and the descending aorta swinging far from the thoracic spine (closed black arrows).

- If the answer to question C is yes, then we're not going to look at the pulmonary vasculature; we're going to look at the configuration of the thoracic aorta.
  - The reason for this is that almost all "C" hearts have normal pulmonary vasculature, so the vasculature won't help to differentiate one cause of a "C" heart from another.
  - What we will use to differentiate one "C" heart from another is the configuration of the thoracic aorta, specifically the ascending aorta, aortic knob, and descending thoracic aorta (Fig. 10-21).
- For the purposes of this system, there are three different configurations of the thoracic aorta: it can be entirely normal, only the ascending aorta may be prominent, or the entire thoracic aorta (ascending, knob, and descending) may be prominent.
- If the answer to question C is "no," then move to the last question, question D.
- Table 10-4 summarizes the different configurations of the aorta in a "C" heart and the diseases that produce them.

D—Is the Heart a Dilated or Delta-Shaped Heart?

- If the answer to question C is "no," then the last question is **"Is the heart a dilated or a delta-shaped heart?"** (D is for dilated or delta).
- A dilated or a delta-shaped heart is usually one that is greater than 65% of the cardiothoracic ratio (a really big heart) and one with smooth contours such that almost the same amount of the heart projects to both the right and the left of the spine (Fig. 10-22).
- The two main entities in the differential diagnosis for a dilated or delta-shaped heart are **cardiomyopathy** and **pericardial effusion.**

Table 10-4

"C" HEART

Type	Remarks
Normal	
Hypertension	Entire aorta prominent
Arteriosclerotic cardiovascular disease	Entire aorta prominent
Aortic regurgitation	Entire aorta prominent
Aortic stenosis	Ascending aorta prominent
Coarctation	Indentation in descending aorta
Cardiomyopathy	Normal aorta
Pulmonary venous hypertension	Presupposes elevated left atrial pressure, which produces an "A" heart
Increased flow	Except in rare truncus, pulmonary artery should be big
Pulmonary arterial hypertension	Presupposes big main pulmonary artery

- Table 10-5 summarizes the causes and findings associated with a dilated cardiac silhouette.

Other Facts

- As you interpret cardiac imaging abnormalities, keep the following principles in mind:

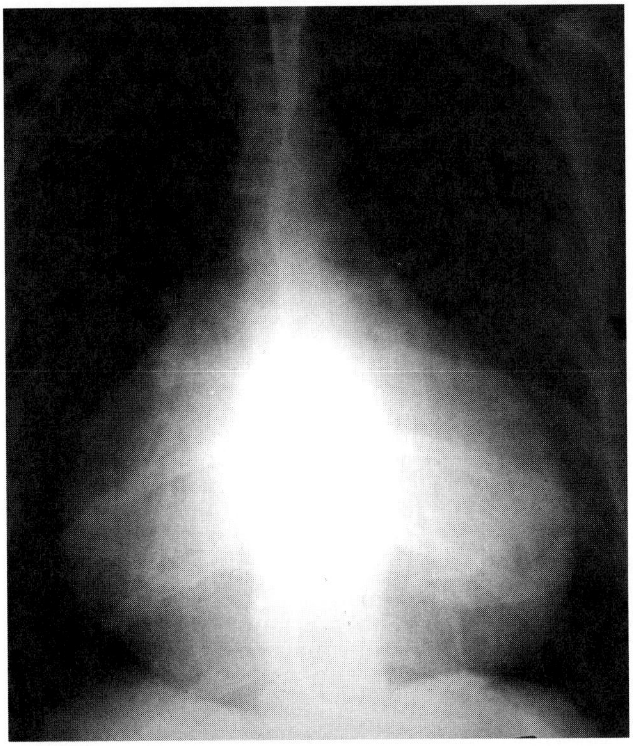

Figure 10-22. **Pericardial effusion.** The cardiac silhouette is markedly enlarged. This heart was more than 65% of the cardiothoracic ratio. This is a dilated or a delta-shaped heart. The main differential diagnosis for such a heart is pericardial effusion versus cardiomyopathy, and they are frequently difficult or impossible to differentiate on conventional radiographs. In this case, though, the globular shape of the heart and the absence of any recognizable cardiac contours leads toward pericardial effusion. The patient had uremic pericarditis. Notice that the soft tissue density of the heart and the pericardial fluid appear as the same radiographic density with conventional radiography. Pericardial effusion is best diagnosed using ultrasound.

- The **ventricles respond to obstruction** to their outflow **by first undergoing hypertrophy** rather than dilation.
  - Therefore, the heart may not be enlarged with lesions such as aortic stenosis, coarctation of the aorta, pulmonary stenosis, or systemic hypertension.

Table 10-5

"D" HEART

Type	Remarks
Pericardial effusion	Causes include uremia, viral, mets, tuberculosis, trauma, post-myocardial infarction
Cardiomyopathy	Causes include alcoholism, beri beri, coronary artery disease
Multiple valve disease	Look for enlarged left atrium
Coronary artery disease	Cardiomyopathy
Ebstein's anomaly	Big right heart; cyanotic

- **Cardiomegaly,** as we usually recognize it, **is primarily produced by ventricular enlargement,** not isolated enlargement of the atria.
  - Therefore, the heart is classically normal in size in early mitral stenosis.
- In general, **the most marked chamber enlargement will occur from volume overload** rather than pressure overload so that the largest chambers, in general, are produced by regurgitant valves rather than stenotic valves.
  - Therefore, the heart will usually be larger with aortic regurgitation than with aortic stenosis.
- The other signs of pulmonary venous hypertension (see Chapter 11, Recognizing Congestive Heart Failure and Pulmonary Edema) are much easier to recognize than cephalization, even for experienced radiologists.

WebLink
More information on The ABCs of Heart Disease is available to registered users on StudentConsult.com.

TAKE-HOME POINTS: The ABCs of Heart Disease in Schematic Form

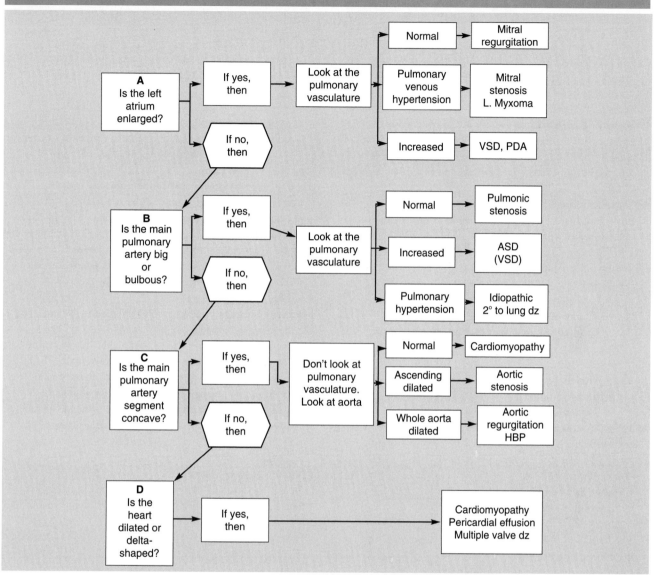

11 Recognizing Congestive Heart Failure and Pulmonary Edema

Congestive Heart Failure—General Considerations
- The incidence of congestive heart failure (CHF) has grown rapidly over the last 15 years and it is now **the most common diagnosis in hospitalized patients over the age of 65.**
- **Causes of congestive heart failure**
  - In the United States, the **two most common causes of CHF are**
    - **Coronary artery disease**
    - **Hypertension**
    - Other causes:
      - **Cardiomyopathy,** such as from longstanding alcohol abuse
      - **Cardiac valvular lesions** such as aortic stenosis and mitral stenosis
      - **Arrythmias**
      - **Hyperthyroidism**
      - **Severe anemia**
      - **Left-to-right shunts**
- Typically, **congestive heart failure** presents as **one of two radiographic patterns,** although not every feature of each pattern is always present and there is overlap between the two patterns.
  - **Pulmonary interstitial edema**
  - **Pulmonary alveolar edema**

Pulmonary Interstitial Edema
- The **four key radiographic signs of pulmonary interstitial edema** are:
  - **Thickening of the interlobular septa**
  - **Peribronchial cuffing**
  - **Fluid in the fissures**
  - **Pleural effusions**
- The key findings in pulmonary interstitial edema are summarized in Box 11-1.

THICKENING OF THE INTERLOBULAR SEPTA—THE KERLEY B LINE
- The interlobular septa is not visible on a normal chest radiograph.
- The septae can become visible if they accumulate excessive fluid, usually at a pulmonary (venous) capillary wedge pressure of about **15 mm Hg.**
- These are **Kerley B lines** (named after Peter James Kerley, an Irish neurologist and radiologist).
- **Recognizing the elusive Kerley B line**
  - Many students believe that Kerley B lines are imaginary, much as I believed the S3 and S4 heart sounds were when auscultating the heart as a medical student.
    - They are, however, real.

- Kerley B lines (also called **septal lines**) will be visible on a frontal radiograph usually **at the lung bases, at or near the costophrenic angles.**
- They are **very short** (1 to 2 cm long), **very thin** (about 1 mm), and **horizontal in orientation,** which means they are **perpendicular to pleural surface.**
- They **usually abut the pleural surface** (Fig. 11-1).
- After repeated episodes of pulmonary interstitial edema, the **septal lines may fibrose** and therefore **remain even after all other signs of pulmonary interstitial edema clear.**
  - These are called **chronic Kerley B lines.**
- **Kerley A lines**
  - Kerley was busy naming other lines seen in congestive heart failure besides the "B" line.
  - **Kerley A** lines appear when connective tissue around the bronchoarterial sheaths in the lung distends with fluid.
  - **Kerley A lines extend from the hila for several centimeters (up to 6 cm) and do not reach the periphery of the lung** like Kerley B lines do (Fig. 11-2).
- Not content with A and B lines, Kerley also described C lines, but there is some doubt that they exist as separate entities.

PERIBRONCHIAL CUFFING
- In adults, bronchi may normally be visible on-end in the hila but are usually not visible *en face* beyond the confines of the pulmonary hila.
- When fluid accumulates in the interstitial tissue around and in the wall of a bronchus as it does in CHF, the **bronchial wall becomes thicker and appears as a ringlike density that can be seen on-end in radiographs.**
- When seen on-end, *peribronchial cuffing* appears as numerous, small, ringlike shadows that look like little *doughnuts* (Fig. 11-3).

Box 11-1

Key Findings in Pulmonary Interstitial Edema

Thickening of the interlobular septa—***Kerley B lines***—and fluid in the central connective tissue of the lungs—***Kerley A lines***

Peribronchial cuffing from fluid-thickened bronchial walls visualized *en face*

Opacification and thickening of the interlobar fissures by fluid

Pleural effusions that are usually bilateral but, when unilateral, are usually right-sided

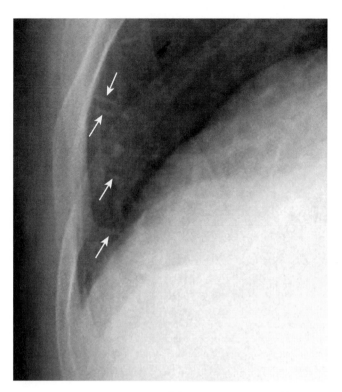

Figure 11-1. **Kerley B lines.** *Interlobular septa are not visible on a normal chest radiograph but can become visible if they accumulate excessive fluid. First described by neurologist/radiologist Peter James Kerley, they are very short (1 to 2 cm long), very thin (about 1 mm) horizontal lines perpendicular to and abutting the pleural surface (closed white arrows).*

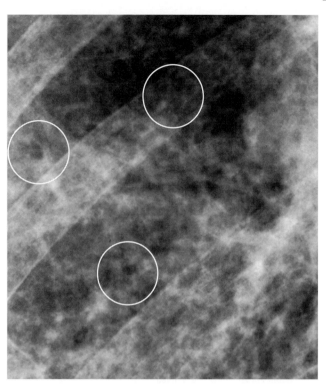

Figure 11-3. **Peribronchial cuffing.** *Normally the bronchus is invisible when seen on-end in the periphery of the lung. When fluid accumulates in the interstitial tissue around and in the wall of a bronchus as it does in CHF, the bronchial wall becomes thicker and can appear as ringlike densities when seen on-end (white circles). Peribronchial cuffing may not always produce perfectly round circles.*

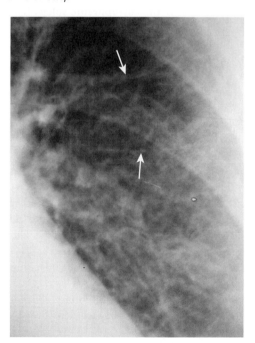

Figure 11-2. **Kerley A lines.** *The A lines (closed white arrows) appear when connective tissue near the bronchoarterial bundle distends with fluid. They extend from the hila for several centimeters (up to 6 cm) in the midlung and do not reach the periphery of the lung like Kerley B lines do. A network of Kerley lines is produced in the lungs in patients with congestive heart failure producing the "prominence of the pulmonary interstitial markings" seen in that disease.*

FLUID IN THE FISSURES

- The major and minor **fissures may be visible normally** but are almost never thicker than a line you could draw with the **point of a sharpened pencil** (Fig. 11-4A).
- **Fluid can collect between the two layers of visceral pleura that form the fissures** of the lung (minor or horizontal, major or oblique) **or in the subpleural space** just beneath the visceral pleura between the visceral pleura and the lung parenchyma.
- The result is that the **fluid** distends the fissure and makes it **thicker,** more **irregular in contour,** and **more visible** than normal (Fig. 11-4B).
- **Fluid may collect in any fissure** including accessory fissures such as the *azygous fissure or inferior accessory fissure.*

PLEURAL EFFUSION

- There are normally only 2 to 5 mL of fluid in the pleural space and this fluid is not visible on a chest radiograph.
- As a result of either increased production or decreased absorption of pleural fluid, additional fluid can collect in the pleural space, typically at a pulmonary capillary wedge pressure of about **20 mm Hg.**
- **Pleural effusions accompanying CHF are usually bilateral,** but can be asymmetrical (Fig. 11-5).
  - When **unilateral,** they are **almost always right-sided.**

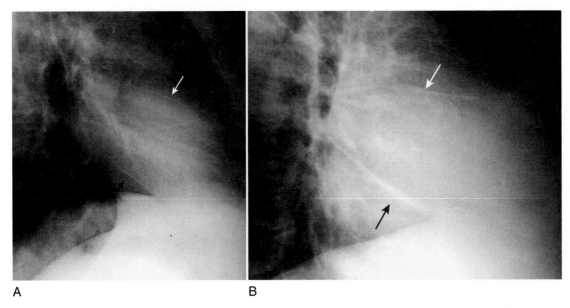

A   B

*Figure 11-4. **Normal fissures and fluid in the fissures.** The major (closed black arrows) and minor fissures (closed white arrows) may be visible normally **(A)** but are almost never thicker than a line you could draw with the point of a sharpened pencil. Fluid can collect in the fissures in congestive heart failure and distend them, making them appear thicker and more irregular in contour and more visible than normal **(B).** When the patient's heart failure clears, the fissures will return to normal appearance, but after repeated and prolonged bouts of failure, fibrosis may result in permanent thickening of the fissures.*

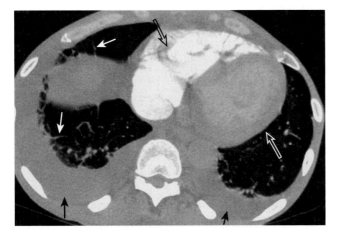

*Figure 11-5. **Bilateral pleural effusions and Kerley B lines on CT.** Axial CT scan of the chest following intravenous injection of contrast material. Note that the right side of the heart is opacified (open black arrow) but the contrast agent has not yet passed through the lungs a sufficient number of times to fully opacify the left side of the heart (open white arrow). There are bilateral pleural effusions present and they layer posteriorly because the patient is being scanned supine (closed black arrows). The thickened interlobular septa (closed white arrows) are Kerley B lines.*

- About 15% of the time, they can be unilateral and on the left, but if you see a unilateral left pleural effusion you should think of other causes before CHF, such as metastases, tuberculosis, or pulmonary thromboembolic disease.

- At times, pleural fluid accumulates in the form of a **laminar effusion** in which the fluid assumes a **thin, bandlike density along the lateral chest wall, beginning near the costophrenic sulcus** but often preserving the sulcus itself.
  - Normally, aerated lung extends to the inside margin of each contiguous rib.
  - Laminar effusions separate the air-filled lung from the inside margin of the ribs at the lung base on the frontal chest radiograph (see Fig. 7–12).
- For more about pleural effusions, see Chapter 7, Recognizing Pleural Effusions.

Pulmonary Alveolar Edema
- When the **pulmonary venous pressure is sufficiently elevated (about 25 mm Hg), fluid spills out of the interstitial tissues of the lung into the airspaces.**
- This results in *pulmonary alveolar edema* (most often shortened to *pulmonary edema* without including "alveolar").
- The **radiographic findings of pulmonary alveolar edema:**
  - **Fluffy, indistinct patchy airspace densities that are usually centrally located.**
    - Outer third of the lung is frequently spared.
    - Lower lung zones more affected than upper.
      - This is called the *bat-wing* or *butterfly* configuration (Fig. 11-6).
      - The key findings in pulmonary alveolar edema are summarized in Box 11-2.

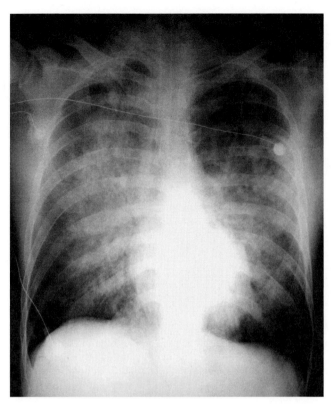

Figure 11-6. **Bat-wing pattern of pulmonary edema.** *The radiographic findings of pulmonary alveolar edema include fluffy, indistinct, and patchy airspace densities frequently centrally located and sparing the outer third of the lung. This is called the **bat-wing (bat's-wing)** or **butterfly** pattern, and it is suggestive of pulmonary edema versus other airspace diseases such as pneumonia. There is considerable overlap in the patterns of cardiogenic and noncardiogenic pulmonary edema, but the absence of pleural effusions, absence of fluid in the fissures, and the normal-sized heart favor a noncardiogenic cause in this case. The patient was in septic shock from an overwhelming urinary tract infection.*

Box 11-2

Key Findings in Pulmonary Alveolar Edema

Fluffy, indistinct patchy airspace densities

Bat-wing or butterfly configuration frequently sparing the outer third of lungs

Pleural effusions are usually present when the edema is cardiogenic in origin

- **What happened to cardiomegaly and cephalization?**
  - Although most patients with congestive heart failure have an enlarged heart, most patients with an enlarged heart are not in congestive heart failure.
  - In any one person, **cardiomegaly itself is not a particularly sensitive indicator for the presence or absence of congestive heart failure.**

- **Cephalization is difficult to identify for most beginners** and is meaningful only if you are sure the patient was upright at the time of the chest exposure.
  - Anyone (even you and me) who undergoes a chest radiograph while supine will demonstrate cephalization, because gravity will exert the same effect on both the upper and lobe vessels in the supine position.
  - Many patients who have portable chest radiographs exposed in the intensive care unit setting are supine at the time of the exposure, so they will all demonstrate cephalization.
- The **essential differences in appearance between pulmonary interstitial edema and pulmonary alveolar edema** are shown in Figure 11-7.
- **How pulmonary edema resolves**
  - Pulmonary edema generally is both **abrupt in onset** and **quick to clear,** typically in a matter of a few hours to a few days (Fig. 11-8).
  - Resolution frequently begins peripherally and moves centrally.
  - Radiologic resolution may lag behind clinical improvement, especially if the patient had large pleural effusions.

Noncardiogenic Pulmonary Edema—General Considerations
- Although congestive heart failure accounts for the majority of cases of pulmonary edema (**cardiogenic pulmonary edema**), there are other, **noncardiogenic causes of pulmonary edema.**
- Among the causes of noncardiogenic pulmonary edema are a diverse group of diseases:
  - **Increased capillary permeability** includes all the various causes of **adult respiratory distress syndrome,** or **ARDS** (see below):
    - **Sepsis**
    - **Uremia**
    - **Disseminated intravascular coagulopathy**
    - **Smoke inhalation**
    - **Near-drowning**
  - **Volume overload**
  - **Lymphangitic spread of malignancy**
  - Other causes
    - **High-altitude pulmonary edema**
    - **Neurogenic pulmonary edema**
    - **Re-expansion pulmonary edema** (Fig. 11-9)
    - **Heroin or other overdoses**

Differentiating Cardiac from Noncardiogenic Pulmonary Edema
- **Adult respiratory distress syndrome (ARDS)** represents **one form of noncardiogenic pulmonary edema.**
  - Characteristically, **patients with ARDS are radiographically normal for 24 to 36 hours** after the initial insult.

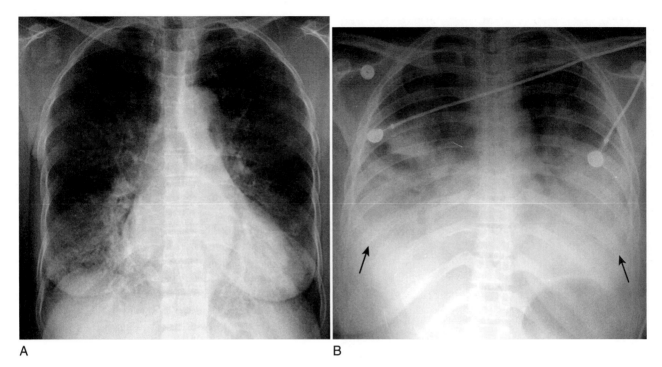

A   B

Figure 11-7. **Pulmonary interstitial versus pulmonary alveolar edema.** *The key findings in pulmonary interstitial edema* **(A)** *include thickening of the interlobular septa (Kerley B lines), peribronchial cuffing, pleural effusion, and fluid in the fissure. The heart is also enlarged in this patient who had congestive heart failure. The key findings in pulmonary alveolar edema* **(B)** *are fluffy airspace densities, frequently perihilar in distribution and sparing the outer third of lungs. Pleural effusions are frequently present when the edema is cardiogenic in origin, as in this case with large, bilateral pleural effusions (closed black arrows).*

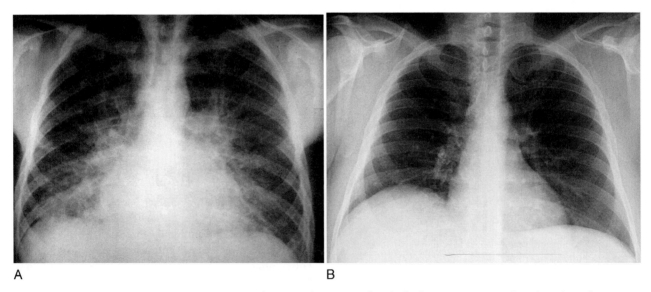

A   B

Figure 11-8. **Rapidly clearing pulmonary edema.** *Pulmonary edema generally is both abrupt in its onset and quick to clear. This patient demonstrates bilateral, perihilar airspace disease with diffuse prominence of the interstitial markings characteristic of pulmonary edema* **(A).** *Four days later* **(B),** *the lungs are clear. Patients with adult respiratory distress syndrome are not likely to clear this quickly, nor are patients who have coexisting diseases such as renal or hepatic failure or superimposed pneumonia.*

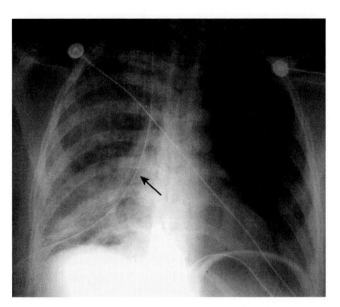

Figure 11-9. **Re-expansion pulmonary edema.** *Unilateral airspace disease affects the entire right lung. In addition, a chest tube (closed black arrow) is seen on the same side. The chest tube was inserted for a large, right-sided, tension pneumothorax that was rapidly re-expanded. Re-expansion pulmonary edema results from the overly rapid expansion of a lung that has typically been chronically collapsed by pneumothorax or a large pleural effusion. Its exact cause is not known. In general, unilateral pulmonary edema can occur either because of an abnormality on the same side as the pulmonary edema (e.g., prolonged positioning with the affected side dependent) or an abnormality on the opposite side (e.g., large pulmonary embolus occluding flow to the opposite lung).*

- Then, pulmonary abnormalities become evident and can appear in the form of **pulmonary interstitial edema** or **patchy airspace disease** or **pulmonary alveolar edema.**
- Clinically, the **patient demonstrates severe hypoxia, cyanosis, tachypnea, and dyspnea.**
- In the later stages of ARDS, a **reticular interstitial pattern may develop,** although the majority of patients who survive tend to have little impairment of lung function.
- The **patterns of cardiogenic and noncardiogenic pulmonary edema overlap considerably** and the patient's **clinical picture is key** to establishing the most likely cause of pulmonary edema.

- In general, **noncardiogenic pulmonary edema** is
  - **Less likely** to demonstrate **pleural effusions** and **Kerley B lines** than cardiogenic pulmonary edema
  - **More likely** to demonstrate a **normal pulmonary capillary wedge pressure (PCWP)** of less than 12 mm Hg than cardiogenic pulmonary edema
  - **More likely** to be associated with a **normal-sized heart** (Fig. 11-10)
- The airspace disease in noncardiogenic pulmonary edema may be more patchy and peripheral than that in cardiogenic pulmonary edema, but this is highly variable.

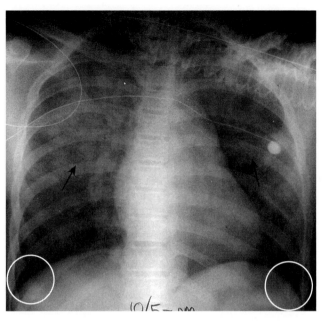

Figure 11-10. **Noncardiogenic pulmonary edema.** *Bilateral airspace disease primarily affects the upper lobes in this patient (closed black arrows). There is no evidence of pleural fluid (white circles). In general, noncardiogenic pulmonary edema is less likely to demonstrate pleural effusions and Kerley B lines, more likely to demonstrate a normal pulmonary capillary wedge pressure (PCWP) of less than 12 mm Hg, and more likely to be associated with a normal-sized heart than cardiogenic pulmonary edema. This patient had taken an overdose of heroin.*

- The key differences between cardiogenic and noncardiogenic pulmonary edema are summarized in Table 11-1.

WebLink
More information on congestive heart failure and pulmonary edema is available to registered users on StudentConsult.com.

Table 11-1

CARDIOGENIC VERSUS NONCARDIOGENIC PULMONARY EDEMA

Imaging Finding	Cardiogenic	Noncardiogenic
Pleural effusions	Common	Infrequent
Kerley B lines	Common	Infrequent
Heart size	Frequently enlarged	May be normal
Pulmonary capillary wedge pressure	Elevated	Normal

TAKE-HOME POINTS: Congestive Heart Failure and Pulmonary Edema

Coronary artery disease and hypertension are the two most common causes of congestive heart failure and the most common diagnosis in hospitalized patients >65 years old.

Two major patterns of CHF are pulmonary interstitial and pulmonary alveolar edema.

The four key findings of pulmonary interstitial edema are thickening of the interlobular septa, peribronchial cuffing, fluid in the fissures, and pleural effusions.

The key findings in pulmonary alveolar edema are fluffy, indistinct, patchy airspace densities; bat-wing or butterfly configuration frequently sparing the outer third of lungs; and pleural effusions, especially with cardiogenic pulmonary edema.

Acute pulmonary edema is generally both abrupt in onset and quick to clear, frequently in less than 72 hours, although radiologic clearing may lag behind patient improvement.

Causes of pulmonary edema can be divided into two major categories: cardiogenic and noncardiogenic causes.

Cardiogenic pulmonary edema is more likely to have pleural effusions and Kerley B lines, more likely to have cardiomegaly, and more likely to have an elevated pulmonary capillary wedge pressure than noncardiogenic pulmonary edema.

The noncardiogenic causes of pulmonary edema are a diverse group of diseases including uremia, disseminated intravascular coagulopathy, smoke inhalation, near-drowning, volume overload, and lymphangitic spread of malignancy.

Noncardiogenic pulmonary edema is less likely to demonstrate pleural effusions, Kerley B lines, and cardiomegaly than the cardiogenic variety.

Adult respiratory distress syndrome can be considered a subset of noncardiogenic pulmonary edema in which the clinical picture is one of severe hypoxia, cyanosis, tachypnea, and dyspnea.

12 Recognizing the Correct Placement of Lines and Tubes and Their Potential Complications: Critical Care Radiology

- Patients in the critical or intensive care units (ICU) are monitored on a frequent basis with portable chest radiography both to check on the position of their multiple assistive devices and to assess their cardiopulmonary status.
  - Diseases commonly seen in critically ill patients are discussed in other chapters (Table 12-1).
- In this chapter, you'll get practical advice for evaluating the successful (or unsuccessful) insertion and ultimate position of multiple tubes, lines, catheters, and other supportive apparatus used in the ICU.
- Most times, a conventional radiograph is obtained after the insertion or attempted insertion of one of these devices to check on its position and to rule out any unintended complications.
- Therefore, **for each tube or device, you'll learn:**
  - **Why they are used**
  - **Where they belong** when properly placed
  - Where such devices can be **malpositioned** and what **complications** may occur from the device.

Endotracheal and Tracheostomy Tubes
ENDOTRACHEAL TUBES (ETTs)
- **Why endotracheal tubes are used**
  - Assist ventilation
  - Isolate the trachea to permit control of airway
  - Prevent gastric distention
  - Provide a direct route for suctioning
  - Administer medications
- **Correct placement of an ETT** (Box 12-1)
  - Endotracheal tubes are usually **wide-bore tubes** (about 1 cm) with a **radiopaque marker stripe** and **no side holes.**
  - The **tip itself is frequently diagonally angled.**
  - With the patient's head in the neutral position (i.e., bottom of mandible is at the level of C5-C6), the **tip of the ETT should be 3 to 5 cm from the carina.**
    - This is roughly **half the distance between the medial ends of clavicles and the carina** (Fig. 12-1).
    - Ideally the **diameter of the endotracheal tube should be one half to two thirds the width of trachea.**
      - An inflated cuff (balloon), if present, may fill—but shouldn't distend—the lumen of the trachea (Fig. 12-2).
- **How to find the carina on a frontal chest radiograph**
  - Follow the right or left main bronchus backward until it meets the opposite main bronchus.

- The carina projects over the T5, T6, or T7 vertebral bodies in 95% of people.
- **Movement of tip with flexion and extension**
  - Neck **flexion** may cause **2 cm of descent** of the tube tip.
  - Neck **extension** from neutral **may cause 2 cm of ascent** of tip.

Table 12-1

COMMON DISEASES IN CRITICALLY ILL PATIENTS

Finding or Disease	Discussed in
Adult respiratory distress syndrome	Chapter 11
Aspiration	Chapter 8
Atelectasis	Chapter 6
Pleural effusion	Chapter 7
Pneumomediastinum	Chapter 9
Pneumonia	Chapter 8
Pneumothorax	Chapter 9
Pulmonary edema	Chapter 11
Pulmonary embolic disease	Chapter 14

Box 12-1

Endotracheal Tubes

The tip should be about 3–5 cm above the carina.

The inflated cuff should not distend the lumen of the trachea.

These tubes are most commonly malpositioned in the right main or right lower lobe bronchi.

If a tube is positioned with the tip in the neck, damage to vocal cords can occur.

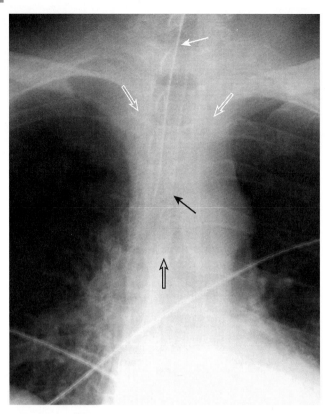

Figure 12-1. Endotracheal tube in satisfactory position.
Endotracheal tubes are usually wide-bore tubes (about 1 cm) with a radiopaque marker stripe (closed white arrow) and no side holes. The tip is frequently diagonally angled (closed black arrow). With the patient's head in the neutral position, the tip of ETT should be 3 to 5 cm from the carina (open black arrow), which is roughly half the distance between the medial ends of clavicles (open white arrows) and the carina.

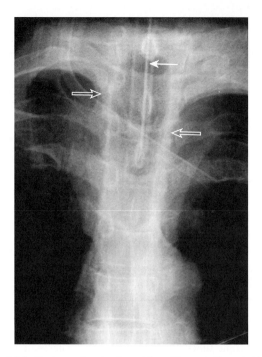

Figure 12-2. Endotracheal tube with cuff overinflated. *Ideally the diameter of the endotracheal tube (closed white arrow) should be one third to one half the width of trachea. An inflated cuff (balloon), if present, may fill—but shouldn't distend—the lumen of the trachea. Here the inflated balloon (open white arrows) is wider than the diameter of the trachea and was deflated. Prolonged compression on the tracheal wall by an overinflated cuff can result in necrosis of the wall and tracheal stenosis.*

- Incorrect placement and complications of an ETT
  - **Most common malposition:** because of a shallower angle and wider diameter, the **tip of the ETT will tend to slide into the right main bronchus** or bronchus intermedius preferentially to the left main bronchus.
    - This can lead to **atelectasis** (especially of the nonaerated right upper lobe and left lung) (see Fig. 6-14A).
    - Intubation of the right main bronchus could also lead to a **right-sided tension pneumothorax.**
  - Inadvertent esophageal intubation will produce a grossly dilated stomach.
  - Tip of the tube should not be positioned in the larynx or pharynx; the tip **should be at least 3 cm distal to level of vocal cords** (Fig. 12-3).
    - Otherwise, tube may damage vocal cords or lead to aspiration.

TRACHEOSTOMY TUBES
- **Why tracheostomy tubes are used**
  - In patients with airway obstruction at or above level of larynx

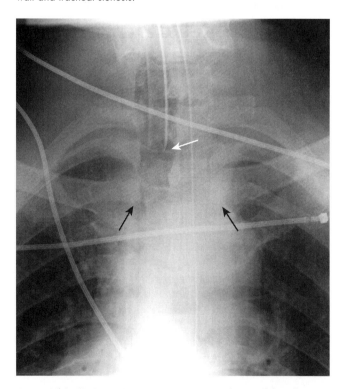

Figure 12-3. Endotracheal tube too high. *The tip of the tube (closed white arrow) should not be positioned in the larynx or pharynx. The tip should be at least 3 cm distal to the level of the vocal cords so that damage to the vocal cords and aspiration do not occur. The medial ends of the clavicles are marked by the closed black arrows.*

- In respiratory failure requiring long-term intubation (>21 days)
- For airway obstruction during sleep apnea
- When there is paralysis of the muscles that affect swallowing or respiration
- **Correct placement of a tracheostomy tube**
  - The **tip should be about half-way between the stoma in which the tracheostomy tube was inserted and the carina.**
    - Usually around **level of T3** (Fig. 12-4)
  - Tracheostomy tube tip placement is not affected by flexion and extension like an ETT.
  - **Width of the tracheostomy tube should be about two-thirds the width of trachea.**
- **Incorrect placement and complications of a tracheostomy tube** (Box 12-2)
  - Immediately after insertion, **look for signs of** inadvertent **perforation of the trachea:**
    - Pneumomediastinum
    - Pneumothorax
    - Subcutaneous emphysema
  - If the tracheostomy tube is equipped with a cuff, the **cuff should generally be inflated to a diameter**

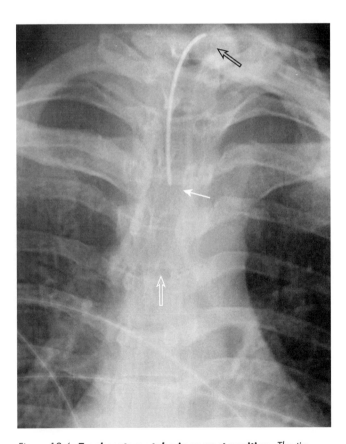

*Figure 12-4. **Tracheostomy tube in correct position.** The tip (closed white arrow) should be about half-way between stoma in which the tracheostomy tube was inserted (open black arrow) and the carina (open white arrow). This is usually around the level of T3. Unlike the tip of an endotracheal tube, tracheostomy tube tip placement is not affected by flexion and extension of the neck.*

Box 12-2

Tracheostomy Tubes

The tip should be halfway between the entrance stoma and the carina.

If so equipped, the cuff is generally not inflated to a size greater than the tracheal lumen.

Short-term complications may include perforation of trachea.

Long-term complications can include tracheal stenosis, usually at site of stoma.

that fills but does not distend the normal tracheal contour.
- **Long-term complications of tracheostomies**
  - **Tracheal stenosis**
    - **Most common late-occurring complication** of tracheostomy tube
    - May occur at entrance stoma, level of cuff, or tip of tube
      - **Most common at stoma**

Intravascular Catheters

CENTRAL VENOUS CATHETERS (CVCs)

- **Why they are used**
  - For venous access to instill chemotherapeutic and hyperosmolar agents not suitable for peripheral venous administration
  - Measurement of central venous pressure
  - To maintain and monitor intravascular blood volume
- **Correct placement of central venous catheters** (Box 12-3)
  - **Central venous catheters are small** (3 mm) and **uniformly opaque without a marker stripe.**
  - The subclavian vein joins the brachiocephalic vein behind **medial end** of clavicle.
  - A central venous catheter should reach the **medial end of clavicle before descending** and its **tip should lie distal to the anterior end of the first rib.**
  - Catheter should **descend lateral to spine** and **tip should be in the superior vena cava** (Fig. 12-5).
    - You should be able to recognize the indentation that marks the junction between the superior vena cava and the right atrium (see Fig. 10-1).

Box 12-3

Central Venous Catheters

The tip should lie in the superior vena cava.

All bends in the catheter should be smooth curves, not sharp kinks.

Most common malpositions are right atrium and internal jugular vein.

Always check for pneumothorax after successful or unsuccessful insertion attempt.

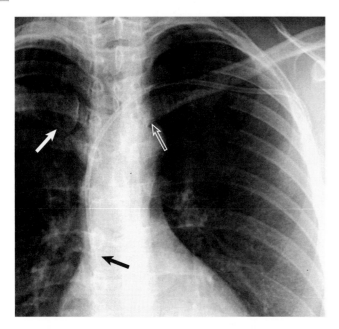

Figure 12-5. Subclavian central venous catheter in correct position. *Central venous catheters are small (3 mm) and uniformly opaque without a marker stripe. The subclavian vein joins the brachiocephalic vein behind the medial end of the clavicle. A central venous catheter should reach the medial end of the clavicle (open white arrow) before descending, and its tip (closed black arrow) should lie distal to the anterior end of the first rib (closed white arrow). The catheter should descend to the right of the thoracic spine, and the tip should be in the superior vena cava.*

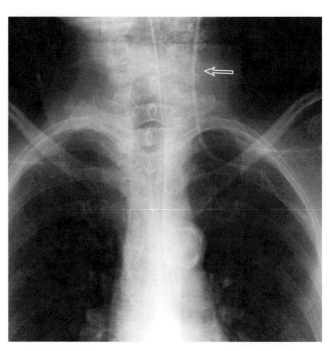

Figure 12-6. Central venous catheter malpositioned in internal jugular vein. *Central venous catheters, especially those placed by the subclavian route, are often malpositioned. They are most often malpositioned with their tips in the right atrium or internal jugular vein (open white arrow). In the right atrium, they can produce cardiac arrythmias. When central venous catheters are malpositioned, they may provide inaccurate central venous pressure measurements.*

- **All bends in the catheter should be smooth curves,** not sharp kinks.
- Other routes of insertion for central venous catheters include the jugular vein and the femoral vein.
- **Incorrect placement and complications of central venous catheters**
  - Central venous catheters, especially those placed by the subclavian route, are often malpositioned.
  - They are **most often malpositioned with their tips in the right atrium or internal jugular vein** (Fig. 12-6).
    - In the **right atrium,** they can **produce cardiac arrythmias.**
    - When central venous catheters are malpositioned, they may provide **inaccurate central venous pressure readings.**
  - **Pneumothorax** can occur in up to 5% of CVC insertions, especially those using the subclavian approach.
  - Occasionally CVCs **may perforate the vein** and lie outside the blood vessel.
    - **Look for sharp bends in the catheter as a clue to a potential perforation.**
  - Sometimes, CVCs may be **inadvertently inserted in the subclavian artery** rather than the subclavian vein.
    - Suspect **arterial placement** if the **flow is pulsatile** and the course of the catheter **parallels the aortic arch** or **fails to descend to the right of the spine** (Fig. 12-7).

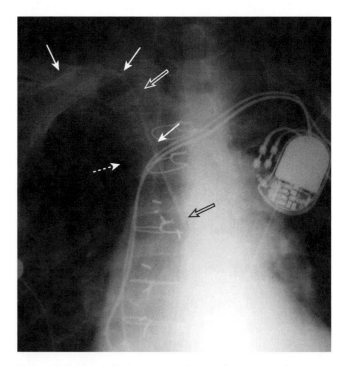

Figure 12-7. Arterial placement of central venous catheter. *Sometimes, central lines may be inadvertently inserted in the subclavian artery rather than the subclavian vein. This catheter (closed white arrows) does not reach the medial end of the clavicle (open white arrow) before descending, and its tip (open black arrow) is oriented over the spine, directed away from the superior vena cava (dotted white arrow). Suspect arterial placement if the flow is pulsatile.*

- Two or more attempts at inserting a CVC
  - A frontal chest radiograph is obtained following placement of a CVC.
  - Should initial placement fail, you should obtain a chest radiograph before trying insertion on the other side to avoid the possibility of producing bilateral pneumothoraces.

PERIPHERALLY INSERTED CENTRAL CATHETERS (PICC LINES)

- **Why they are used**
  - For long-term venous access (months)
    - To administer medications such as chemotherapy or antibiotics
    - For frequent blood sampling
      - Because of their small size, they can be inserted into an antecubital vein.
- **Correct placement of PICC lines** (Box 12-4)
  - **Tip** should lie **within** the **superior vena cava** but may be placed in an axillary vein.
  - Because the lines are so small, they may be difficult to visualize (Fig. 12-8)

Box 12-4

PICC Lines
The tip should lie in the superior vena cava or axillary vein.
They may be difficult to visualize because of their small size.
Thrombosis of the line may occur over time.

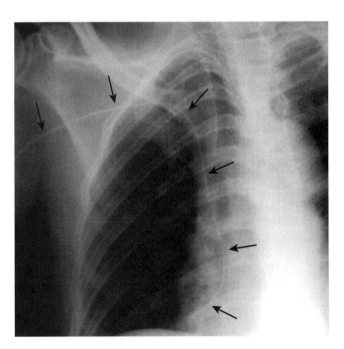

Figure 12-8. **Peripherally inserted central catheter (PICC line) in right atrium.** PICC lines (closed black arrows) can be used for long-term venous access. Because the lines are so small, they may be difficult to visualize. The tip should lie within the superior vena cava but may be placed in an axillary vein. In this case, the tip is in too far, residing in the region of the right atrium.

- **Incorrect placement and complications of PICC lines**
  - Tips may become malpositioned over time.
  - Thrombosis of the line may occur because of its small lumen size.

PULMONARY ARTERY CATHETERS: SWAN-GANZ CATHETERS

- **Why they are used**
  - Monitor hemodynamic status of critically ill patients
  - Help in differentiating cardiac from noncardiac pulmonary edema
- **Correct placement of Swan-Ganz catheters** (also known as *pulmonary capillary wedge pressure catheters*)
  - Swan-Ganz catheters have the **same appearance as central venous lines but are longer.**
  - Inserted via the subclavian vein or internal jugular vein, their tips are floated out into the **proximal right or proximal left pulmonary artery.**
    - The **tip should be about 2 cm from the hilum** (Fig. 12-9).
  - Balloon is temporarily inflated only when pressure measurements are made and should then be deflated.
- **Incorrect placement and complications of Swan-Ganz catheters** (Box 12-5)
  - **Serious complications are uncommon.**
  - Most common significant complication is **pulmonary infarction.**

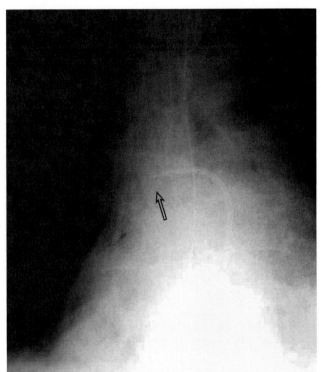

Figure 12-9. **Swan-Ganz catheter in correct position.** Swan-Ganz catheters have the same appearance as central venous lines but are longer. They are inserted via the subclavian vein or internal jugular vein and their tips are floated out into the proximal right (open black arrow) or proximal left pulmonary artery. The tip should be no more than 2 cm from the hilar shadow.

Box 12-5

Pulmonary Artery Catheters (Swan-Ganz Catheters)

Tip should be about 2 cm from the hilum in either the right or left pulmonary artery.

Balloon should be inflated only when pressure measurements are performed.

The tip of the catheter should not lie within a peripheral pulmonary artery.

Box 12-6

Double Lumen Catheters

The tip should be in either the superior vena cava or the right atrium: some catheters are designed with separate lumens so that one tip is in the superior vena cava and the other is in the right atrium.

The right internal jugular vein has the lowest incidence of clotting, so it is the preferred access route.

Complications include pneumothorax, thrombosis, and infection.

* From occlusion of pulmonary artery by catheter
* From emboli arising from catheter
* Make sure the catheter tip does not lie in a distal branch of a pulmonary artery because this increases the risk of infarction (Fig. 12-10).

DOUBLE LUMEN CATHETERS: "QUINTON CATHETERS," HEMODIALYSIS CATHETERS

* **Why double lumen catheters are used** (Box 12-6).
  * Hemodialysis
  * Simultaneous ports for administration of medication and blood sampling
* **Correct placement of double lumen catheters for hemodialysis**
  * These **large-bore catheters** are **typically marked with a central stripe.**
  * There are many variations in design among different commercial brands, but all have at least two lumens arranged coaxially inside a single catheter with the goal to minimize the amount of recirculation that occurs between the two ports.
    * The **"arterial" port** from which blood is **withdrawn from the patient is proximal to the "venous" port** through which **blood is returned to the patient** to minimize recirculation of blood.
* The **right internal jugular route is most often used for access.**
* Those that are used temporarily (2–3 weeks) usually have their tips in the superior vena cava while the tips of the more permanent catheters may be in the right atrium.
* Some catheters are designed as two, separate single lumen catheters with one catheter tip in the superior vena cava and the other catheter tip in the right atrium (Fig. 12-11).
* **Incorrect placement and complications of double lumen catheters**
  * **Immediate complications** can include **pneumothorax** or **malposition or perforation of the tip.**
  * **Long-term complications** include **infection** and **thrombosis** of the vein containing the catheter or **occlusion** of the catheter itself.

PLEURAL DRAINAGE TUBES (CHEST TUBES, THORACOTOMY TUBES)

* **Why thoracotomy tubes are used**
  * To remove either air or abnormal collections of fluid from the pleural space
* **Correct placement of pleural drainage tubes** (Box 12-7)
  * Chest tubes are **wide-bore tubes with a radiopaque stripe** used as a marker.
    * **The stripe "breaks" at the site of the side hole.**
  * Ideal position is **anterosuperior for evacuating a pneumothorax** and **posteroinferior for draining an effusion** (Fig. 12-12).
    * Chest tubes usually work well no matter where positioned.
  * **None of the side holes should lie outside the thoracic wall** (Fig. 12-13).
    * An air leak can develop leading to persistence of the underlying condition and possible subcutaneous emphysema.
* **Incorrect placement and complications of pleural drainage tubes**
  * Most malpositions lead to **inadequate drainage** rather than serious complication.

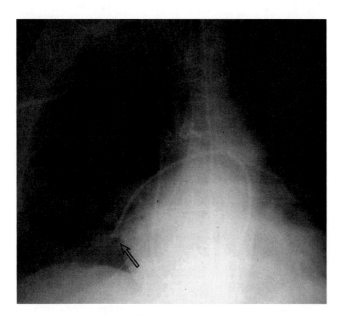

*Figure 12-10. **Swan-Ganz catheter with tip too peripheral.** The tip of a Swann-Ganz catheter should lie within 2 cm of the hilar shadow. The tip of this catheter (open black arrow) lies in a peripheral branch of the right descending pulmonary artery. This increases the risk of complication, such as pulmonary infarction.*

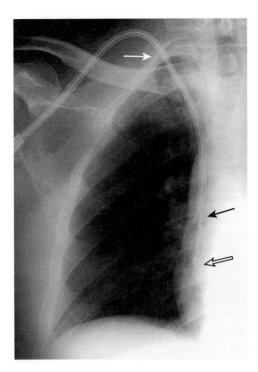

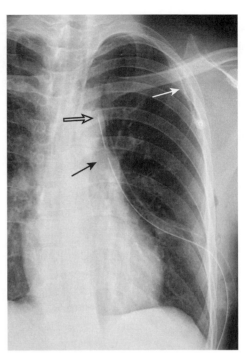

Figure 12-11. ***Double lumen catheter in correct position.*** *These large-bore catheters are typically marked with a central stripe (closed white arrow). All have at least two lumens arranged coaxially inside a single catheter with the tip for blood withdrawal (closed black arrow) farther from the heart than the tip for blood return (open black arrow) to the patient in order to minimize recirculation. The right internal jugular route is most often used for access. Some catheters, such as this one, are designed as two, separate single lumen catheters with one tip in the superior vena cava and the other in the right atrium.*

Figure 12-12. ***Chest tube in correct position.*** *Chest tubes are wide-bore tubes with a radiopaque stripe used as a marker (open black arrow). The stripe "breaks" at the site of the side hole (closed black arrow). Ideal position is anterosuperior, such as in this patient, for evacuating a pneumothorax and posteroinferior for draining an effusion. Chest tubes usually work well no matter where positioned. In this patient, there is a small pneumothorax still present as demonstrated by visualization of the visceral pleural line (closed white arrow).*

Box 12-7

Pleural Drainage Tubes (Chest Tubes)
For a pleural effusion, they work best with their tip placed posteriorly and inferiorly.
For a pneumothorax, they work best with their tip placed anteriorly and superiorly.
In general, chest tubes work well no matter where they are positioned but malpositioning can result in inadequate drainage.
Rapid drainage of a large pleural effusion or large pneumothorax can produce re-expansion pulmonary edema in the underlying lung.

- This includes malpositions in which the tube is inadvertently placed in the major fissure (Fig. 12-14).
- **If the side hole extends outside the chest wall,** this can lead to an ***air leak*** causing both inadequate drainage and subcutaneous emphysema.
- **Serious complications are uncommon:**
  - **Bleeding secondary to laceration of intercostal artery**

- **Laceration of liver or spleen on insertion**
- **Rapid re-expansion of a collapsed lung** caused either by a large pneumothorax or a large pleural effusion may lead to unilateral, ***re-expansion pulmonary edema*** (see Fig. 11-9).

Cardiac Devices: Pacemakers, AICD, IABP

PACEMAKERS
- **Why they are used**
  - Cardiac conduction abnormalities
  - Certain conditions refractory to medical treatment (e.g., congestive heart failure)
- **Correct placement of cardiac pacemakers** (Box 12-8)
  - All **pacemakers consist of a pulse generator** usually implanted subcutaneously in the left anterior chest wall **and at least one lead (electrode)** inserted percutaneously most often into the subclavian vein.
    - The **tip of one lead is almost always located in the apex of the right ventricle.**
      - Remember that **in the frontal projection, the apex of the right ventricle lies to the left of the spine** and **on the lateral film the apex of the right ventricle is anterior** (Fig. 12-15).
  - Some pacemakers have two leads (usually their tips are in the right atrium and right ventricle) while others may have three leads (with their tips usually in the right atrium, right ventricle and coronary sinus).

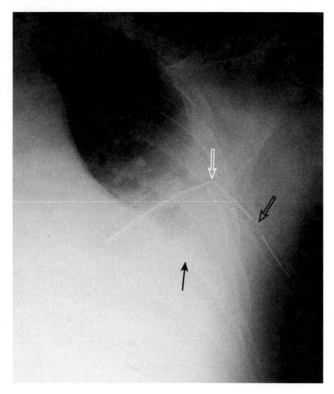

Figure 12-13. ***Side hole of chest tube extends outside thorax.***
*Chest tubes typically have one or more side holes marked by a
discontinuity in the marker stripe. None of the side holes should lie
outside the thoracic wall as it does (open black arrow) in this patient.
An air leak can develop leading to persistence of the pleural effusion
(closed black arrow). The tube is also kinked as it enters the chest
(open white arrow), which may further reduce its efficiency.*

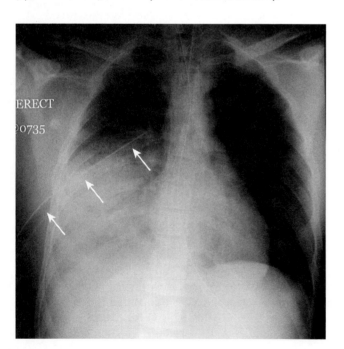

Figure 12-14. ***Chest tube in fissure.*** *Suspect insertion of a chest
tube into one of the interlobar fissures (closed white arrows) when the
tip is directed toward the hilum, as in this case, where the tube lies
within the major fissure. Malpositions like this can lead to inadequate
drainage rather than serious complication.*

Box 12-8

Pacemakers

Pacemakers are usually placed in the left anterior chest wall; at least one lead should be in right ventricular apex.

Remember that the right ventricle projects to the left of the spine on the frontal view and anteriorly on the lateral view of the chest.

Complications are infrequent but include fractures in the lead wires and pneumothorax.

Ectopically placed leads may result in pacemaker failure.

- **All leads should have gentle curves.**
  - **There should be no sharp kinks in the electrodes.**
- **Incorrect placement and complications of cardiac pacemakers**
  - **Pneumothoraces** are infrequent complications of either pacemaker or AICD insertion.
  - **Fracture of the leads** may occur at any of three places: the pacer itself, the tip of the lead, or the site of venous access.
    - Breaks in the lead can be **recognized by discontinuity in the wire lead itself** (Fig. 12-16).
  - **Leads can perforate the heart** producing cardiac tamponade.
    - **Look for sharp bends in leads** secondary to perforation of a blood vessel.
  - **Leads may retract from normal contact with the ventricular wall** because the patient twists or twiddles the pacemaker generator under the skin, unknowingly winding the leads around the pacer causing retraction of the tips *(Twiddler's syndrome)* (Fig. 12-17) or from subcutaneous migration of the pacer.
  - **Leads may be ectopically placed, e.g., in the hepatic vein.**

AUTOMATIC IMPLANTABLE CARDIAC DEFIBRILLATORS (AICDs)
- **Why they are used**
  - To prevent sudden death, usually from tachyarrhythmias like ventricular fibrillation or ventricular tachycardia
- **Correct placement of automatic implantable cardiac defibrillators** (Box 12-9)
  - AICDs can usually **be differentiated from pacemakers by the wider and more opaque segment of at least one of the electrodes** (Fig. 12-18).
    - One electrode is usually placed in the superior vena cava or brachiocephalic vein.
    - If present, the other electrode tip is placed in the apex of the right ventricle.
  - **All bends in the leads should be smooth curves, not sharp kinks.**
- **Incorrect placement and complications of automatic implantable cardiac defibrillators**
  - Leads may migrate and become dislodged.
  - Leads may fracture.

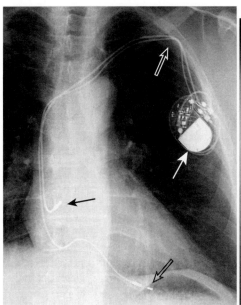

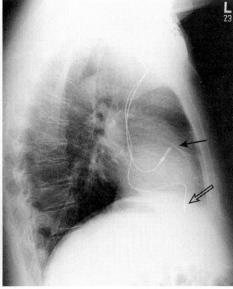

A   B

Figure 12-15. **Dual-lead pacemaker in correct position.** Pacemakers consist of a pulse generator (closed white arrow) usually implanted in the left chest wall and one or more electrode leads usually inserted into the subclavian vein (open white arrow). This patient has a dual-lead pacemaker. One of the leads is in the apex of the right ventricle (open black arrows) while the other lead is in the right atrium (closed black arrows). Notice that the right ventricular lead (open black arrows) projects to the left of the midline **(A)** and anteriorly **(B)**, and the right atrial lead typically curls upward **(A).**

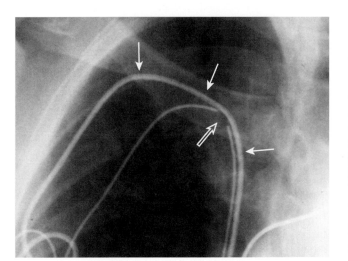

Figure 12-16. **Fractured pacemaker lead.** Fractures of pacemaker or automatic implantable cardiac defibrillator (AICD) leads may occur at any of three places: the generator itself, the tip of the lead, or the site of venous access. Breaks in the lead can be recognized by discontinuity in the wire lead itself (open white arrow) which, in this patient, occurred at the site of venous access to the subclavian vein. The broken lead had been discovered earlier and a second, intact lead is already in place (closed white arrows).

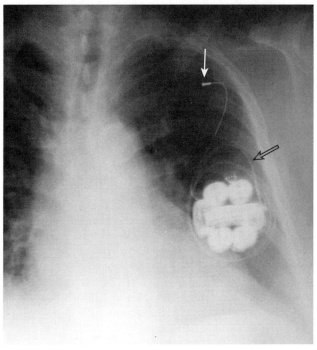

Figure 12-17. **Twiddler's syndrome.** Some patients inadvertently "twiddle" with their subcutaneous pulse generator and, if the subcutaneous tissue allows, may rotate the generator many times on its own axis, curling the lead(s) around the device (open black arrow). This can retract the tip of the electrode from the inner wall of the right ventricle, rendering the pacemaker useless. This lead has retracted to the left subclavian vein (closed white arrow).

INTRA-AORTIC COUNTERPULSATION BALLOON PUMP (IACB OR IABP)

- **Why they are used**
  - To improve cardiac output and improve perfusion of the coronary arteries following surgery or in patients with cardiogenic shock or refractory ventricular failure.
    - Placed in descending thoracic aorta, **the balloon is inflated in diastole and deflated in systole.**

- **Correct placement of intra-aortic balloon pumps** (Box 12-10)
  - **Tip can be identified by small, linear metallic marker.**

Box 12-9

Automatic Implantable Cardiac Defibrillator

AICDs can be differentiated from pacemakers by the presence of a thicker electrode on at least one lead.

AICDs may have one (right ventricular), two (right atrium and right ventricle), or three leads (right atrium, right ventricle, and coronary sinus).

Bends in the leads should be smooth curves, not sharp kinks.

Visible complications can include lead breakage and dislodgement.

Box 12-10

Intra-aortic Balloon Pumps

The tip has a metallic marker which should lie distal to origin of left subclavian artery.

When inflated, the balloon will be visible as an air-containing "sausage" in thoracic aorta.

Catheters placed too proximally may occlude the great vessels.

Catheters placed too distally may be ineffective.

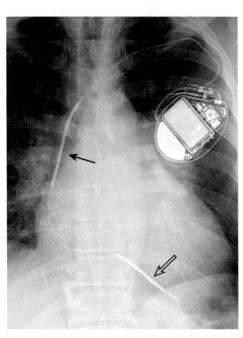

Figure 12-18. ***Automatic implantable cardiac defibrillator (AICD).*** *AICDs can usually can be differentiated from pacemakers by the wider and more opaque segment of at least one of the electrodes (open and closed black arrows). One electrode is usually placed in the superior vena cava (closed black arrow) or brachiocephalic vein and the other electrode tip is placed in the apex of the right ventricle (open black arrow). All bends in the leads should be smooth curves, not sharp kinks.*

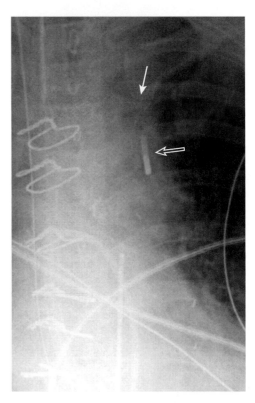

Figure 12-19. ***Intra-aortic counterpulsation balloon pump (IABP).*** *The tip of this assistive device can be identified by a small, linear metallic marker in the region of the descending thoracic aorta (open white arrow). The tip should lie distal to origin of the left subclavian artery so as not to occlude it. In this case, the tip is about 2 cm from the top of the aortic knob (closed white arrow), which is satisfactory. The metallic marker may point slightly toward the right in the region of the arch.*

- **The tip should lie distal to origin of the left subclavian artery** so as not to occlude it.
- Metallic **marker may point slightly toward the right** in region of aortic arch (Fig. 12-19).
- When inflated, the sausage-shaped balloon may be visualized as an air-containing structure in the descending thoracic aorta.
- **Incorrect placement and complications of intra-aortic balloon pumps**
  - If catheter is **too proximal, balloon may occlude great vessels** leading to stroke.
  - If balloon is **too distal, device has decreased effectiveness.**

- Aortic dissection and arterial perforation may occur infrequently.

Gastrointestinal Tubes and Lines: Nasogastric Tubes, Feeding Tubes

NASOGASTRIC TUBES (NGTs)
- **Why they are used**
  - Short-term feeding
  - Gastric sampling and decompression through suction
  - Administering medication

- **Correct placement of nasogastric tubes** (Box 12-11)
  - Nasogastric tubes are **wide tubes** (about 1 cm) marked **with a radiopaque stripe** that "breaks" at the **side hole,** usually about **10 cm from the tip.**
  - **Tip and all side holes** of the tube should **extend about 10 cm into the stomach beyond the esophagogastric (EG) junction** to prevent aspiration from administration of the feeding into esophagus.
  - **How to recognize the location of the EG junction**
    - The **EG junction** is usually **located at the junction of the left hemidiaphragm and the left side of the thoracic spine** (this is called the *left cardiophrenic angle*) (Fig. 12-20).

Box 12-11

Nasogastric Tube (Levin Tube)
The tip of a nasogastric tube should extend into the stomach about 10 cm past the EG junction.
NG tubes are the most commonly malpositioned of all tubes; always check with an x-ray to confirm location.
When malpositioned, NG tubes most frequently coil in the esophagus.
If inserted in the trachea, NG tubes can extend into a bronchus and to the periphery of lung.

- **Incorrect placement and complications of nasogastric tubes**
  - **Most commonly malpositioned of all tubes and lines**
    - **Coiling of the NG tube in the esophagus is the most common malposition.**
    - A tube **may be inadvertently inserted into the trachea** and enter a bronchus (Fig. 12-21).
    - **Perforation caused by an NG tube is rare,** but when it occurs, it usually occurs in the cervical esophagus.
    - **Long-term indwelling NG tube can lead to gastroesophageal reflux.**
      - May cause **esophagitis and stricture**
  - Always obtain a confirmatory radiograph before feeding the patient or administering any medication through the tube.

FEEDING TUBES (DOBBHOFF TUBES, DHT)

- **Why they are used**
  - To provide nutrition
- **Correct placement of feeding tubes** (Box 12-12)
  - **Tip of feeding tube should be in duodenum** so as to reduce risk of aspiration after feeding (Fig. 12-22).
    - The tip is recognizable by a weighted, metallic end.

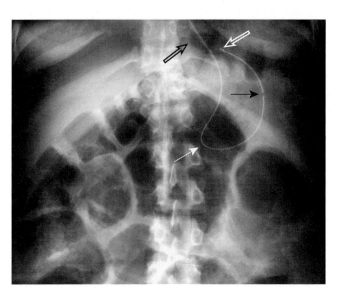

*Figure 12-20. **Nasogastric tube in stomach.** Nasogastric tubes are wide-bore tubes marked with a radiopaque stripe that "breaks" in the position of the side hole, usually about 10 cm from the tip (closed black arrow). The tip and all side holes of the tube should extend about 10 cm into the stomach beyond the esophagogastric (EG) junction to prevent aspiration from administration of the feeding into esophagus. This tube is coiled back upon itself (closed white arrow) and the tip (open white arrow) is too close to the EG junction (open black arrow). The EG junction is usually located at the junction of the left hemidiaphragm and the left side of the thoracic spine (the **left cardiophrenic angle**).*

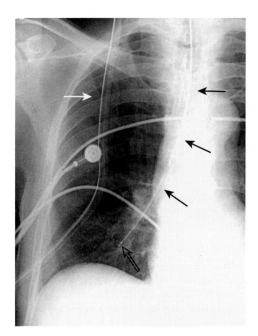

*Figure 12-21. **Nasogastric tube in right lower lobe bronchus.** Nasogastric tubes are the most commonly malpositioned of all tubes and lines. Coiling of the NG tube in the esophagus is the most common malposition. In this patient, the nasogastric tube (closed black arrows) entered the trachea instead of the esophagus and its tip extends to the right lower lobe (open black arrow). It is important to obtain a radiograph to confirm positioning of a nasogastric tube before using it for feeding. A portion of the NG tube that lies outside the patient is superimposed on the chest (closed white arrow), as are several heart monitor leads.*

Box 12-12

Feeding Tubes (Dobbhoff Tubes)

The tip should ideally be in the duodenum, although most lie in the stomach.

The tip is recognizable by a metallic marker.

If inadvertently inserted into the trachea, the tip may extend into the lung.

Always obtain a confirmatory radiograph before using the tube for feedings.

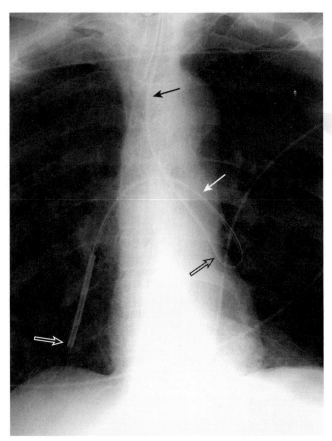

Figure 12-23. **Dobbhoff tube in left and right lower lobe bronchi.** *In this case, the Dobbhoff tube inadvertently entered the trachea* (closed black arrow), *entered the left lower lobe bronchus* (open black arrow), *then coiled back on itself* (closed white arrow) *to cross the midline and end in the right lower lobe bronchus* (open white arrow). *It is important to obtain a confirmatory radiograph prior to using the tube for feedings.*

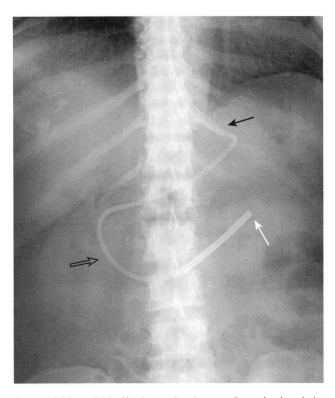

Figure 12-22. **Dobbhoff tube in duodenum.** *Correctly placed, the tip of a Dobbhoff feeding tube should be in the duodenum so as to reduce risk of aspiration after feeding. The tip is recognizable by a weighted, metallic end* (closed white arrow). *This Dobbhoff tube enters the stomach* (closed black arrow), *courses around the duodenal sweep* (open black arrow), *and ends at the junction between the fourth portion of the duodenum and the jejunum. Placement in the stomach rather than the duodenum is very common.*

- **Incorrect placement and complications of feeding tubes.**
  - **Placement in the stomach** rather than the duodenum **is very common.**
  - **Placement in the trachea** rather than the esophagus may lead to tip entering the lung.
    - Always obtain a confirmatory radiograph before feeding the patient (Fig. 12-23).
  - **Perforation of the esophagus by the guidewire** is an uncommon complication.
    - Once the guidewire is removed, it is not reinserted.
- Weblink: More information on the correct placement of tubes and lines is available to registered users on StudentConsult.com.

TAKE-HOME POINTS: Recognizing the Correct Location of Lines and Tubes

Line or Tube	Desired Position
ETT	Tip 3–5 cm from carina
Tracheostomy tube tip	Halfway between stoma and carina
Central venous catheter	Tip in SVC
PICC Line	Tip in SVC
Swan-Ganz catheter	Tip in proximal R or L pulmonary artery
Hemodialysis (Quinton) catheters	Tips in either SVC or right atrium (or both) depending on type of catheter
Pleural drainage tube	Anterosuperior for pneumothorax; posteroinferior for effusion
Pacemaker	Tip at apex of R ventricle; other leads in RA or coronary sinus
AICD	One lead in SVC or RA; other leads in R ventricle or coronary sinus
Nasogastric (Levin) tube	Tip in stomach 10 cm from EG junction
Feeding (Dobbhoff) tube	Tip in the duodenum

13 Recognizing Mediastinal and Lung Masses and Metastases

- In this chapter, you'll learn how to recognize mediastinal masses and lung neoplasms, both benign and malignant, and determine whether they are primary or metastatic to the lung.
- We'll begin with mediastinal masses and work our way outward to the lungs.

Mediastinal Masses

- The mediastinum is an area whose **lateral margins are defined by the medial borders of each lung,** whose **anterior margin** is the **sternum and anterior chest wall** and whose **posterior margin is the spine,** usually including the paravertebral gutters.

- The mediastinum can be arbitrarily subdivided into three compartments—the ***anterior, middle, and posterior*** compartments—and each contains its favorite set of diseases (Fig. 13-1).
  - The ***superior mediastinum,*** roughly the area above the plane of the aortic arch, is a division that is now usually combined with one of the other three compartments.
- **Pitfall:** Because these compartments have no true anatomic boundaries, **diseases from one compartment may extend into another compartment.**
  - When a mediastinal abnormality becomes extensive or a mediastinal mass becomes quite large, it is frequently

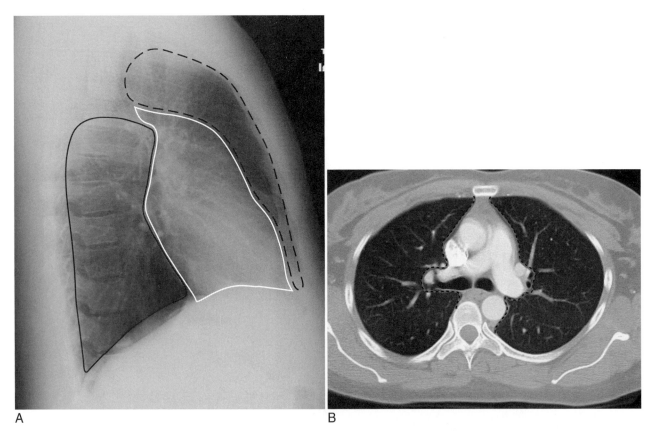

A   B

Figure 13-1. **The mediastinum can be arbitrarily subdivided into three compartments: anterior, middle, and posterior, with each containing its favorite set of diseases. A,** *The anterior mediastinum is the compartment that extends from the back of the sternum to the anterior border of the heart and great vessels (broken black outline). The middle mediastinum is the compartment that extends from the anterior border of the heart and aorta to the posterior border of the heart and the origins of the great vessels (white outline). The posterior mediastinum is the compartment that extends from the posterior border of the heart to the anterior border of the vertebral column (solid black outline). For practical purposes, however, it is considered to extend into the paravertebral gutters.* **B,** *An axial CT scan shows the mediastinal structures contained within the broken black outline.*

impossible to determine which compartment was its site of origin.

- **Differentiating a mediastinal from a parenchymal lung mass on frontal and lateral chest radiographs**
  - **Mediastinal masses will originate in the mediastinum** (makes sense, doesn't it?), although large masses may be difficult to place.
  - If a **mass is surrounded by lung tissue in both the frontal and lateral projections, it lies within the lung;** if a **mass is surrounded by lung tissue in one but not both projections, it may be in either the lung or the mediastinum.**
    - Unfortunately, masses may not be surrounded by lung tissue in either projection and still originate within the lung.
  - In general (and this is a generalization), **the margin of a mediastinal mass** is **sharper** than that for a mass originating in the lung.
  - Mediastinal masses frequently **displace, compress, or obstruct** other mediastinal structures.

Anterior Mediastinum

- The **anterior mediastinum** is the compartment that extends from the **back of the sternum** to the **anterior border of the heart and great vessels.**
- **Differential diagnosis for anterior mediastinal masses:**
  - Substernal **thyroid masses**
  - **Lymphoma**
  - **Thymoma**
  - **Teratoma**
    - Lymphoma is sometimes called "terrible lymphoma" so that all the diseases in this list start with the letter "T" (Table 13-1).

THYROID MASSES

- On occasion, the isthmus or lower pole of either lobe of the thyroid may enlarge but project downward into the upper thorax rather than anteriorly into the neck.

- About 75% of thyroid masses extend in front of the trachea; the remaining 25% descend posterior to the trachea (almost all of which are right-sided).
- In **everyday practice, enlarged substernal thyroid masses** are the **most frequently encountered anterior mediastinal mass.**
- The vast majority of these masses are **multinodular goiters** and the mass is called a *substernal goiter* or *substernal thyroid* or *substernal thyroid goiter.*
- Classically, **substernal goiters do not extend below the top of the aortic arch.**
- **Substernal goiters** are anterior mediastinal masses that **characteristically displace the trachea** either to the left or right **above the level of the aortic arch,** a tendency the other anterior mediastinal masses do not typically demonstrate (Fig. 13-2).
  - Therefore, you should **think of an enlarged substernal thyroid goiter** whenever you see **an anterior mediastinal mass that displaces the trachea.**
- Radioisotope **thyroid scans are the study of first choice** in confirming the diagnosis of a substernal thyroid as virtually

Table 13-1

ANTERIOR MEDIASTINAL MASSES ("3 T'S AND AN L")

Mass	What to Look for
Thyroid goiter	The only anterior mediastinal mass that routinely deviates the trachea
Lymphoma (lymphadenopathy)	Lobulated, polycyclic mass, frequently asymmetrical, that may occur in any compartment of the mediastinum
Thymoma	Look for a well-marginated mass that may be associated with myasthenia gravis
Teratoma	Well-marginated masses that may contain fat and calcium on CT scans

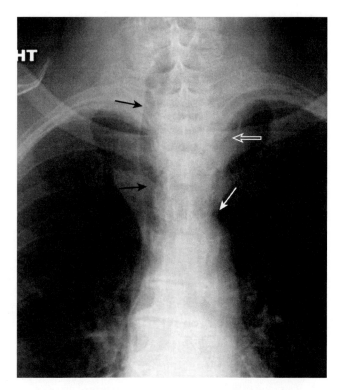

*Figure 13-2. **Substernal thyroid mass.** Sometimes, the lower pole of the thyroid may enlarge but project downward into the upper thorax (open white arrow) rather than anteriorly into the neck. Classically, substernal thyroid goiters produce mediastinal masses that do not extend below the top of the aortic arch (closed white arrow). Substernal goiters characteristically displace the trachea (closed black arrows) either to the left or right above the aortic knob, a tendency the other anterior mediastinal masses do not typically demonstrate. Therefore, you should think of an enlarged substernal thyroid goiter whenever you see an anterior mediastinal mass that displaces the trachea.*

all thyroid goiters will display some uptake of the radioactive tracer which can then be imaged and recorded with a special camera.

- **On CT scans,** substernal thyroid masses are **contiguous with the thyroid gland, frequently contain calcification,** and **avidly take up intravenous contrast material but with a mottled, inhomogeneous appearance** (Fig. 13-3).

LYMPHOMA

- Lymphadenopathy, whether from lymphoma, metastatic carcinoma, sarcoid, or tuberculosis, is the most common cause of a mediastinal mass overall.
- **Anterior mediastinal lymphadenopathy is most common in Hodgkin's disease, especially the nodular sclerosing variety.**
- Unlike teratomas and thymomas, which are presumed to arise from a single abnormal cell from which they uniformly expand outward, lymphomatous masses are frequently composed of several contiguously enlarged lymph nodes.
- As such, **lymphadenopathy frequently presents with a border that is lobulated or polycyclic in contour** owing to the conglomeration of enlarged nodes.
  - This finding **may help differentiate lymphadenopathy from other mediastinal masses.**
  - *Mediastinal lymphadenopathy* in Hodgkin's disease is usually **bilateral and asymmetrical** (Fig. 13-4).
  - **Asymmetrical hilar adenopathy** is associated with mediastinal adenopathy in many patients with Hodgkin's disease.
- **On CT scans,** lymphomas will **produce multiple, lobulated soft tissue masses** or a **large, soft tissue mass** from lymph node aggregation.
  - The **mass is usually homogeneous** in density but **may be heterogeneous** when it achieves a sufficient size to

undergo **necrosis (areas of lower attenuation, i.e., blacker)** or **hemorrhage (areas of higher attenuation, i.e., whiter)** (Fig. 13-5).

- In general, **mediastinal lymph nodes that exceed 1 cm** measured along their **short axis** on CT scans of the chest are **considered to be enlarged.**
- Some findings of lymphoma may mimic those of sarcoid because both produce thoracic adenopathy. The accompanying chart helps to differentiate the two (Table 13-2).

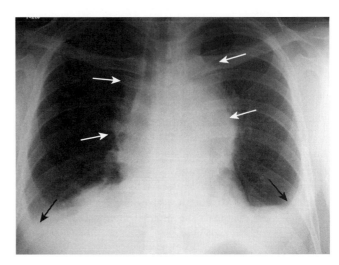

Figure 13-4. **Mediastinal adenopathy from Hodgkin's disease.** *Lymphadenopathy frequently presents with a lobulated or polycyclic border owing to the conglomeration of enlarged nodes that produce the mass (closed white arrows). This finding may help differentiate lymphadenopathy from other masses. Mediastinal lymphadenopathy in Hodgkin's disease is usually bilateral and asymmetrical, as in this case. Pleural effusions (closed black arrows) are common, occurring in up to 33% of patients with the disease.*

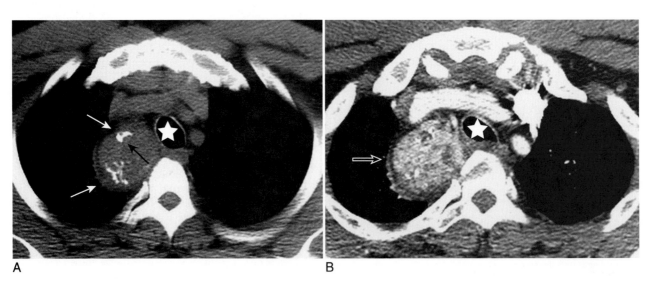

A
B

Figure 13-3. **CT of a substernal thyroid goiter without and with contrast enhancement.** *These two images were taken at the same level in a patient who was scanned both before **(A)** and then after intravenous contrast administration **(B).** On CT scans, substernal thyroid masses (closed white arrows in **A**) are contiguous with the thyroid gland, frequently contain calcification (closed black arrow) and avidly take up intravenous contrast but with a mottled, inhomogeneous appearance (open white arrow in **B**). This mass is displacing the trachea (white stars) slightly to the left.*

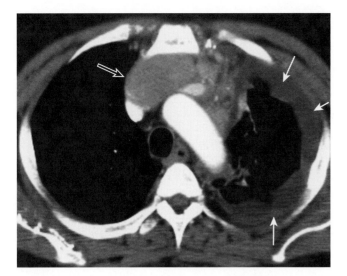

Figure 13-5. **CT of anterior mediastinal adenopathy in Hodgkin's disease.** On CT, lymphomas will produce multiple, lobulated soft tissue masses or a large soft tissue mass from lymph node aggregation (open white arrow). The mass is usually homogeneous in density, as in this case, but may be heterogeneous when the nodes achieve a sufficient size to undergo necrosis (areas of low attenuation, i.e., blacker) or hemorrhage (areas of high attenuation, i.e., whiter). There is a malignant pleural effusion present in this patient (closed white arrows) as evidenced by the nodular and irregular appearance of the pleural disease.

THYMIC MASSES

- **Normal thymic tissue can be visible on CT throughout life,** although the gland begins to **involute after age 20.**

Table 13-2

SARCOIDOSIS VS. LYMPHOMA

Feature	Sarcoid	Lymphoma
Adenopathy	Bilateral hilar and right paratracheal adenopathy classic combination; anterior mediastinal adenopathy is uncommon	More often mediastinal adenopathy, associated with asymmetrical hilar enlargement; anterior mediastinal adenopathy is common
Nodes	Bronchopulmonary nodes more peripheral	Hilar nodes more central
Pleural effusion	Pleural effusion in about 5%	Pleural effusion much more common in 30%

- **Thymomas** are **neoplasms of thymic epithelium and lymphocytes.**
- They occur most often in **middle-aged adults,** generally at an **older** age than those with **teratomas** (Fig. 13-6).
  - Most thymomas are benign.
- Thymomas are **associated with myasthenia gravis about 35% of the time.**
  - About **15% of patients with** clinical **myasthenia gravis will** be found to **have a thymoma.**
  - The importance of identifying a thymoma in patients with myasthenia gravis lies in the **favorable prognosis** for patients with myasthenia **after thymectomy.**
- On **CT scans, thymomas** classically present as a **smooth or lobulated mass** that arises near the **junction of the heart**

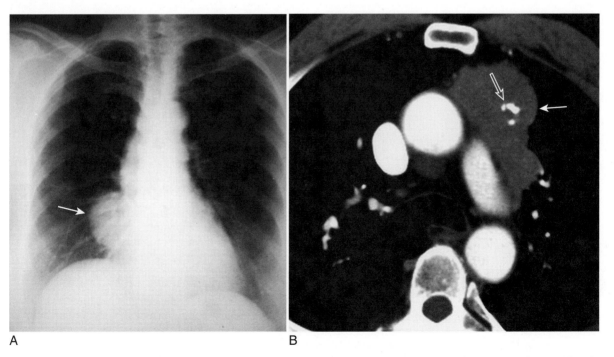

A   B

Figure 13-6. **Thymomas, conventional radiograph (A) and CT scan (B).** Thymomas are neoplasms of thymic epithelium and lymphocytes that occur most often in middle-aged adults, generally at an older age than those with teratomas. The patient in **A** has a smoothly contoured anterior mediastinal mass seen on the frontal view (closed white arrow). This patient had myasthenia gravis and improved following resection of the thymoma. Another patient with a thymoma **(B)** has an anterior mediastinal mass (closed white arrow) that contains some amorphous calcification (open white arrow).

and great vessels and which **may contain calcification,** just as a teratoma would.

- Other lesions that can produce enlargement of the thymus include thymic cysts, thymic hyperplasia, thymic lymphoma, carcinoma, and lipoma.

TERATOMA

- Teratomas are **germinal tumors** that typically **contain all three germ layers** (ectoderm, mesoderm, and endoderm).
- The most common variety of teratoma is **cystic;** it produces a **well-marginated mass** near the origin of the great vessels and **characteristically contains fat, cartilage, and possibly bone on CT** (Fig. 13-7).
- Most teratomas are benign.

Middle Mediastinal Masses

- The **middle mediastinum** is the compartment that extends from the **anterior border of the heart and aorta** to the **posterior border of the heart and contains the origins of the great vessels.**
  - It contains the **heart and proximal great vessels, trachea** and **main bronchi,** and **lymph nodes** (see Fig. 13-1A).
- **Lymphadenopathy produces the most common mass in this compartment.**
  - Although lymphoma is the most likely cause of mediastinal adenopathy, other malignancies and several benign diseases can produce such findings.
  - Other malignancies that produce mediastinal lymphadenopathy include **small cell lung carcinoma** and **metastatic disease** from a primary tumor such as **breast carcinoma** (Fig. 13-8).

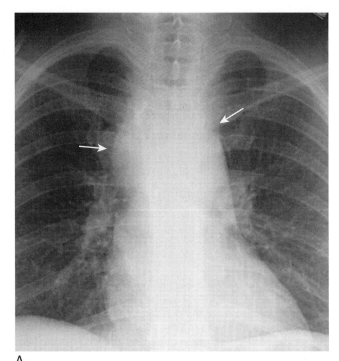

A

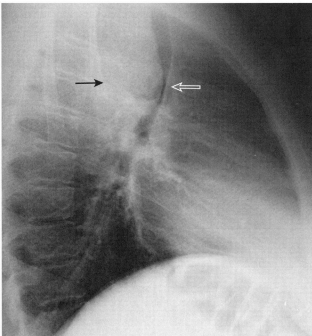

B

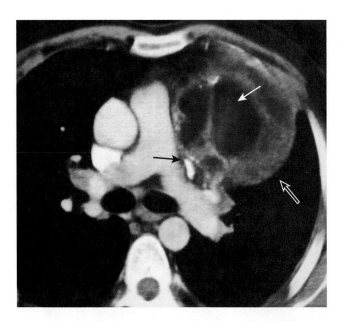

Figure 13-7. ***Mediastinal teratoma.*** *Teratomas are germinal tumors that typically contain all three germ layers. They tend to be discovered at a younger age than thymomas. The most common variety of teratoma is cystic (closed white arrow), as in this case. As shown here, they usually produce a well-marginated mass (open white arrow) near the origin of the great vessels. They characteristically contain fat, cartilage, and sometimes bone (closed black arrow) on CT.*

Figure 13-8. ***Middle mediastinal lymphadenopathy.*** *Although lymphoma is the most likely cause of mediastinal adenopathy in the middle mediastinal compartment, other malignancies, such as small cell lung carcinoma and metastatic disease from tumors such as breast carcinoma, as well as several benign diseases can produce these findings. This patient has a mediastinal mass demonstrated on both the frontal (**A**) (closed white arrows) and lateral (**B**) views (closed black arrow). The mass is pushing the trachea forward (open white arrow) on the lateral view. The biopsied lymph nodes in this patient demonstrated small cell carcinoma of the lung.*

- Benign causes of mediastinal lymphadenopathy include **infectious mononucleosis** and **tuberculosis, the latter usually producing unilateral mediastinal adenopathy.**

Aortic Aneurysms

- Aneurysms are **defined as enlargement of a vessel greater than 50% of its original size.**
- **Atherosclerosis is the most common cause** of a descending thoracic aortic aneurysm.
  - **Most patients are also hypertensive.**
- Most patients are **asymptomatic** and the **aneurysm is discovered serendipitously.**
  - When the **aneurysm expands**, it **may cause** pain which classically, but not always, **radiates to the back** (from a **descending aortic aneurysm).**
  - The **normal appearance of the thoracic aorta** is discussed in Chapter 10 and summarized in Table 13-3.

AORTIC ANEURYSMS—GENERAL CONSIDERATIONS

- As measured on CT or MRI scans, the **ascending aorta is usually < 3.5 cm** and the **descending aorta is < 3 cm.**
- An **aneurysm** of the thoracic aorta is usually defined as a **persistent enlargement of > 4 cm.**
- In general, **aneurysms of 5 to 6 cm are at risk to rupture** and will require surgical intervention.
- The **rate of growth** of an aneurysm is also important in determining the need for surgical intervention and repair.
  - Annual aneurysm growth rates should be < 1 cm/year or elective resection is considered.

RECOGNIZING A THORACIC AORTIC ANEURYSM

- The **appearance** of a thoracic aortic aneurysm **will depend, in part, from which portion of the thoracic aorta it arises.**
  - Aneurysms of the **ascending aorta** may extend **anteriorly and to the right.**
  - Aneurysms of the **aortic arch** produce a **middle mediastinal mass.**
  - Aneurysms of the **descending aorta** project **posteriorly, laterally,** and to the **left** (Fig. 13-9).

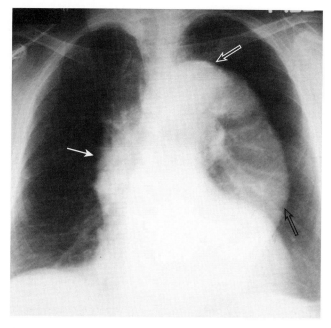

Figure 13-9. Aortic aneurysm. *The entire thoracic aorta is enlarged in this 67-year-old man. The ascending aorta (closed white arrow) should normally not project farther to the right than the right heart border on a nonrotated chest radiograph. The aortic knob (open white arrow) should be <35 mm in diameter measured from the air in the trachea to the lateral border of the knob on a frontal chest radiograph. The descending thoracic aorta (open black arrow) normally parallels and almost disappears with the thoracic spine; as it becomes larger, it swings farther away from the spine. Calcification in the wall of an aneurysm (open white arrow) is common.*

- **Calcification** in the wall of an aneurysm is **common,** but calcification in the wall of the aorta is common in atherosclerosis in general.
- **Contrast-enhanced CT** is the modality **most often used** to diagnose a thoracic aortic aneurysm because it is **accurate, relatively inexpensive,** and **readily available;** MRI is also excellent at demonstrating aneurysms but is less available and more expensive (Fig. 13-10).
- On **CT,** aneurysms can appear as **fusiform (long)** or **saccular (globular)** in shape.
- Their anatomy will be **more readily delineated on contrast-enhanced studies** using iodinated contrast material injected intravenously as a bolus, but may be visible on noncontrast studies as well.
- Frequently **calcification is seen in the intima,** which may be **separated** from the **contrast-filled lumen** by **varying amounts of clot.**

AORTIC DISSECTION

- **Aortic dissections most often originate in the ascending aorta (Stanford type A)** or may involve only the **descending aorta (Stanford type B).**
  - They **result from a tear** that **allows blood to dissect in the wall, usually along the media** for varying lengths of the aorta.
    - They are associated with tears in the **intima.**

Table 13-3

Portion	Appearance on Conventional Radiographs	CT/MRI Findings
NORMAL THORACIC AORTA		
Ascending aorta	Should not project farther to the right than the right heart border on a nonrotated chest radiograph	< 3.5 cm normally; > 4 cm considered an aneurysm; 5–6 cm at risk for rupture
Aortic knob	Should be less than 35 mm in diameter measured from the air in the trachea to the lateral border of the knob on a frontal chest radiograph	< 3 cm normally; > 4 cm considered an aneurysm; 5–6 cm at risk for rupture
Descending thoracic aorta	Normally parallels and almost disappears with the thoracic spine; as it becomes larger, it swings further away from the spine	< 3 cm normally; > 4 cm considered an aneurysm; 5–6 cm at risk for rupture

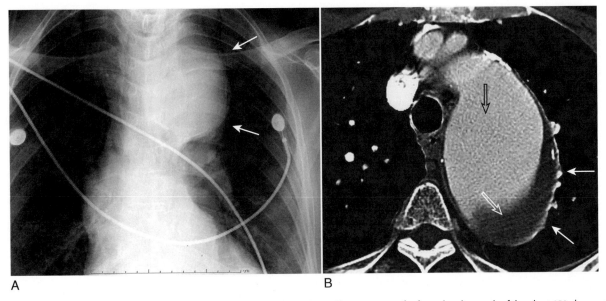

A   B

Figure 13-10. ***Aortic aneurysm, conventional chest radiograph and CT.*** *Close-up view of a frontal radiograph of the chest* **(A)** *demonstrates a large mediastinal soft tissue mass with a calcified rim (closed white arrows). This soft tissue density represents a large aneurysm of the proximal descending aorta seen also in the CT scan to the right* **(B).** *The aneurysm measured 6.7 cm, which placed it at significant risk for rupture. Calcification in the wall of an aneurysm is common (closed white arrows). Contrast material mixes with blood flowing in the lumen of the aorta (open black arrow), but the flowing blood is separated from the intimal calcification (closed white arrows) by a considerable amount of non-contrast-containing thrombus adherent to the wall (open white arrow).*

- In general, **patients with aortic dissection have been hypertensive** and may have an **underlying condition that can predispose to dissection,** such as cystic medial degeneration, atherosclerosis, Marfan syndrome, Ehlers-Danlos syndrome, trauma, syphilis, or crack cocaine abuse.
- In many patients, **abrupt onset** of **ripping or tearing chest pain,** which is **maximal at its time of origin,** is the characteristic history.
- **Conventional radiographs** are **not significantly sensitive to be diagnostically reliable,** but they **may point to the diagnosis** when several imaging findings occur together, especially in the proper clinical setting.
  - "Widening of the mediastinum" is a **poor means of establishing the diagnosis** because (a) it is commonly overinterpreted on portable supine radiographs, while on the other hand, (b) it occurs in only about 1 in 4 cases of aortic dissection.
  - **Left pleural effusion** (which **frequently represents a transudate** caused by pleural irritation, although transient hemorrhage from the aorta can also produce a hemothorax) (Fig. 13-11)
  - **Left apical pleural cap** of fluid or blood
  - **Loss of the normal shadow of the aortic knob**
  - **Deviation of the trachea or esophagus to the right**
- **MRI is probably more sensitive** than CT at detecting a dissection, but **CT is usually more readily available.**
  - Transesophageal ultrasound is also used to establish the diagnosis.

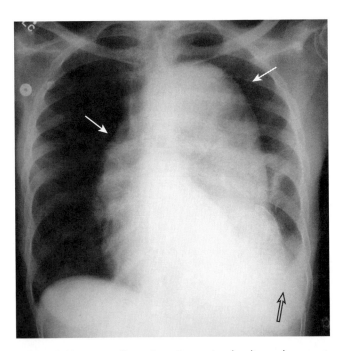

Figure 13-11. ***Aortic dissection.*** *Conventional radiographs are not sensitive enough to be diagnostically reliable for aortic dissection, but they may point to the diagnosis when several imaging findings occur together, especially in the proper clinical setting. "Widening of the mediastinum" is frequently not present and is a poor means of establishing the diagnosis, although in this patient the mediastinum is clearly widened by an enlarged aorta (closed white arrows). Also, a left pleural effusion is present (open black arrow). The combination of a widened mediastinum and a left pleural effusion in a patient with chest pain should alert you to the possibility of an aortic dissection.*

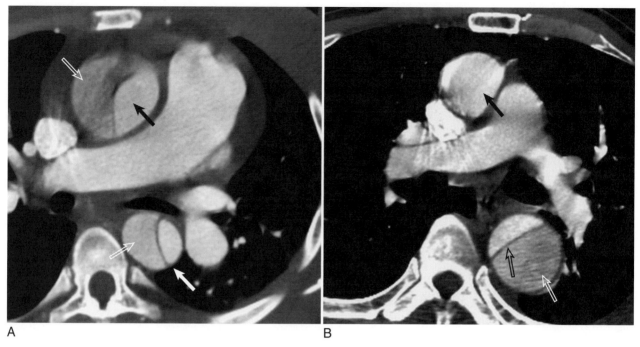

Figure 13-12. **Aortic dissections, types A and B. A,** *An intimal flap is seen to traverse both the ascending* (closed black arrow) *and descending aorta* (closed white arrow). *This is a type A dissection.* **B,** *There is a normal appearing ascending aorta* (closed black arrow) *while there is an intimal flap noted by the black line traversing the descending aorta* (open black arrow). *The intimal flap is the characteristic lesion of an aortic dissection. The smaller lumen is usually the true (original) lumen and the larger, false lumen* (open white arrows) *is actually a channel that has been produced by blood dissecting through the media.*

- On both **MRI and CT,** the **diagnosis rests on identification** of the **intimal flap** that separates the **true (original)** from the **false lumen** (canal created by the dissection) (Fig. 13-12).
- In general, **type A (ascending aortic) dissections are treated surgically** whereas **type B (descending aortic dissections) are treated medically.**

Posterior Mediastinal Masses

- The **posterior mediastinum** is the compartment that extends from the **posterior border of the heart** to the **anterior border of the vertebral column** (see Fig. 13-1A).
  - For practical purposes, however, it is **considered to extend into the paravertebral gutters.**
- It contains the **descending aorta, esophagus, and lymph nodes;** is the site of masses representing **extramedullary hematopoiesis;** and most important, is the home of **tumors of neural origin.**
  - Although neurogenic tumors produce the largest percentage of posterior mediastinal masses, none of these lesions is particularly common.

NEUROGENIC TUMORS

- Neurogenic tumors include such entities as **neurofibroma, schwannoma (neurilemmoma), ganglioneuroma,** and **neuroblastoma.**
- **Nerve sheath tumors** (schwannoma or neurilemmoma) **are** the most **common** and are usually **benign.**
  - Neoplasms that arise from nerve elements **other than the sheath** are usually **malignant.**

- **Imaging findings of neurogenic tumors**
  - They will produce a **mass, usually sharply marginated,** of soft tissue density in the paravertebral gutter (Fig. 13-13).
  - Both benign and malignant tumors **may erode ribs** (Fig. 13-14A).
  - They may **enlarge the neural foramina** producing *dumbbell*-shaped lesions that arise from the spinal canal but project through the neural foramen into the mediastinum (Fig. 13-14B).
  - They may produce **scalloping** of the posterior aspect of vertebral bodies (Fig. 13-15).
  - They may produce a **scoliosis,** especially a sharp angle scoliosis.
  - **Pleural effusions** may occur with **benign** as well as **malignant** neural tumors.
- **Neurofibromas** can occur as an **isolated tumor** arising from the Schwann cell of the nerve sheath **or as part of a syndrome** called *neurofibromatosis.*
  - As part of the latter, they are part of a neurocutaneous bone dysplasia that can cause numerous abnormalities including **erosion of adjacent bone (***rib notching***), scalloping** of the vertebral bodies, **absence** of the **sphenoid wings, pseudarthroses,** and **sharp-angled kyphoscoliosis** at the thoracolumbar junction.

Solitary Nodule or Mass in the Lung

- **What is the difference between a** *nodule* **and a** *mass?*
  - Size: under 3 cm, it is usually called a *nodule;* over 3 cm it is usually called a *mass.*

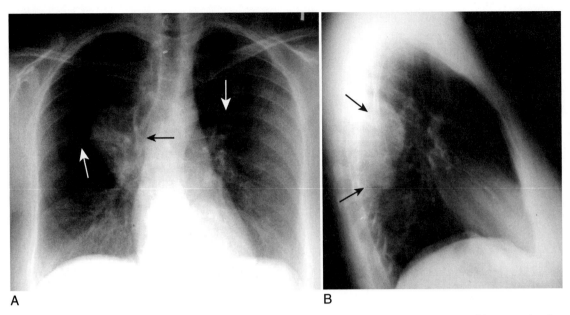

A   B

Figure 13-13. **Neurofibromatosis.** *Neurofibromas can occur as an isolated tumor arising from the Schwann cell of the nerve sheath or as part of the syndrome* **neurofibromatosis,** *as in this case. A large neurofibroma (closed black arrows) is seen on the frontal* **(A)** *and lateral* **(B)** *views. Also, multiple nodules (closed white arrows) are superimposed on the lung but actually represent cutaneous neurofibromas.*

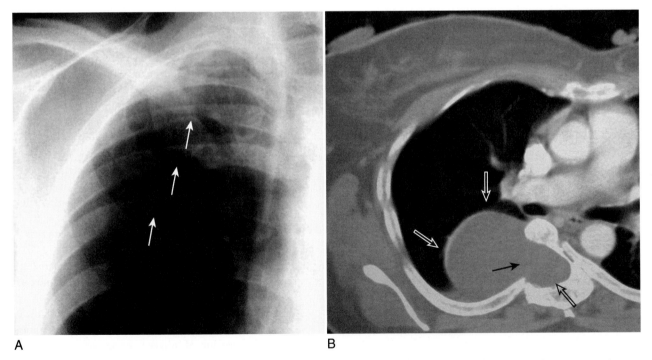

A   B

Figure 13-14. **Rib-notching and a dumbbell-shaped lateral meningocele. A,** *Plexiform neurofibromas can produce erosions along the inferior borders of the ribs (where the intercostal nerves are located) and produce either notching or a wavy appearance called* **ribbon ribs** *(closed white arrows)* **B,** *Another patient demonstrates a lateral meningocele associated with neurofibromatosis that is enlarging the neural foramen producing a dumbbell-shaped lesion that arises from the spinal canal (open black arrow) but projects through the foramen into the posterior mediastinum (open white arrows). The right half of the vertebral body (closed black arrow) has been eroded by the tumor.*

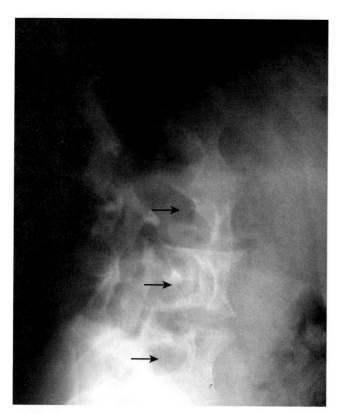

*Figure 13-15. **Scalloping of the vertebral bodies in neurofibromatosis.** Neurofibromatosis is a neurocutaneous disorder associated with a skeletal dysplasia. There may be numerous skeletal abnormalities associated with the disease including scalloping of posterior vertebral bodies (closed black arrows), especially in the thoracic or lumbar spine (as shown here). This is produced by diverticula of the thecal sac caused by dysplasia of the meninges that leads to erosion of adjacent bone through the pulsations transmitted via the spinal fluid.*

- Much has been written about the workup of a patient in whom a single nodular density is discovered in the lung on imaging of the thorax, i.e., the *solitary pulmonary nodule.*
- In evaluating a solitary pulmonary nodule, the **critical question** to be answered is: **is the nodule most likely benign or most likely malignant?**
  - If it is most likely benign, it can be watched (or in some cases ignored), whereas if it is most likely malignant, it will almost certainly be treated aggressively with therapies which themselves carry some risks for morbidity and possibly death.
- The answer to the question of benign versus malignant will depend on many factors including the availability of **prior imaging studies**, which **can help greatly in establishing stability of a lesion over time.**

SIGNS OF A BENIGN VERSUS MALIGNANT SOLITARY PULMONARY NODULE

- **Size of the lesion**—larger than 5 cm has a 95% **chance of malignancy** (Fig. 13-16).

- **Calcification**—the **most important determinant** in distinguishing benign from malignant, the presence of calcification is usually determined by CT.
  - **Lesions containing calcium tend to be benign.**
- **Margin**—lobulation, shagginess, and spiculation all suggest malignancy (Fig. 13-17).
- **Change in size over time**—obtaining a previous study or a follow-up study of a suspicious nodule will provide a basis of comparison of size over time.
  - **Malignancies** tend to **increase in size at a rate that is not so brief as to suggest an inflammatory etiology** (changes in weeks) **nor so prolonged as to suggest benignity** (no change for over a year).
    - **Adenocarcinomas,** as a cell type, grow the **most slowly.**
    - **Squamous cell carcinomas** and **small cell carcinomas** tend to grow **rapidly.**
    - **Large cell carcinomas grow extremely rapidly.**
- **Solitary pulmonary nodules** that are found on mass **screenings of asymptomatic** patients prove to be **cancer less than 5%** of the time.
- **Solitary pulmonary nodules** that are **surgically removed** (meaning there were clinical signs or symptoms and imaging findings that suggested malignancy) are **malignant 50% of the time in men over the age of 50.**

BENIGN CAUSES OF SOLITARY PULMONARY NODULES

- **Granulomas**—tuberculosis and histoplasmosis usually produce calcified nodules < 1 cm in size, although tuberculomas and histoplasmomas can reach up to 4 cm.
  - **When calcified, they are clearly benign.**
    - **Tuberculous** granulomas are usually **homogeneously calcified** (Fig. 13-18A).
    - **Histoplasmomas** may contain a **central** or "**target**" **calcification** or may have a **laminated calcification,** which is diagnostic (Fig. 13-18B).
  - If the nodule is large enough, **CT densitometry** can be used to help differentiate between a calcified and a noncalcified pulmonary nodule.
    - CT densitometry involves detection of occult calcification within nodules using calculations based on numerical density measurements.
  - **Positron emission tomographic** scans (PET scans) can also help in differentiating benign from malignant nodules and provide insight into the presence of any metastatic disease.
    - Usually, the nodules must be >1 cm in size for the most reliable evaluation.
- **Hamartomas** are peripherally located tumors of **disorganized lung tissue** that characteristically **contain fat and calcification** on CT scan.
  - The **classical calcification** of a hamartoma is called *popcorn calcification* (Fig. 13-19).
- Other, uncommon lesions that can produce solitary pulmonary nodules include rheumatoid nodules, fungal diseases such as nocardiosis, arteriovenous malformations, and Wegener's granulomatosis.

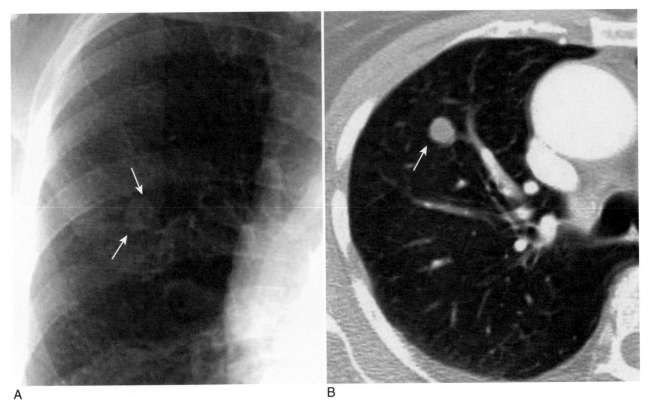

A   B

Figure 13-16. **Solitary pulmonary nodule, conventional radiograph (A) and CT (B).** *A 1.8-cm nodule is in the right upper lobe (closed white arrows) in this 53-year-old man with an episode of hemoptysis. The critical question to be answered in evaluating any solitary pulmonary nodule is whether the lesion is benign or malignant. The answer to the question will depend on many factors, including the availability of prior imaging studies, which can help greatly in establishing stability of a lesion over time. This patient had no prior studies and the presence of symptoms led to a biopsy that revealed an adenocarcinoma of the lung.*

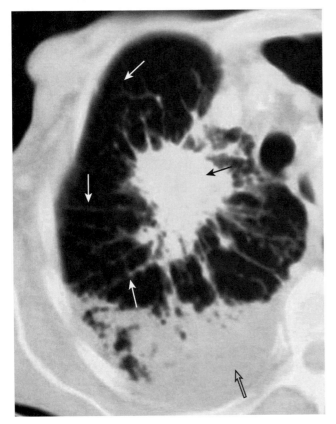

Figure 13-17. **Bronchogenic carcinoma with lymphangitic spread.** *A spiculated mass in the right upper lobe (closed black arrow) with an irregular margin and extension of tumor along the bronchovascular bundles (closed white arrows) to the pleural space (open black arrow) all point to a bronchogenic carcinoma. This was a squamous cell carcinoma of the lung.*

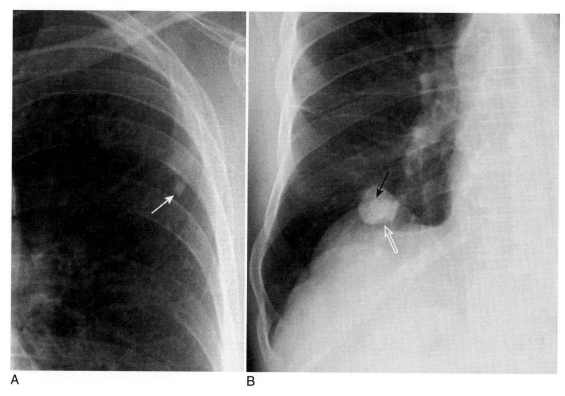

A   B

Figure 13-18. **Calcified tuberculous granuloma and histoplasmoma.** *When a solitary pulmonary nodule is calcified, it is almost always benign. Tuberculous granulomas are common sequelae of prior, usually subclinical, tuberculous infection and are usually homogeneously calcified (closed white arrow in **A**). Histoplasmomas (open white arrow in **B**) may contain a central or "target" calcification (closed black arrow) or may have a laminated calcification, either of which is diagnostic. CT can be used to differentiate between a calcified and a noncalcified pulmonary nodule with greater sensitivity than conventional radiography.*

- Round atelectasis may mimic a solitary pulmonary nodule and is discussed in Chapter 6, Recognizing Atelectasis.

Bronchogenic Carcinoma

- In the United States, **lung cancer is the most common fatal malignancy in men** and the **second most common** (to breast cancer) **in women.**
- For malignancies presenting as pulmonary nodules, **primary lung cancer** usually presents as a **solitary pulmonary nodule,** whereas **metastatic disease** to the lung from another organ characteristically produces **multiple nodules.**
- Table 13-4 summarizes the classical manifestations and growth tendencies of the four types of bronchogenic carcinoma by cell type.
- **Recognizing a bronchogenic carcinoma**
  - They may be recognized by visualization of the **tumor itself:** that is, a **nodule/mass in the lung.**
  - They may be suspected by recognizing the **effects of bronchial obstruction:** that is, **pneumonitis** or **atelectasis.**
  - They may be suspected by recognizing the results of either their **direct extension or metastatic spread** to the lung itself or to other organs.

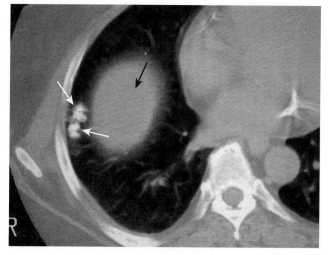

Figure 13-19. **Hamartoma of the lung.** *Hamartomas of the lung are peripherally located tumors of disorganized lung tissue that classically contain fat and calcification on CT scans. The characteristic calcification of a hamartoma is called **popcorn calcification** (closed white arrows). The small island of soft tissue in the middle of the right lung (closed black arrow) is the uppermost part of the right hemidiaphragm.*

Table 13-4

CARCINOMA OF THE LUNG—CELL TYPES

Cell Type	Graphic Representation	Classical Manifestation
Squamous cell carcinoma		Primarily central in location
		Arise in segmental or lobar bronchi
		Invariably produce bronchial obstruction leading to obstructive pneumonitis or atelectasis
		Tend to grow rapidly
Adenocarcinoma, including bronchoalveolar cell carcinoma		Primarily peripheral in location
		Usually solitary except in the case of diffuse bronchoalveolar cell carcinoma, which can present as multiple nodules
		Slowest growing
Small cell, including oat cell carcinoma		Primarily central in location
		May contain neurosecretory granules that lead to an association of small cell carcinoma with paraneoplastic syndromes such as Cushing's syndrome, inappropriate secretion of antidiuretic hormone
		Highly aggressive, grows rapidly, usually has metastasized on presentation
Large cell carcinoma		Diagnosis of exclusion for lesions that are non–small cell and not squamous or adenocarcinoma
		Large peripheral lesions
		Grows extremely rapidly

BRONCHOGENIC CARCINOMAS PRESENTING AS A NODULE OR MASS IN THE LUNG

- Most often this type is an **adenocarcinoma.**
- The nodule may have **irregular** and **spiculated margins** (see Fig. 13-17).
- It **may cavitate,** especially if it is of squamous cell origin (also occurs with adenocarcinoma), producing a **relatively thick-walled** cavity with a **nodular and irregular inner margin** (see Fig. 14-16).
- Table 13-5 summarizes the key findings in differentiating **three commonly occurring cavitary lesions in the lung** (Fig. 13-20).

BRONCHOGENIC CARCINOMA PRESENTING WITH BRONCHIAL OBSTRUCTION

- Endobronchial lesions produce varying degrees of bronchial obstruction leading to

- **Obstructive pneumonitis and atelectasis** (see Fig. 6-12)
  - It is called *pneumonitis* because the obstructed lung is consolidated but frequently not infected (though it can be).
  - **Atelectasis** secondary to an endobronchial obstructing lesion features the usual shifts of the fissures or mobile mediastinal structures toward the side of the atelectasis (Chapter 6) in addition to visualization of the obstructing mass.
- **Bronchial obstruction is most often caused by a squamous cell carcinoma.**
  - Large, squamous cell carcinomas may undergo central necrosis and cavitation (see Table 13-4).

BRONCHOGENIC CARCINOMA PRESENTING WITH DIRECT EXTENSION OR METASTATIC LESIONS

- **Rib destruction by direct extension:** *Pancoast tumor* is the eponym for a tumor arising from the superior sulcus of the lung, frequently producing destruction of one or more of the first three ribs on the affected side (Box 13-1 and Fig. 13-21).

Table 13-5

DIFFERENTIATING THREE CAVITATING LUNG LESIONS

Lesion	Thickness* of the Cavity Wall	Inner Margin of Cavity
Bronchogenic carcinoma (Fig. 13-20A)	Thick	Nodular
Tuberculosis (Fig. 13-20B)	Thin	Smooth
Lung abscess (Fig. 13-20C)	Thick	Smooth

*Thick = more than 5 mm; thin = less than 5 mm.

Box 13-1

Pancoast Tumor—Apical Lung Cancer*
Manifests as a soft tissue mass in the apex of the lung
Most often squamous cell carcinoma or adenocarcinoma
Frequently produces adjacent rib destruction
May invade brachial plexus or cause Horner's syndrome on affected side
On the right side, may produce superior vena caval obstruction

*See Figure 13-21.

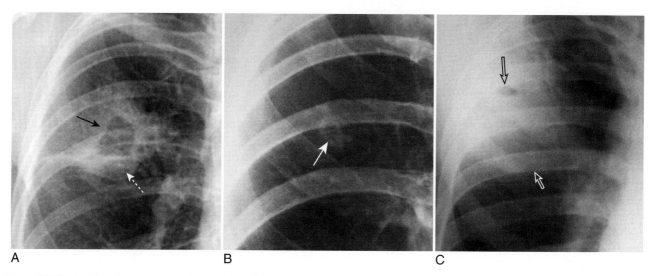

Figure 13-20. **Cavitary lesions of the lung.** *Three of the most common cavitary lesions of the lung can frequently be differentiated from each other by noting the thickness of the wall of the cavity and the smoothness or nodularity of its inner margin.* **A,** *A cavitary squamous cell bronchogenic carcinoma with a thick wall* (dotted white arrow) *and a nodular inner margin* (closed black arrow); **B,** *upper lobe tuberculosis has a thin-walled cavity with a smooth inner margin* (closed white arrow); **C,** *a staphylococcal lung abscess demonstrating a characteristic markedly thickened wall* (open white arrow) *and a small but smooth inner margin* (open black arrow).

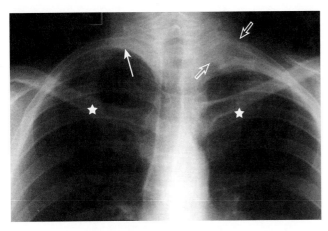

Figure 13-21. **Pancoast tumor, left upper lobe.** *A soft tissue density is seen in the apex of the left lung (compare the two sides). It is associated with rib destruction. The stars are placed on the anterior first rib on each side. On the normal right side, you can follow the first rib posteriorly to its junction with the spine (closed white arrow). On the left side, the posterior first rib is invisible because it has been destroyed by tumor. The posterior second and third ribs are also partially destroyed on the left (open white arrows). The finding of an apical soft tissue mass with associated rib destruction is classical for a Pancoast or superior sulcus tumor.*

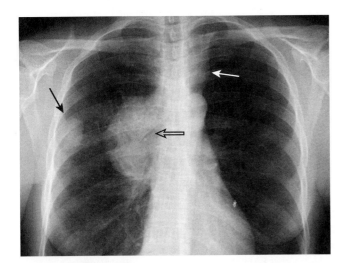

Figure 13-22. **Bronchogenic carcinoma with hilar and mediastinal adenopathy.** *This peripheral lung mass (closed black arrow) shows evidence of ipsilateral hilar and mediastinal adenopathy (open black arrow) and contralateral mediastinal adenopathy (closed white arrow). Bronchogenic carcinoma may present with metastatic lesions that can manifest in distant organs or in the thorax itself. This was an adenocarcinoma of the lung.*

- **Hilar adenopathy** is usually unilateral on the same side as the tumor (Fig. 13-22).
- **Mediastinal adenopathy** may be the sole manifestation in small cell carcinoma, the peripheral nodule being invisible (see Fig. 13-8).
- **Other nodules in the lung:** one of the manifestations of diffuse bronchoalveolar cell carcinoma may be multiple nodules throughout both lungs and, as such, may mimic metastatic disease.

- **Pleural effusion,** frequently from lymphangitic spread
- **Metastases to other bones** tend to be mixed osteolytic and osteoblastic lesions.

Metastatic Neoplasms in the Lung

MULTIPLE NODULES

- Multiple nodules in the lung are most often metastatic lesions that have traveled through the bloodstream from a distant primary site (*hematogenous spread*).
- Multiple metastatic nodules are **usually of slightly differing sizes** indicating tumor embolization that occurred at different times.
- They are **frequently sharply marginated,** varying in size from **micronodular** to "cannonball" masses (see Fig. 4-15).
- For all practical purposes it is **impossible to determine the primary lesion** by the **appearance of the metastatic nodules;** i.e., all metastatic nodules appear similar.
- Tissue sampling, whether by bronchoscopic or percutaneous biopsy, is the best means of determining the organ of origin of the metastatic nodule.
- Table 13-6 summarizes the primary malignancies most likely to metastasize to the lung hematogenously.

LYMPHANGITIC SPREAD OF CARCINOMA

- In lymphangitic spread of carcinoma, tumor grows in and obstructs lymphatics in the lung producing a pattern that is **radiologically similar to pulmonary interstitial edema** from heart failure **including Kerley B lines, thickening of the fissures,** and **pleural effusions.**
- **Unilateral** findings of pulmonary interstitial edema should alert you to the possibility of lymphangitic spread rather than congestive heart failure (Fig. 13-23).
- The **most common primary malignancies to produce lymphangitic spread** are those that arise around the thorax: **breast, lung, and pancreatic carcinoma.**

WebLink

More information on chest and mediastinal masses is available to registered users on StudentConsult.com.

Table 13-6

SOME COMMON PRIMARY SITES OF METASTATIC LUNG NODULES	
Males	**Females**
Colorectal carcinoma*	Breast cancer*
Renal cell carcinoma	Colorectal carcinoma
Head and neck tumors	Renal cell carcinoma
Testicular and bladder carcinoma	Cervical or endometrial carcinoma
Malignant melanoma	Malignant melanoma
Sarcomas	Sarcomas

*Most common

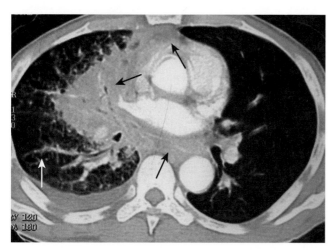

Figure 13-23. **Bronchogenic carcinoma with lymphangitic spread of tumor.** *In lymphangitic spread of carcinoma, tumor grows in and obstructs lymphatics in the lung producing a pattern that is radiologically similar to pulmonary interstitial edema from heart failure, including Kerley B lines, thickening of the fissures, and pleural effusions. The findings may be unilateral, as in this case, which should alert you to the possibility of lymphangitic spread rather than congestive heart failure. In this case, there is extensive hilar and mediastinal adenopathy (closed black arrows)* from a bronchogenic carcinoma of the lung with extension along the bronchovascular bundles to the periphery of the lung (closed white arrow). A right pleural effusion is present.

TAKE-HOME POINTS: Recognizing Chest Masses

The mediastinum lies in the central portion of the thorax between the two lungs and is arbitrarily divided into anterior, middle, and posterior compartments.

The anterior compartment gives rise to substernal thyroid masses, lymphoma, thymoma, and teratoma.

The middle mediastinal compartment gives rise primarily to lymphadenopathy from lymphoma and metastatic disease (e.g., small cell carcinoma of the lung) as well as benign entities (e.g., tuberculosis).

The posterior mediastinal compartment gives rise to neurogenic tumors, which originate either from the nerve sheath (tend to be benign) or tissues other than the sheath (tend to be malignant).

Aortic aneurysms are defined as enlargement of the aorta greater than 50% of its original size; for the thoracic aorta, that is usually considered > 4 cm, with 5–6 cm aneurysms posing a significant risk for rupture.

Aortic dissection occurs when blood dissects through the wall of the aorta, usually in the media; they usually originate just distal to the root of the ascending aorta (Stanford type A) or just distal to the origin of the left subclavian artery (Stanford type B). They are usually associated with tears in the intima.

Type A dissections are surgical emergencies; type B dissections are usually treated medically.

Solitary pulmonary nodules are smaller than 3 cm and are only infrequently cancerous when found on screening studies; nevertheless, the key question is to determine whether the nodule is most likely benign or most likely malignant in any given individual.

Criteria on which an evaluation of benignity can be made include absolute size of the nodule upon discovery, presence of calcification within it, the margin of the nodule, and change in the size of the nodule over time.

Bronchogenic carcinomas present in one of three ways: by visualization of the tumor itself; by recognizing the effects of bronchial obstruction such as pneumonitis or atelectasis; or by recognizing the results of either their direct extension or metastatic spread to the chest or to distant organs.

Bronchogenic carcinomas presenting as a solitary nodule/mass in the lung are most often adenocarcinomas; bronchoalveolar cell carcinoma is a subset of adenocarcinoma that may present with multiple nodules, mimicking metastatic disease.

Bronchogenic carcinoma presenting with bronchial obstruction is most often due to squamous cell carcinoma that produces obstructive pneumonitis or atelectasis; squamous cell carcinomas are most apt to cavitate.

Small cell carcinomas are highly aggressive, centrally located peribronchial tumors, the majority of which have already metastasized at the time of initial presentation; they can be associated with paraneoplastic syndromes such as inappropriate secretion of antidiuretic hormone and Cushing's syndrome.

Multiple nodules in the lung are most often metastatic lesions that have traveled through the bloodstream from a distant primary lesion (**hematogenous spread**); common sites of primary lesions for such metastases include colorectal, breast, renal cell, head and neck, bladder, uterine and cervical, soft tissue sarcomas and melanoma.

In lymphangitic spread of carcinoma, tumor grows in and obstructs lymphatics in the lung, producing a pattern that is radiologically similar to pulmonary interstitial edema; primary tumors that metastasize to the lung in this fashion include breast, lung, and pancreatic cancer.

14 Recognizing the Basics on CT of the Chest

- A computed tomographic image is composed of a matrix of thousands of tiny squares called *pixels,* each of which is computer-assigned a *CT number* from −1000 to +1000 measured in *Hounsfield units (HU),* named after Sir Godfrey Hounsfield, the British electrical engineer credited with developing the first CT scanner.
  - A *tomogram* is a **slice** (measured in **millimeters**) through the body that allows for the accurate localization of objects in that section, unlike conventional radiographs that superimpose all structures within a given field of view.
  - **A CT scanner uses x-rays** transmitted to multiple *detectors* connected to a **computer,** which processes the data though various **algorithms** to produce **images** of diagnostic quality.
- The CT number will **vary according to the density of the tissue** scanned and is a **measure of how much of the x-ray beam is absorbed** by the tissues at each point in the scan.
  - By convention, **air is assigned a Hounsfield number of −1000 HU** and bone is about 400 to 600 HU (fat is −40 to −100, water is 0, and soft tissue 20 to 100)
- CT images are displayed or viewed using a range of Hounsfield numbers preselected to best demonstrate the tissues being studied (for example, from −100 to +300) and anything within that range of CT numbers is displayed over the levels of density in the available gray scale.
- This range of densities is called the *window* or *window-width* **setting** and the number within that range that is arbitrarily chosen to be the **center of the gray scale** is called the *center* or the *window level.*
- **Denser substances** that absorb more x-rays have **high CT numbers,** are said to demonstrate *increased attenuation,* and are displayed as **whiter densities** on CT scans.
  - On conventional radiographs, these substances (e.g., **metal** and **calcium**) would also appear whiter and be said to have *increased density* or be *more opaque.*
- **Less dense substances** that absorb fewer x-rays have **low CT numbers,** are said to demonstrate *decreased attenuation,* and are displayed as **blacker densities** on CT scans.
  - On conventional radiographs, these substances (e.g., air and fat) would also appear as blacker densities and be said to have *decreased density* (or *increased lucency*).
- **High-resolution computed tomography (HRCT)** uses an x-ray beam that is collimated to be extremely thin (1–1.5 mm compared to 5–7 mm for conventional CT) and a special computer algorithm that makes HRCT

particularly useful for the study and characterization of diffuse parenchymal lung diseases.
- **Spiral CT** (helical CT) uses a continuously rotating x-ray source and detector array combined with constant table movement to permit data acquisition through the chest or abdomen so fast it can be done in a single breath-hold by the patient.
  - This results in an extremely **rapid acquisition** of data that has **no "gaps"** between slices and, in turn, allows for seamless reconstruction of those images in almost any plane.
  - Traditionally, CT images were viewed mostly in the axial plane.
    - With volumetric data acquisition and seamless reconstruction, CT scans now provide **diagnostically useful images** in the **coronal** and **sagittal planes** as well as **three-dimensional reconstructions** that can be viewed at any angle.
- **Multislice CT** (also called *multidetector CT*) makes use of multiple rows of detectors that allow for images to be reconstructed in a range of **slice thicknesses after the scan is completed** without reimaging the patient.
  - Because of increasingly sophisticated arrays of detectors and acquisition of as many as 64 slices simultaneously, **multislice CT scanners permit very fast imaging** (head to toe in less than 30 seconds) that has allowed for development of new applications for CT such as *virtual colonoscopy* and *virtual bronchoscopy, cardiac calcium scoring,* and *CT coronary angiography.*
    - Such examinations can contain a thousand or more images so that the older convention of filming each image for study on a viewbox is impractical and such examinations are almost always viewed on computer workstations.
- So, you might ask, why not scan everyone at the thinnest possible slice thickness from head to toe?
  - The radiation dose delivered by CT studies is dependent on many factors including the type of equipment, the energy of the x-rays used to produce the images, and the size of the patient.
  - Dose-reducing measures are being employed that include use of optimized CT settings, reduction in the x-ray energy used, limiting the number of repeat scans, and assuring—through appropriate consultation—that the benefits derived from obtaining the study outweigh any potential risks of the radiation exposure.
- CT scans of the chest **can be performed with or without the intravenous administration of iodinated contrast**

material (and are frequently obtained both without and then with IV contrast material) but, in general, **they yield more diagnostic information** that is more easily recognizable **when intravenous contrast can be used.**

- Radiographic contrast agents, in general, are **administered to increase the differences in density between two tissues.**
- CT scans done **with intravenous contrast** agents are called *contrast-enhanced* or simply *enhanced.*
- While it might sound like a wonderful idea to give everyone contrast material, keep in mind that **iodinated contrast** can have **adverse effects** and produce **serious reactions** in **susceptible individuals** (Box 14-1).

- Table 14-1 outlines, in general, **when intravenous contrast studies are indicated and when they are not used** for particular problems.
  - You will probably not be required to make the decision of when or if to use contrast because **the radiologist will usually tailor the examination to the clinical question being asked** in most clinical settings, so it is always important to provide as much clinical information as possible when requesting a study.

- By convention, **CT scans of the chest,** like most other radiologic studies, **are viewed with the patient's right on your left and the patient's left on your right.**
  - If the patient is scanned in the supine position, as most usually are, the **top** of each image is **anterior** and the **bottom** of each image is **posterior.**

Table 14-1

CT SCANS OF THE CHEST— INDICATIONS FOR INTRAVENOUS CONTRAST STUDIES
Intravenous Contrast Study Indicated
CT-PA for pulmonary embolism
Evaluation of the mediastinum or hila for mass or adenopathy
Detect aortic aneurysm or dissection
Evaluate blunt or penetrating trauma
Characterize pleural disease (metastases, empyema)
CT densitometry of pulmonary masses
Evaluate the coronary arteries
Intravenous Contrast Study Usually Not Indicated
Evaluation of diffuse infiltrative lung diseases using HRCT
Confirmation of the presence of a nodule suspected from conventional radiographs
Detect pneumothorax/pneumomediastinum
Calcium scoring for the coronary arteries
Known allergies to contrast agents or renal failure

Box 14-1

Contrast Reactions and Renal Failure

Intravenous contrast materials available today are nonionic, low osmolar solutions containing a high concentration of iodine which circulate through the bloodstream, opacify those tissues and organs with high blood flow, are absorbed by x-ray (and therefore appear "whiter" on images), and are finally excreted in the urine by the kidneys.

In some patients (diabetes, dehydration, multiple myeloma) with compromised renal function (evidenced by creatinine >1.5 mg/dL), iodinated contrast agent can produce a nephrotoxic effect that can range from transient renal dysfunction to acute renal failure; therefore, iodinated contrast material should be used with caution, if at all, in these patients.

All iodinated contrast agents can rarely produce mild side effects including nausea and vomiting, local irritation at the site of injection, itching and hives; these side effects usually require no treatment.

Asthmatics and those with a history of severe allergies or prior reactions to IV contrast agent have a higher likelihood of contrast reactions (but still very low overall) and may benefit from steroids, benadryl, and cimetidine administered prior to and/or after injection.

In about 0.01–0.04% of all patients, severe and idiosyncratic reactions to contrast material can occur that can produce intense bronchospasm, laryngeal edema, circulatory collapse and, very rarely, death (1 in 200,000 to 300,000).

- Chest CT scans are usually "windowed" and **displayed in** at least **two formats** designed to be viewed as parts of the same study in order to optimize anatomic definition.
  - *Lung windows* are chosen to maximize our ability to image abnormalities of the **lung parenchyma** and to identify **normal and abnormal bronchial anatomy.**
    - The mediastinal structures usually appear as a homogeneous white density on lung windows.
  - *Mediastinal windows* are chosen to display the **mediastinal, hilar, and pleural structures** to best advantage.
    - The lungs usually appear completely black when viewed with mediastinal windows.
  - *Bone windows* are also utilized quite often as a third way of displaying the data, demonstrating the bony structures to their best advantage.
  - It is important to know that the displays of these different windows are **manipulations of the data** obtained during the **original scan** and **do not require rescanning the patient** (Fig. 14-1).

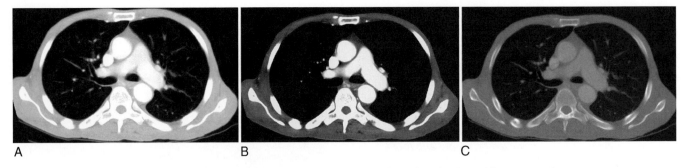

Figure 14-1. Windowing the thorax. *Chest CT scans are usually "windowed" and displayed in several formats in order to optimize anatomic definition. Lung windows (A) are chosen to maximize our ability to image abnormalities of the lung parenchyma and to identify normal and abnormal bronchial anatomy. Mediastinal windows (B) are chosen to display the mediastinal, hilar, and pleural structures to best advantage. Bone windows (C) are utilized as a third way of displaying the data, visualizing the bony structures to their best advantage. It is important to recognize that the displays of these different windows are manipulations of the data obtained during the original scan and do not require rescanning the patient.*

Normal Chest CT Anatomy

- We will cover only a few of the major anatomic landmarks demonstrable on chest CT, and all the scans utilized will be *contrast-enhanced;* i.e., the patient will have received intravenous contrast to opacify the blood vessels.
- It is best to read the text in conjunction with its associated photograph.
  - Any references to "right" or "left" mean the patient's right or left side, not yours.
- We will start at the top of the chest and progress inferiorly, highlighting the major structures visible at **six key levels.**
  - Those levels are (from top to bottom):
    - Five-vessel level
    - Aortic arch level
    - Aorto-pulmonary window level
    - Main pulmonary artery level
    - High cardiac level
    - Low cardiac level
  - This is a good way to systematically examine every CT study of the chest.

FIVE-VESSEL LEVEL

- For this discussion, refer to Figure 14-2.
- At this level, you should be able to identify the **lungs, the trachea, and the esophagus.**
  - The **trachea** is black because it contains air, is usually oval, and is about 2 cm in diameter.
  - The **esophagus** lies posterior and either to the left or to the right of the trachea.
    - It is usually collapsed but may contain swallowed air.
  - Depending on the exact level of the image, several of the great vessels will be visible:
    - The **venous structures** tend to be **more anterior than the arterial.**
      - The **brachiocephalic veins** lie just posterior to the sternum.
    - From the patient's **right** to the patient's **left,** the visible arteries may include the **innominate artery, left common carotid artery,** and **left subclavian arteries.**

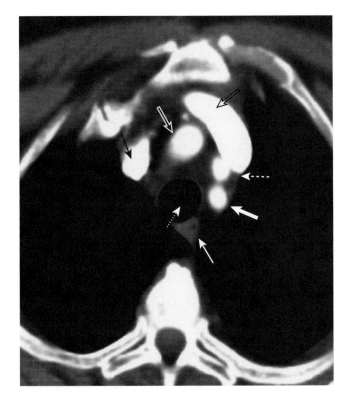

Figure 14-2. Five-vessel level. *At this level, you should be able to identify the lungs, the trachea (dotted white arrow), and the esophagus (thin white arrow). Depending on the exact level of the image, several of the great vessels will be visible. The venous structures tend to be more anterior than the arterial. The superior vena cava is the large vessel to the right of the trachea (closed black arrow). The brachiocephalic vein lies just posterior to the sternum (open black arrow). From the patient's right to the patient's left, the arteries you see may include the innominate artery (open white arrow), left common carotid (dashed white arrow), and left subclavian arteries (thick white arrow).*

AORTIC ARCH LEVEL

- For this discussion, refer to Figure 14-3.
- At this level, you should be able to identify the **aortic arch, superior vena cava, and azygous vein.**

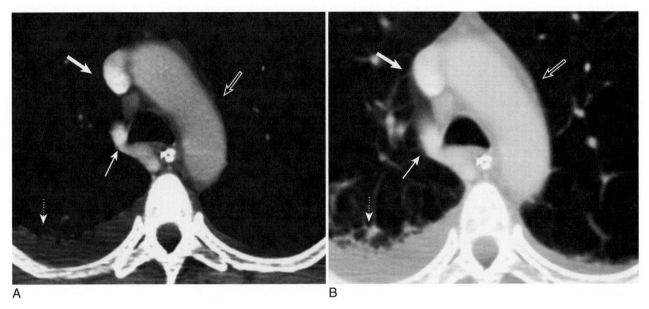

A   B

Figure 14-3. **Aortic arch level, mediastinal window and lung window. A,** *At this level, you should be able to identify the aortic arch (open white arrow), superior vena cava (thick white arrow), and azygous vein (thin white arrow). There is a nasogastric tube in the esophagus (white circle behind trachea). The aortic arch is an upside-down U-shaped tube. If the scan skims the top of the arch, it will appear as a comma-shaped tubular structure with roughly the same diameter anteriorly as posteriorly. This patient has a small right pleural effusion (dotted white arrow).* **B,** *The same image shown in* **A,** *but windowed to best visualize lung anatomy. Lung windows are chosen to maximize our ability to image abnormalities of the lung parenchyma and to identify normal and abnormal bronchial anatomy.*

- The *aortic arch* is an upside-down U-shaped tube.
- If the scan skims the very top of the arch, it will appear as a comma-shaped tubular structure with roughly the same diameter anteriorly as posteriorly.
- To the right of the trachea will be the *superior vena cava* into which the *azygous vein* enters.

AORTO-PULMONARY WINDOW LEVEL
- For this discussion, refer to Figure 14-4.
- At this level you should be able to identify the **ascending and descending aorta, superior vena cava,** and **uppermost aspect of the left pulmonary artery** (maybe).
- As we scan lower and scan through the opening of the upside-down U-shaped aortic arch, the **ascending aorta** will appear as a rounded density **anteriorly** while the descending aorta will appear as a rounded density **posteriorly** and to the **left** of the spine.
  - The **ascending aorta** usually measures 2.5 to 3.5 cm in diameter, and the descending aorta is slightly smaller at 2 to 3 cm.
- In most people, there is a space visible just underneath the arch of the aorta but above the pulmonary artery called the *aorto-pulmonary window.*
  - The aorto-pulmonary window is an important landmark because it is a common location for **enlarged lymph nodes to appear.**
- At or slightly below this level, the trachea bifurcates at the **carina** into the **right and left main bronchi.**

MAIN PULMONARY ARTERY LEVEL
- For this discussion, refer to Figure 14-5.

- At these levels (it may require more than one image to see all of these structures), you should be able to identify the **main, right, and left pulmonary arteries,** the **right and left main bronchi,** and the **bronchus intermedius.**
- The **left pulmonary artery** is higher than the right and appears as if it were a continuation of the main pulmonary artery.
- The **right pulmonary artery** originates at a 90° angle to the main pulmonary artery and crosses to the right side.
- The **right main bronchus** will appear as a circular, air-containing structure that will then become tubular as the **right upper lobe** bronchus comes into view.
  - There should be nothing but lung tissue posterior to the bronchus intermedius.
- The **left main bronchus** will appear as an air-containing circular structure on the left.

HIGH CARDIAC LEVEL
- For this discussion, refer to Figure 14-6.
- At this level, you should be able to identify the **left atrium, right atrium, aortic root,** and **right ventricular outflow tract.**
  - The **left atrium** occupies the posterior and central portion of the heart.
    - One or more **pulmonary veins** may be seen to enter the left atrium.
  - The **right atrium** forms the right heart border and lies immediately to the right of the left atrium.
  - The **right ventricular outflow tract** lies anterior, lateral, and superior to the root of the aorta.

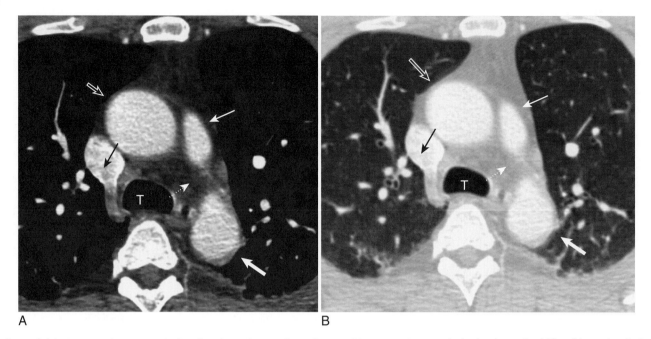

Figure 14-4. ***Aorto-pulmonary window level, mediastinal window and lung window. A,*** *At this level you should be able to identify the ascending and descending aorta, superior vena cava (closed black arrow), and uppermost aspect of the left pulmonary artery (sometimes) (thin white arrow). As we scan lower and scan through the opening of the upside-down U-shaped aortic arch, the ascending aorta will appear as a rounded density anteriorly (open white arrow) and the descending aorta will appear as a rounded density posteriorly and to the left of the spine (thick white arrow). The ascending aorta usually measures 2.5 to 3.5 cm in diameter and the descending aorta is slightly smaller at 2 to 3 cm. In most people, there is a space visible just under the arch of the aorta and above the pulmonary artery called the aorto-pulmonary window (dotted white arrow).* ***B,*** *At or slightly below this level, the trachea (T) bifurcates at the carina into the right and left main bronchi.*

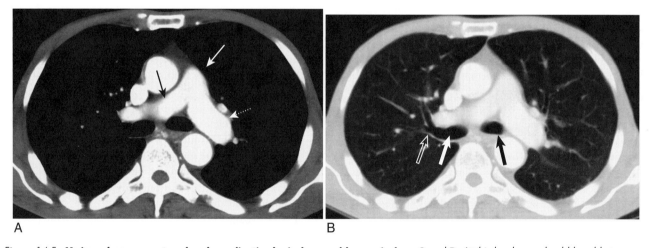

Figure 14-5. ***Main pulmonary artery level, mediastinal window and lung window. A*** *and* ***B,*** *At this level, you should be able to identify the main, right, and left pulmonary arteries, the right and left main bronchi, and the bronchus intermedius (thick white arrow). The left pulmonary artery (dotted white arrow) is higher than the right and appears as if it were a continuation of the main pulmonary artery. The right pulmonary artery (thin black arrow) originates at a 90° angle to the main pulmonary artery (thin white arrow) and crosses to the right side. The posterior wall of the right upper lobe bronchus is 2 to 3 mm in thickness with only lung behind it (open white arrow). The left main bronchus will be seen as an air-containing circular structure on the left (thick black arrow).*

- The **p**ulmonary valve lies **a**nterior, **l**ateral, and **s**uperior to the aortic valve (you can remember that if you can remember the acronym PALS).

LOW CARDIAC LEVEL

- For this discussion, refer to Figure 14-7.

- At this level, you should be able to identify the **right atrium, right ventricle, left ventricle, interventricular septum,** and **pericardium.**
  - The **right atrium** continues to form the right heart border.

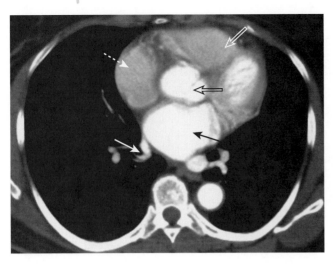

Figure 14-6. **High cardiac level.** At this level, you should be able to identify the left atrium, right atrium, aortic root, and right ventricular outflow tract. The left atrium occupies the central portion of the heart posteriorly (closed black arrow). One or more pulmonary veins may be seen to enter the left atrium (closed white arrow). The right atrium produces the right heart border and lies immediately to the right of the left atrium (dotted white arrow). The right ventricular outflow tract (open white arrow) lies anterior, lateral, and superior to the root of the aorta (open black arrow).

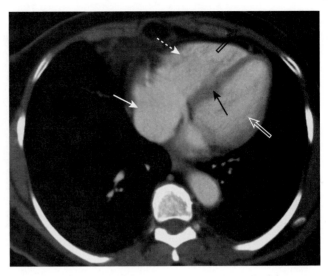

Figure 14-7. **Low cardiac level.** At this level, you should be able to identify the right atrium, right ventricle, left ventricle, pericardium, and interventricular septum. The right atrium continues to form the right heart border (closed white arrow). The right ventricle is anteriorly located, just behind the sternum (dotted white arrow). The left ventricle produces the left heart border (open white arrow). The interventricular septum is visible between the right and left ventricles (closed black arrow). The normal pericardium is about 2 mm thick and is usually outlined by mediastinal fat (outside the pericardium) and epicardial fat (on its inner surface) (open black arrow).

- The **right ventricle** is anteriorly located, just behind the sternum.
- The **left ventricle** produces the left heart border and normally has a thicker wall than the right ventricle.
- With IV contrast material, you should be able to see the **interventricular septum** between the right and left ventricles.
- The **normal pericardium** is about **2 mm thick** and is usually outlined by **mediastinal fat** (outside the pericardium) and **epicardial fat** (on its inner surface).

The Fissures

- Depending on slice thickness, the **major fissures** will be visible either as thin white lines or by an avascular band about 2 cm thick that they produce as they travel obliquely through the lungs **from posterosuperior to anteroinferior** (Fig. 14-8A).
- The **minor fissure** travels in the same plane as an axial CT image so that it is normally not visible.
  - Like the major fissures, though, the **location of the minor fissure can be inferred by an avascular zone** between the right upper and middle lobes (Fig. 14-8B).
  - On thin-collimation scans, the minor fissure may be visible as one or more thin white lines, with some variability in its appearance, depending on the exact plane of the minor fissure.

Selected Abnormalities Visible on Chest CT Scans

- A complete discussion of all abnormalities visible on chest CT scan is beyond the scope of this text.
- Several diseases have already been discussed in other chapters (Table 14-2).

- We will, instead, concentrate on a few abnormalities not yet covered in other chapters in which chest CT scans play a major role.

Pulmonary Thromboembolic Disease

- **Over 90% of pulmonary emboli (PE) develop from thrombi in the deep veins of the leg,** especially above the level of the popliteal veins.
- They are usually a **complication of surgery** or **prolonged bedrest** or **cancer.**
  - Because of the **dual** circulation of the lungs (pulmonary and bronchial), **most pulmonary emboli do not result in infarction.**
- **Conventional chest radiography** has a **high false negative rate.**
  - Although conventional chest radiographs are frequently abnormal in patients with PE, they demonstrate nonspecific findings such as **subsegmental atelectasis, small pleural effusions,** and **elevation of the hemidiaphragm.**
  - Chest radiographs **infrequently manifest one of the "classic" findings for pulmonary embolism:**
    - Wedge-shaped peripheral air-space disease (*Hampton's hump*) (Fig. 14-9)
    - Focal oligemia (*Westermark's sign*)
    - **A prominent central pulmonary artery (*Knuckle sign*)**
- **Ventilation/perfusion (V/Q) lung scans** had been the imaging study of first choice for patients with suspected

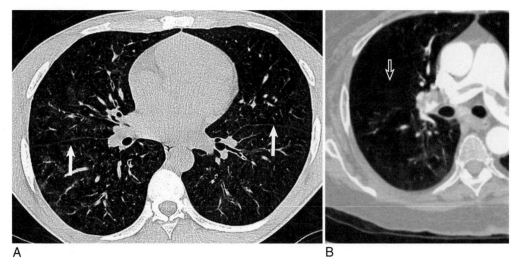

A   B

Figure 14-8. ***Minor fissure and major fissures.*** *The major fissures will be visible either as thin white lines (closed white arrows seen in* **A)** *or by the avascular band about 2 cm thick they produce as they travel obliquely through the lungs from posterosuperior to anteroinferior. The minor fissure travels in the same plane as the axial CT scan so that it is normally not visible. Like the major fissures, though, the location of the minor fissure can be inferred by an avascular zone between the right upper and middle lobes (open white arrow in* **B).** *On thin-collimation scans, the minor fissures may be visible as thin white lines.*

Table 14-2

CHEST CT TOPICS DISCUSSED ELSEWHERE IN THIS TEXT

Topic	Appears in
Atelectasis	Chapter 6
Pleural effusion	Chapter 7
Pneumonia	Chapter 8
Pneumothorax, pneumomediastinum, and pneumopericardium	Chapter 9
Mediastinal masses, bronchogenic carcinoma, and thoracic aortic aneurysms	Chapter 13

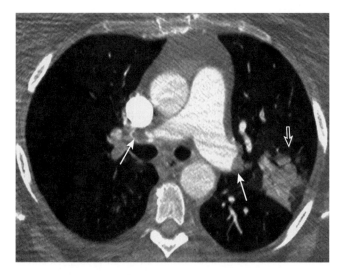

Figure 14-9. ***Hampton's hump.*** *A wedge-shaped, peripheral airspace density is present (open white arrow)* and associated with filling defects in the left and right pulmonary arteries (closed white arrows). The wedge-shaped infarct is called **Hampton's hump.** Without the associated emboli being present, the pleural-based density of airspace disease would have a differential diagnosis that includes pneumonia, lung contusion, and aspiration.

thromboembolism but have, for the most part, been replaced by CT pulmonary arteriograms.

- **CT pulmonary angiography (CT-PA)** is made possible by **the fast data acquisition** of **spiral CT** scanners (one breath hold) combined with **thin slices** and **rapid bolus intravenous injection of iodinated contrast** that produces maximal opacification of the pulmonary arteries with little or no motion artifact.
  - Acute **pulmonary emboli** appear as **partial or complete filling defects centrally-located** within the **contrast-enhanced** lumina of the **pulmonary arteries** (Fig. 14-10).
  - CT-PA has a **sensitivity in excess of 90%** and has replaced, in many instances, the use of nuclear medicine

ventilation-perfusion scan, especially in patients with **chronic obstructive pulmonary disease** or a **positive chest radiograph** in whom a V/Q scan is known to be less sensitive.
  - CT-PA has the **additional benefit** of **demonstrating other diseases** that may be present, like pneumonia, even if the study is negative for pulmonary embolism.

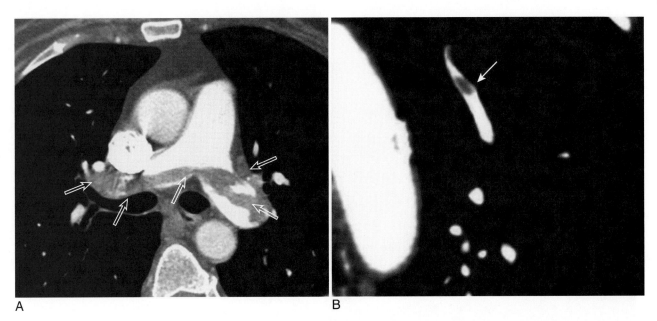

A   B

Figure 14-10. **Saddle and peripheral pulmonary emboli.** *Acute pulmonary emboli appear as partial or complete filling defects centrally located within the contrast-enhanced lumens of the pulmonary arteries.* **A,** *A large pulmonary embolus almost completely fills both the left and right pulmonary arteries (open white arrows). This is a* **saddle embolus.** **B,** *A small, central filling defect is seen in a more peripheral pulmonary artery (closed white arrow). This pulmonary artery seems to be floating disconnected in the lung because the plane of this particular image does not include its connection to the right pulmonary artery.*

Chronic Obstructive Pulmonary Disease

- Chronic obstructive pulmonary disease (COPD) is defined as a disease of **airflow obstruction due to chronic bronchitis or emphysema.**
- **Chronic bronchitis** is defined **clinically** by **productive cough** whereas **emphysema** is defined **pathologically** by the presence of **permanent and abnormal enlargement and destruction of the airspaces distal to the terminal bronchioles.**
- **Emphysema has three pathologic patterns:**
  - **Centriacinar (centrilobular) emphysema** (Fig. 14-11A)
    - Features focal destruction limited to the respiratory bronchioles and the central portions of acinus.
    - **Associated with cigarette smoking**
    - Most severe in the **upper lobes**
  - **Panacinar emphysema** (Fig. 14-11B)
    - Involves the entire alveolus distal to the terminal bronchiole
    - Most severe in the **lower lung zones** and generally develops in patients with homozygous α_1-**antitrypsin deficiency.**
  - **Paraseptal emphysema** (Fig. 14-11C)
    - **Least common** form
    - Involves distal airway structures, alveolar ducts, and sacs
    - Localized to fibrous septa or to the pleura and leads to formation of bullae, which **may cause pneumothorax.**
    - Not associated with airflow obstruction
- Conventional radiographs can display several **imaging findings of COPD:**

- **Hyperinflation,** including **flattening of the diaphragm,** especially on the **lateral** exposure (Fig. 14-12)
- **Increase** in the **retrosternal clear space**
- **Hyperlucency** of the lungs with fewer than normal vascular markings visible
- **Prominence of the pulmonary arteries** from pulmonary arterial hypertension
- **CT findings of COPD**
  - **Focal areas of low density** in which the cystic areas lack visible walls except where bounded by interlobular septa.
  - CT is helpful in evaluating the extent of emphysematous disease and in planning for surgical procedures designed to remove bullae to reduce lung volume.

Blebs and Bullae, Cysts and Cavities

- Blebs, bullae (singular: bulla), cysts, and cavities are all **air-containing lesions in the lung** of differing **size, location,** and **wall composition.**
- Almost any of these lesions can contain **fluid** instead of, or in addition to, air.
  - Fluid usually develops as a result of **infection, hemorrhage,** or **liquefaction necrosis.**
  - When these lesions are **completely filled with fluid,** they will **appear solid** on conventional radiographs and CT scans, but they will typically demonstrate a **low CT number** that will differentiate them from a solid tumor.
  - When they contain some fluid and some air, they will manifest an **air-fluid level** on a conventional radiograph (exposed with a horizontal x-ray beam) or on CT scans (Fig. 14-13).

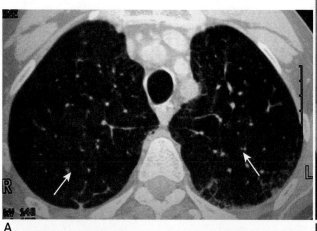

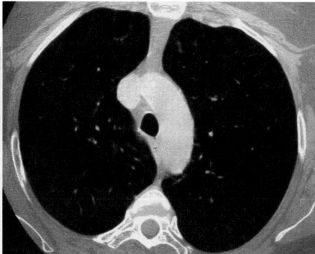

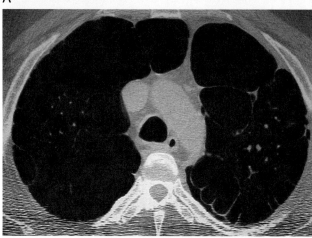

Figure 14-11. **Types of emphysema.** **Centriacinar (centrilobular) emphysema (A)** *features focal destruction limited to the respiratory bronchioles and the central portions of the acinus (closed white arrows). It is associated with cigarette smoking and is most severe in the upper lobes.* **Panacinar (panlobular) emphysema (B)** *involves the entire alveolus distal to the terminal bronchiole, is most severe in the lower lung zones and generally develops in patients with homozygous α₁-antitrypsin deficiency.* **Paraseptal emphysema (C)** *is the least common form; it involves distal airway structures, alveolar ducts, and sacs; tends to be subpleural, and may cause pneumothorax.*

BLEBS

- **Blebs are very small.**
- They are located **within** the **visceral pleura,** usually at the **apex** of the lung.
- They are **very thin-walled** and usually too small to be visible.

BULLAE

- Bullae measure **more than 1 cm.**
  - They can **grow to fill the entire hemithorax** and compress the lung to such an extent on the affected side, the lung seems to disappear (*vanishing lung syndrome*).
- They occur in the **lung parenchyma.**
- They have a **very thin wall** (<1 mm) that is frequently **only partially visible** on conventional radiography (Fig. 14-14).
  - On **conventional radiographs** their **presence is often inferred** by a localized paucity of lung markings.
- Although they usually contain only air, bullae can develop an **air-fluid level** through infection or hemorrhage.
- They are usually **associated with emphysema.**

CYSTS

- Cysts are either congenital or acquired.

- They can occur in either the **lung parenchyma** or the **mediastinum.**
- They have a **thin wall** but usually thicker than a bulla (< 3 mm).
  - *Pneumatoceles* represent **thin-walled cysts** that usually develop after a lung infection caused by such organisms as *Staphylococcus* or *Pneumocystis* or following trauma (Fig. 14-15).

CAVITIES

- Cavities can **vary in size** from a few millimeters to many centimeters.
  - They usually **result from a process that results in necrosis** of the central portion of the lesion.
- They occur in the **lung parenchyma.**
- Cavities usually have **the thickest wall** of any of these four air-containing lesions **with a wall thickness from 3 mm to several centimeters** (Fig. 14-16).
  - Differentiation between three of the most frequent causes of cavities (carcinoma, pyogenic abscess, and tuberculosis) is discussed in Chapter 13 (see Fig. 13-20).

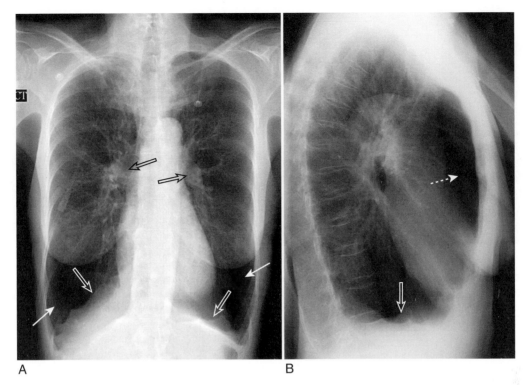

Figure 14-12. Emphysema. *On conventional radiographs, the imaging findings of chronic obstructive pulmonary disease (COPD) are hyperinflation, including flattening of the diaphragm, especially on the lateral exposure* **(B)** *(open white arrows),* increase in the retrosternal clear space *(dotted white arrow), hyperlucency of the lungs with fewer than normal vascular markings (closed white arrows)* **(A),** *and prominence of the pulmonary arteries secondary to pulmonary arterial hypertension (open black arrows).*

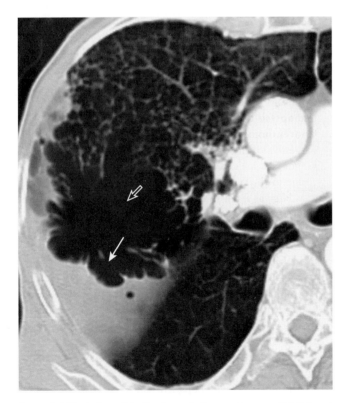

Figure 14-13. Infected bulla. *Large bulla contains some fluid (closed white arrow) and some air (open white arrow). Bullae normally contain air but can become partially or completely fluid-filled if they become infected or there is hemorrhage into them.*

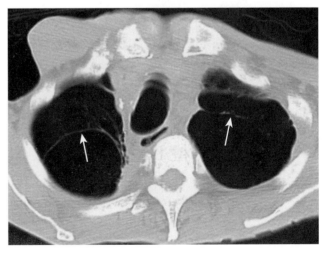

Figure 14-14. Bullous disease. *Bullae measure larger than 1 cm. They have a very thin wall (<1 mm) (closed white arrows) that is often only partially visible on conventional radiography. Characteristically, they contain no blood vessels but there may be septa that appear to traverse the bullae. On conventional radiographs their presence is often inferred by a localized paucity of lung markings (see Fig. 9-5).*

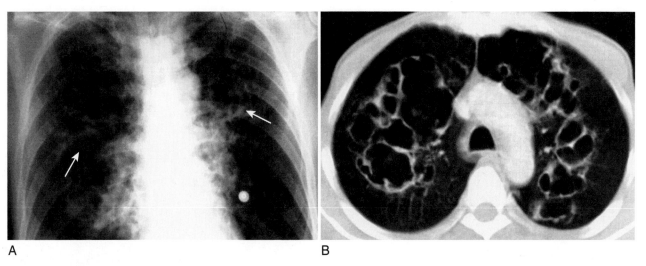

A   B

Figure 14-15. **Cysts (pneumatoceles) in Pneumocystis pneumonia (PCP).** *Cysts are visible on chest radiographs in 10% of patients with PCP (closed white arrows in* **A**), *and far more frequently with HRCT scans (up to 33%). They may occur in the acute or in the postinfective phase of the disease. They have a predilection for the upper lobes and are commonly multiple* **(B).** *Their etiology is unclear.*

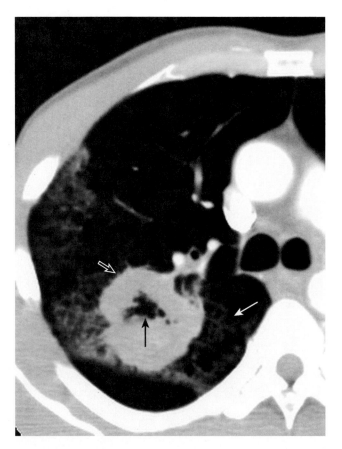

Figure 14-16. **Cavitary bronchogenic carcinoma.** *There is a thick-walled cavitary lesion in the right upper lobe (open white arrow). The inner margin of the cavity is nodular and irregular (closed black arrow). There is pneumonia surrounding a portion of the mass (closed white arrow). This was a squamous cell carcinoma of the lung.*

Bronchiectasis
- Bronchiectasis is defined **as localized irreversible dilatation of part of the bronchial tree.**
- Although it can be associated with many other diseases, it is **usually caused by necrotizing bacterial infections** such as those of *Staphylococcus* and *Klebsiella* and it usually affects the lower lobes.
  - Bronchiectasis also occurs with cystic fibrosis, primary ciliary dyskinesia (***Kartagener's syndrome***), allergic bronchopulmonary aspergillosis, and ***Swyer-James syndrome*** (unilateral hyperlucent lung).
- Clinically, **chronic productive cough** and associated **hemoptysis** are the major symptoms.
- **Conventional radiographs** may demonstrate findings suggestive of the disease but are **usually not specific.**
  - Findings include parallel-line opacities (***tram-tracks***) due to thickened, dilated bronchial walls, **cystic lesions** as large as 2 cm in diameter due to cystic bronchiectasis, and **tubular densities** from fluid-filled bronchi (Fig. 14-17).
- Today, **HRCT is the study of choice in diagnosing bronchiectasis.**
  - The hallmark lesion is the ***signet ring sign*** in which the **bronchus,** frequently with a thickened wall, **becomes larger than its associated pulmonary artery,** which is the opposite of the normal relationship between the two (Fig. 14-18).
  - The bronchus may also show a failure to taper normally.

Chest Trauma
- Chest injuries in trauma patients are **very common** and are responsible for 25% of trauma-related deaths.
  - Trauma-related chest injuries are classified by the two major mechanisms that produce them:

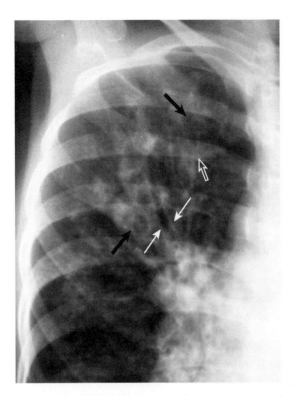

Figure 14-17. ***Bronchiectasis in cystic fibrosis.*** *Conventional radiographs may demonstrate parallel line opacities called* **tramtracks** *due to thickened walls of dilated bronchi (closed white arrows), cystic lesions as large as 2 cm in diameter due to cystic bronchiectasis (closed black arrows), and tubular densities from fluid-filled bronchi (open white arrow). Bilateral upper lobe bronchiectasis in children is highly suggestive of cystic fibrosis.*

- **Blunt trauma,** in which the chest wall remains intact, is usually the result of motor vehicle accidents and is the more common of the two.
  - **Penetrating trauma** is usually the result of accidental or criminal stabbings and gunshot wounds.
- Table 14-3 summarizes some of the injuries that may result from chest trauma and the chapter in which they are discussed; *pulmonary contusions* and *hematomas* along with *aortic trauma* will be discussed in this chapter.

PULMONARY CONTUSIONS

- Pulmonary contusions are the most frequent complications of blunt chest trauma.
- They **represent hemorrhage into the lungs,** usually at the point of impact.
- **Recognizing a pulmonary contusion** (Fig. 14-19)
  - The **history of trauma** is of **paramount importance** as contusions present as **airspace disease** that is **indistinguishable from other airspace diseases** (e.g., pneumonia or aspiration).
  - They tend to be **peripherally placed** and **frequently occur at the point of maximum impact.**
  - **Air bronchograms** are usually **not present** because blood fills the bronchi as well as the airspaces.
- Classically, they **appear within 6 hours after the trauma** and, because blood in the airspaces tends to be reabsorbed quickly, **disappear within 72 hours,** frequently sooner.
- Airspace disease that **lingers more than 72 hours** should **raise suspicions** of another process such as **aspiration pneumonia** or a **pulmonary laceration** (see the next topic).

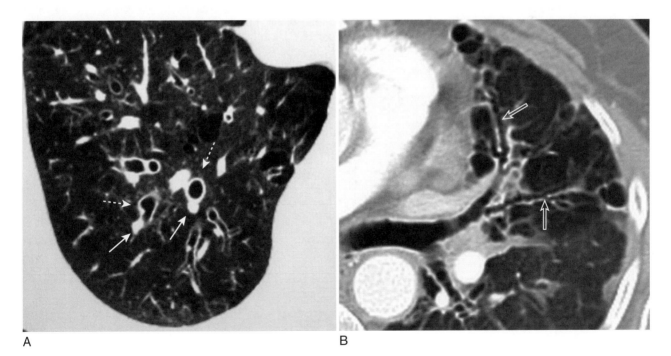

A   B

Figure 14-18. ***Bronchiectasis.*** *HRCT is the study of choice in diagnosing bronchiectasis. The hallmark lesion is the* **signet ring sign,** *seen in this patient with bronchiectasis* **(A)** *in which the bronchus with a thickened wall (dotted white arrows) becomes larger than its associated pulmonary artery (closed white arrows), which is the opposite of the normal relationship between the two. The bronchus may also show* **tram-tracking,** *thickened walls, and a failure to taper normally* **(B)** *(open white arrows).*

Table 14-3

PULMONARY ABNORMALITIES IN CHEST TRAUMA

Injury	Discussed in
Pleural effusion/hemothorax	Chapter 7
Aspiration	Chapter 8
Pneumothorax, pneumomediastinum, and pneumopericardium	Chapter 9
Pulmonary contusion, laceration (hematoma), and aortic trauma	Chapter 14
Rib fractures	Chapter 22

PULMONARY LACERATIONS (HEMATOMA OR TRAUMATIC PNEUMATOCELE)

- Pulmonary hematomas result from a **laceration of the lung parenchyma** and, as such, may accompany more severe **blunt trauma or penetrating chest trauma.**
- The laceration has been variously called a *traumatic pneumatocele* or *hematoma.*

- They are sometimes masked, at least for the first few days, by the airspace disease in a surrounding pulmonary contusion.
- **Recognizing a pulmonary laceration** (Fig. 14-20)
  - Their **appearance will depend on whether they contain blood and, if so, how much** blood fills the pneumatocele.
    - If they are **completely filled** with **blood,** they will appear as an **ovoid mass.**
    - If they are **partially filled with blood** and **partially filled with air,** they may contain a visible **air-fluid level** or demonstrate a *crescent sign* as the blood begins to form a clot and pull away from the wall of the pneumatocele.
    - If they are **completely filled with air,** they will appear as an **air-containing cyst-like structure** in the lung.
- Unlike pulmonary contusions that clear rapidly, **pulmonary lacerations,** especially if they are blood-filled, **may take weeks or months to completely clear.**

AORTIC TRAUMA

- Most frequently the result of **deceleration injuries in motor vehicle accidents;** only those with incomplete tears in which the **adventitial lining prevents exsanguination** survive to be imaged.

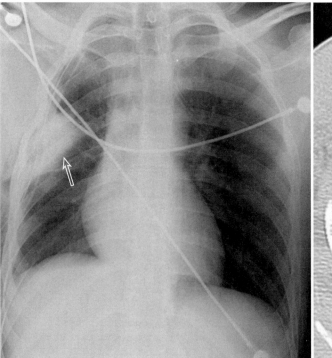
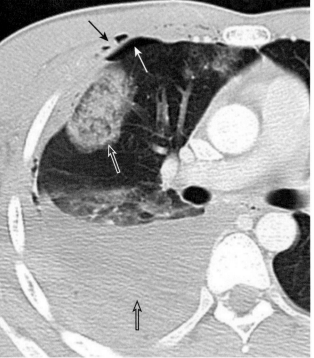

A   B

Figure 14-19. **Pulmonary contusion, chest radiograph and CT.** *Pulmonary contusions tend to be peripherally placed and frequently at the point of maximum impact (open white arrows in **A** and **B**). Air bronchograms are usually not present because blood fills the bronchi as well as the airspaces. This patient, who was an unrestrained passenger in an automobile accident, also has a large hemothorax (open black arrow) and a small pneumothorax (closed white arrow) seen on CT. The fluid has collected in a subpulmonic location and is not as evident on the frontal chest radiograph. A small amount of subcutaneous emphysema is present (closed black arrow in **B**).*

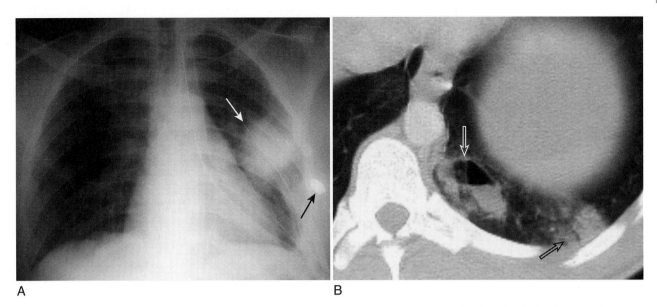

A   B

Figure 14-20. **Laceration, conventional radiograph and CT.** *Lacerations are sometimes masked, at least for the first few days, by the airspace disease in a surrounding pulmonary contusion. If they are completely filled with blood, as in this patient* **(A),** *they will appear as an ovoid mass (closed white arrow). Notice the bullet that produced the laceration (closed black arrow). If they are partially filled with blood and partially filled with air* **(B),** *lacerations may contain a visible air-fluid level (open white arrow). Unlike pulmonary contusions (open black arrow) that clear rapidly, pulmonary lacerations, especially if they are blood-filled, may take weeks or months to completely clear.*

- The most common site of injury is the **aortic isthmus,** which is the portion of the **aorta just distal to the origin of the left subclavian artery.**
- Only emergency repair will prevent approximately 50% from dying within the first 24 hours if left untreated.
- **Recognizing aortic trauma**
  - **Findings seen on conventional radiographs of the chest** are the same as those discussed under "Aortic Dissection" in Chapter 13.
    - "Widening of the mediastinum" is a **poor means of establishing the diagnosis** because it is difficult to assess on a supine, portable chest radiograph and it is commonly overinterpreted.
    - **Left pleural effusion** (see Fig. 13-11)
    - **Left apical pleural cap** of fluid or blood
    - **Loss of the normal shadow of the aortic knob**
    - **Deviation of the trachea or esophagus to the right**
  - **Findings on contrast-enhanced CT scans of the chest**
    - These findings are **frequently subtle** (those with the more obvious findings will not have survived to be imaged) and require experience to recognize.
    - They include **mediastinal hemorrhage,** delineation of a **contrast-filled collection outside the normal confines of the aorta** representing extravasation, and **hemopericardium** (Fig. 14-21).
  - Patients with **equivocal** CT findings may go on to a catheter study of the aorta (**aortography**).

Pericardial Effusion

- CT scanning can demonstrate pericardial effusions, although pericardial sonography would be the imaging study of first choice.

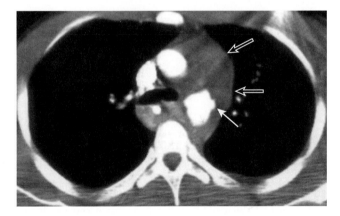

Figure 14-21. **Aortic tear.** *Findings of aortic trauma on contrast-enhanced CT scans of the chest are frequently subtle, as those with the most obvious findings will probably not have survived. In this patient involved in a motor vehicle collision, the findings are not subtle. There is mediastinal hemorrhage (open white arrows) and, in the region of the aortic isthmus, an irregular contrast-filled collection projecting outside the normal confines of the aorta. This collection represents a confined perforation or a* **pseudoaneurysm** *of the aorta (closed white arrow).*

- Fluid first begins to accumulate in the **dependent portions of the pericardial space,** which in a supine individual means that it will be visible **posterior to the left ventricle** (Fig. 14-22A).
- As it increases in size, it tends to appear **more along the right heart border** until it fills the pericardial space and **encircles the heart** (Fig. 14-22B).

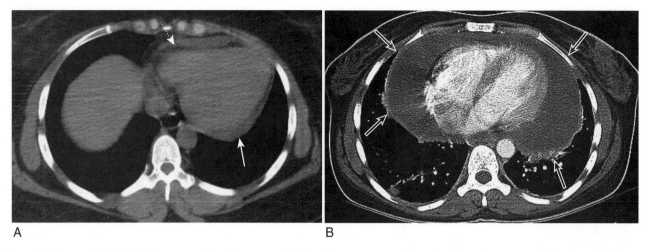

A   B

Figure 14-22. **Pericardial effusions, small and large. A,** *Fluid first begins to accumulate in the dependent portions of the pericardial space, which in a supine individual means that it will be visible posterior to the left ventricle (closed white arrow). There is also fluid anterior to the right ventricle (dotted white arrow). As the effusion increases in size, it fills the pericardial space and encircles the heart (**B**) (open white arrows). Conventional chest radiographs (see Fig. 10-22) show the enlarged cardiac silhouette but cannot differentiate the density of the heart from the effusion.*

Box 14-2

Causes of Pericardial Effusion
Congestive heart failure
Infection (tuberculosis, viral)
Metastatic malignancy (lung and breast, especially)
Uremic pericarditis
Collagen vascular disease (lupus)
Trauma
Post-pericardiotomy syndrome

- **Pericardial thickening** from inflammation **can produce a similar picture.**
  - **Pericardial thickening will enhance with intravenous contrast,** which helps to differentiate it from pericardial effusion.
- The appearance of pericardial effusion on conventional radiographs is discussed in Chapter 10, The ABCs of Heart Disease.
- Some of the causes of pericardial effusions are outlined in Box 14-2.

Cardiac CT

- Faster multislice CT scanners and ECG-gated acquisition to reduce motion artifact, along with powerful computer algorithms, now allow for the imaging and three-dimensional reconstruction of the coronary arteries, including measurement of the amount of **coronary artery calcium,** evaluation for **vessel patency,** and identification of the presence of **thrombus** in the lumen or **plaque** in the vessel wall following the administration of intravenous contrast agent.

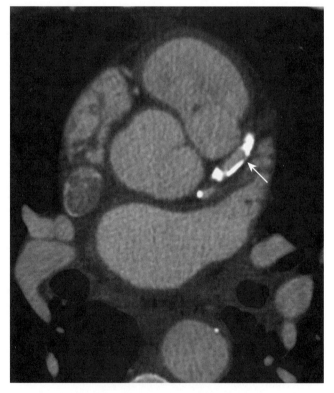

Figure 14-23. **Coronary artery calcification.** *There is dense calcification (closed white arrow) in the left anterior descending coronary artery arising from the aorta. It is now possible to image the coronary arteries, measure the amount of coronary artery calcium and, following the administration of intravenous contrast material, evaluate for vessel patency and identify the presence of thrombus in the lumen or plaque in the vessel wall.*

- By reconstructing multiple phases of the cardiac cycle, it is also possible to analyze wall motion and evaluate ejection fraction and myocardial perfusion.

- **Calcium scoring** is based on the premise that the amount of calcium in the coronary arteries is related to the degree of atherosclerosis and that quantifying the amount of calcium may help predict future cardiac events related to coronary artery disease.
  - The scoring is done by calculations that include the amount of calcium present in the coronary arteries visualized (Fig. 14-23).
  - The **absence** of coronary artery calcification has a high negative predictive value for significant luminal narrowing.

- It may be possible to perform an ultrafast CT scan in the emergency department that will allow for the simultaneous evaluation of **coronary artery disease, aortic dissection,** and **pulmonary thromboembolic disease,** the so-called *triple scan* for patients who present with **acute chest pain.**

WebLink
More information on recognizing the basics on CT of the chest is available to registered users on StudentConsult.com.

 TAKE-HOME POINTS: Recognizing the Basics on CT of the Chest

CT scanners produce a computer-generated representation of human anatomy based on measurements of the density of the tissue scanned, which is determined by the amount the x-ray beam is absorbed or transmitted by the tissues at each point in the scan

High-resolution computed tomography (HRCT) uses a finely collimated x-ray beam and a special computer algorithm which makes it particularly useful for the study and characterization of diffuse parenchymal lung diseases

Spiral CT scanners use a continuously rotating x-ray detector combined with constant table movement to permit rapid and "gapless" data acquisition that can be obtained in a single breath-hold by the patient thus allowing for diagnostically useful images in the coronal and sagittal planes as well as 3D reconstructions that can be viewed at any angle

CT scans can be performed without and/or with intravenous contrast and displayed in any number of **windows** that allow the original data acquired to be viewed with optimum density settings for the lungs, mediastinum, or bone without the need for re-scanning the patient

Normal anatomy of major structures is described at 6 levels in the chest from top to bottom: five-vessel view, aortic arch, aorto-pulmonary window, main pulmonary artery, upper cardiac and lower cardiac levels

Conventional radiography has a high false negative rate in pulmonary thromboembolic disease because demonstration of "classic" findings like Hampton's Hump, Westermark's sign, and the Knuckle sign is infrequent

CT pulmonary angiography (CT-PA), made possible by the fast data acquisition of spiral CT scanners (one breath hold) combined with rapid bolus intravenous injection of iodinated contrast, produces images of the pulmonary arteries with little or no motion artifact

Chronic obstructive pulmonary disease (COPD) consists of emphysema and chronic bronchitis; of the two, chronic bronchitis is a clinical diagnosis, while emphysema is defined pathologically and has findings that can be seen on both conventional radiographs and CT scans

Blebs, bullae, cysts and cavities are all air-containing lesions in the lung which differ in size, location and wall composition; bullae, cysts and cavities are seen on CT and may also be seen on conventional radiographs

Although bronchiectasis may be seen on conventional radiographs in the form of tram-tracks, cystic lesions and tubular densities, HRCT is the study of choice in diagnosing bronchiectasis

Chest injuries are responsible for 25% of the trauma-related deaths and are generally divided into two major mechanisms: *blunt trauma* (the more common) usually the result of motor vehicle accidents, and *penetrating trauma* which is usually the result of accidental or criminal stabbings and gunshot wounds

Findings of pulmonary contusion, pulmonary laceration, and traumatic aortic injuries are described in this chapter; other findings that can occur in trauma to the chest are discussed in other chapters (see *Table 14-3*)

There are many causes of a pericardial effusion, but all effusions tend to first accumulate in the dependent portions of the pericardial space (on CT) and then, with increasing size, finally encircle the heart

Faster multislice CT scanners allow for the measurement of the amount of coronary artery calcium, can evaluate for vessel patency, and identify the presence of thrombus in the lumen or plaque in the vessel wall following the administration of intravenous contrast

15 Recognizing the Normal Abdomen: Conventional Radiographs

- Although imaging of the abdomen is now largely performed utilizing CT, ultrasound, or MRI, many patients have "plain films" of the abdomen as a first step before other imaging studies are performed or as a method of following up on findings demonstrated by other modalities.
  - As always, the principles that guide the interpretation of conventional radiographs apply to the modalities of CT, MRI, and ultrasound.
- In order to recognize *abnormal* findings on conventional radiographs of the abdomen, you must familiarize yourself with the appearance of *normal* findings first.

What to Look for

- **First,** look at the **overall gas pattern** (Box 15-1).
  - You are looking for the overall pattern, so don't spend too much time trying to identify every bubble of bowel gas you see.
- **Second,** check to see if there is **extraluminal air.**
- **Third,** look for **abnormal abdominal calcifications.**
- **Fourth,** look for any **soft tissue masses.**

Normal Bowel Gas Pattern

- Virtually all gas in the bowel comes from swallowed air.
  - Only a fraction comes from the bacterial fermentation of food.
- **Stomach**
  - There is almost **always air in the stomach,** unless
    - The patient has recently vomited.
    - There is a nasogastric tube in the stomach and the tube is attached to suction.
- **Small bowel**
  - There is usually a small amount of **air in about two to three loops of nondistended small bowel** (Fig. 15-1).
    - The **normal diameter of small bowel is less than 2.5 cm,** which is about 1 inch or the diameter of one United States quarter.

- Loops of bowel that contain a sufficient amount of air to fill the lumen completely are said to be ***distended.***
  - ***Distention*** of bowel is **normal.**
- Loops of bowel that are filled beyond their normal size are said to be ***dilated.***
  - ***Dilatation*** of the bowel is **not normal.**
- **Large bowel**
  - There is **almost always air in the rectum or sigmoid.**
  - There may be **varying amounts of gas** in the remainder of the **colon** (Fig. 15-2).
  - Use this rule to decide if the large bowel is dilated or not:

Box 15-1

Recognizing the Normal Abdomen—What to Look For
The gas pattern
Extraluminal air
Calcifications
Soft-tissue masses

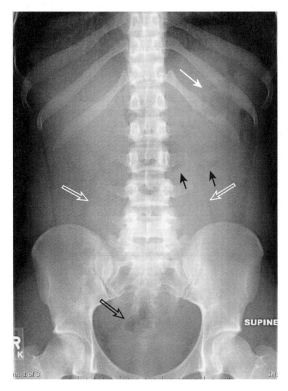

Figure 15-1. **Normal supine abdomen.** This is the "scout" film of the abdomen, the one that gives you a general idea of the bowel gas pattern, allows you to search for radiopaque calculi, and helps detect organomegaly. There is usually a small amount of air in about two to three loops of nondistended small bowel (closed black arrows). There will almost always be air in the stomach (closed white arrow) and in the rectosigmoid (open black arrow). Depending on the amount of fat around the visceral organs, their outlines may be partially visible on conventional radiographs. The psoas muscles are outlined by fat (open white arrows), making them visible on this exposure.

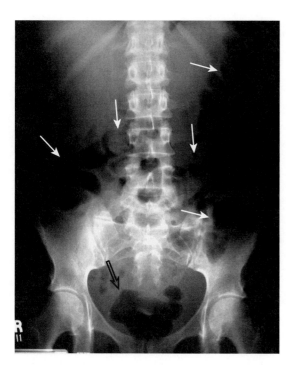

Figure 15-2. **Normal prone abdomen.** In the prone position, the ascending and descending colon as well as the rectosigmoid, all posterior structures, are most posterior and thus most likely to fill with air. There is air in the S-shaped rectosigmoid (open black arrow). Air is also seen throughout the remainder of the colon (closed white arrows). The liver occupies the right upper quadrant and normally displaces bowel from this region.

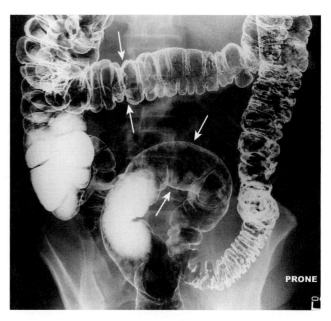

Figure 15-3. **What is normal colonic distention?** Look at a few barium enema studies. The diameter of the colon you see on a barium enema is the size to which the colon can distend (closed white arrows), beyond which it would be considered dilated. This patient has had a **double-contrast barium enema** examination in which both air and barium are instilled as contrast agents. The combination allows for excellent visualization of the mucosal surface of the colon.

- **The large bowel can normally distend to about the same size as it does on a barium enema examination.**
- How large is that? Look at Figure 15-3.
- Stool is recognizable by the **multiple, small bubbles of gas** present within a semisolid-appearing mass (Fig. 15-4).
  - Recognizing the appearance of stool will help in localizing the large bowel.
- Individuals who swallow large quantities of air may develop *aerophagia,* characterized by numerous polygonal, air-containing loops of bowel, none of which are dilated (Fig. 15-5).

Normal Fluid Levels in the Abdomen
- **Stomach**
  - There is almost always fluid in the stomach so there is **almost always an air-fluid level in the stomach** on an upright abdominal or upright chest radiograph or if the patient is in the decubitus position.
    - **To see an air-fluid level, the x-ray beam must be directed horizontally,** parallel to the floor (see Chapter 1, Recognizing Anything).
- **Small bowel**
  - **Two or three air-fluid levels** may be seen normally on an upright or decubitus view of the abdomen.

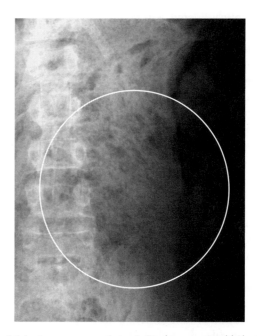

Figure 15-4. **Appearance of stool.** Stool is recognizable by the multiple, small bubbles of gas present within a semisolid-appearing mass (white circle). Stool marks the location of the large bowel and can help in identification of individual loops of bowel on conventional radiographs. This patient has a markedly dilated sigmoid colon from chronic constipation.

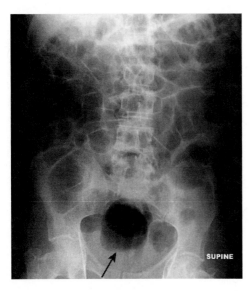

Figure 15-5. **Aerophagia.** *Virtually all bowel gas comes from swallowed air. Swallowing large quantities of air may produce a picture called **aerophagia**, characterized by numerous polygonal, air-containing loops of bowel, none of which is dilated. Notice that there is gas in the rectosigmoid (closed black arrow).*

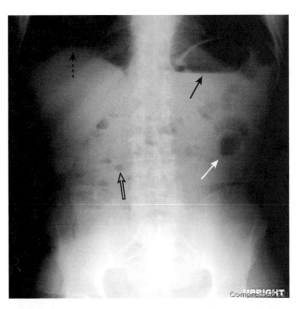

Figure 15-6. **Normal upright abdomen.** *There are two things to look for on an upright view of the abdomen: air-fluid levels and free intraperitoneal air. Normally, there is an air-fluid level in the stomach (closed black arrow). There may be short, air-fluid levels in two or three nondilated loops of small bowel (open black arrow). There are usually very few or no air-fluid levels in the colon (closed white arrow). Free air, if present, should be visible just below the hemidiaphragm (dotted black arrow) and would be easier to recognize on the right than the left, because the stomach bubble is usually present on the left.*

- **Large bowel**
  - The large bowel functions, in part, to remove fluid so **there are usually no, or very few, air-fluid levels in the colon** (Fig. 15-6).
    - There may be **many air-fluid levels** present in the colon if the patient has had a **recent enema** or if the patient is **taking medication with a strong anticholinergic, antiperistaltic effect.**
  - The normal distribution of bowel gas and fluid is summarized in Table 15-1.

Differentiating Large from Small Bowel
- **Large bowel**
  - **Large bowel is peripherally placed** around the perimeter of the abdominal cavity, except for the right upper quadrant, which is occupied by the liver (Fig. 15-7).
  - **Haustral markings usually do not extend completely across the large bowel** from one wall to the other.
    - If they do connect one wall with another, **haustral markings are spaced more widely apart** than the valvulae conniventes of the small bowel (Fig. 15-8).
- **Small bowel**
  - **Small bowel is centrally placed** in the abdomen.
  - **Valvulae markings typically extend across lumen** of small bowel from one wall to the other.
  - The **valvulae are spaced much closer together** than the haustra of the large bowel (Fig. 15-9).
  - **Small bowel can achieve a maximum diameter, even when dilated, of about 5 cm.**
    - **Large bowel can dilate to several times that size.**

Acute Abdominal Series
- Almost every department of radiology has a series of images (a protocol) that is routinely obtained in patients who have acute abdominal pain.

Table 15-1

NORMAL DISTRIBUTION OF GAS AND FLUID IN THE ABDOMEN

Organ	Normally Contains Gas	Normally Has Air Fluid Levels
Stomach	Yes	Yes
Small bowel	Yes, 1–2 loops	Yes
Large bowel	Yes, especially rectosigmoid	No

- These series are sometimes called "obstructions series" or "complete abdominal series" or "acute abdominal series" or the like.
- For the purposes of this book, we'll call such series "acute abdominal series."
- **Views included in the acute abdominal series.**
  - **Supine view** of the abdomen
    - Almost always needed

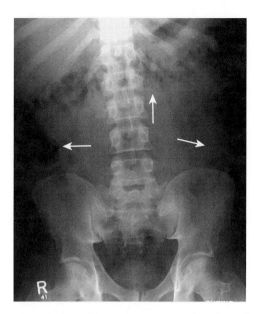

Figure 15-7. **Location of large bowel.** *Large bowel usually occupies the periphery of the abdomen. The small bowel is located more centrally. Here, large bowel (closed white arrows) contains a normal amount of air. There is no air visible in the small bowel.*

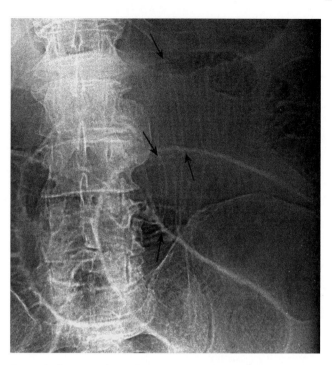

Figure 15-9. **Normal small bowel valvulae.** *Markings representing the valvulae typically do extend across the lumen of the small bowel to extend from one wall to the other. In addition, the valvulae are spaced much closer together than the haustra of the large bowel, even when the bowel is dilated. The closed black arrows point to valvulae that traverse the entire lumen in this enhanced close-up of abnormally dilated small bowel.*

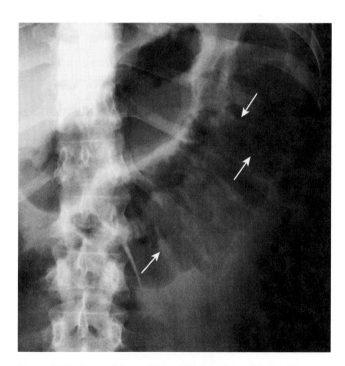

Figure 15-8. **Normal large bowel haustral markings.** *Most haustral markings in the colon do not traverse the entire lumen to extend from one wall to the opposite wall (closed white arrows). This is unlike the appearance of the valvulae conniventes in the small bowel. If the haustral markings do connect one wall with another, they are spaced more widely apart than the valvulae of the small bowel (see Fig. 15-9).*

- **Prone or lateral rectum view**
  - The inclusion of these views is the most variable in different hospital's acute abdominal series.
- **Upright or left-side down (left lateral) decubitus view**
  - One or the other is almost always included.
- **Chest, upright or supine view**
  - Inclusion depends on hospital practices.
- Table 15-2 summarizes **what to look for on each of the views** in an acute abdominal series.

Table 15-2

ACUTE ABDOMINAL SERIES— THE VIEWS AND WHAT TO LOOK FOR

View	Look for
Supine abdomen	Bowel gas pattern, calcifications, masses
Prone abdomen	Gas in the rectosigmoid
Upright abdomen	Free air, air-fluid levels in the bowel
Upright chest	Free air, pneumonia, pleural effusions

SUPINE VIEW ("SCOUT RADIOGRAPH")

- **What it's good for**
  - Showing the **overall appearance of the gas pattern**
    - The **overall appearance of the bowel gas pattern**, including amounts of air and fluid and their most likely location, is **more important** than identifying every small bubble of air on the radiograph.
  - Identifying the **presence or absence of calcifications**
  - Identifying the **presence of soft tissue masses** (see Fig. 15-1)
- **How it's obtained**
  - The patient lies on his or her back on the x-ray table or stretcher and the x-ray beam is directed vertically downward (Fig. 15-10).
- **Substitute view**
  - No other view substitutes for a supine view of the abdomen.
    - Virtually all patients, regardless of their condition, can tolerate this part of the examination.

PRONE VIEW

- **What it's good for**
  - **Identifying gas in the rectum and sigmoid**
    - Because the rectum and sigmoid are the **highest points of the large bowel** with the person lying prone on the x-ray table, air will rise into the rectosigmoid.
    - By the way, almost no air is introduced during the course of a routine rectal examination.
  - **Identifying gas in ascending and descending colon**
    - Because these two parts of the large bowel, along with the rectosigmoid, are also posteriorly placed, air will collect in them when the patient is lying prone (see Fig. 15-2).
- **How it's obtained**
  - The patient lies on his or her abdomen on the x-ray table or stretcher and the x-ray beam is directed vertically downward (Fig. 15-11).

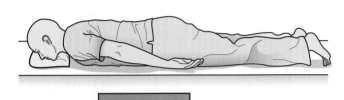

Figure 15-11. **Positioning for prone view of the abdomen.** *The patient lies on his or her abdomen on the x-ray table or stretcher and the x-ray beam is directed vertically downward. The camera icon represents the x-ray tube, which would actually be positioned about 40 inches above the cassette, represented by the thick line.*

- **Substitute view**
  - Frequently, patients are **unable to lie prone** because of their physical condition (recent surgery, severe abdominal pain).
  - These patients can turn on their **left side** and have a **lateral view of the rectum** exposed with a **vertical beam** to substitute for the prone radiograph (Fig. 15-12).
    - The lateral view of the rectum will usually demonstrate the presence or absence of air in the rectum and sigmoid (Fig. 15-13).

UPRIGHT VIEW

- **What it's good for**
  - Seeing **free air in the peritoneal cavity** (i.e., extraluminal air)
  - Seeing **air-fluid levels within the bowel** (see Fig. 15-6)
- **How it's obtained**
  - The patient stands or sits up and exposure is made with the **x-ray beam directed horizontally**, parallel to the plane of the floor (Fig. 15-14).

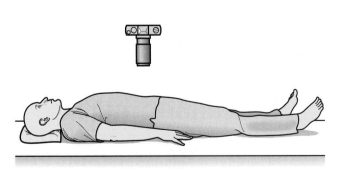

Figure 15-10. **Positioning for supine view of the abdomen.** *The patient lies on his or her back on the x-ray table or stretcher and the x-ray beam is directed vertically downward. The camera icon represents the x-ray tube, which would actually be positioned about 40 inches above the cassette, represented by the thick line.*

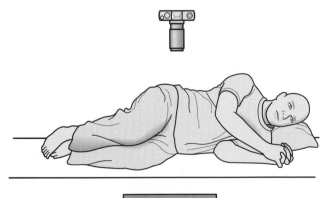

Figure 15-12. **Positioning for the lateral rectum view.** *Patients who cannot lie prone can turn on their left side and have a lateral view of the rectum exposed with a vertical beam to substitute for the prone radiograph. The camera icon represents the x-ray tube, which would actually be positioned about 40 inches above the cassette, represented by the thick line.*

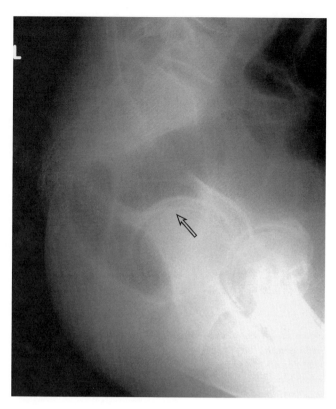

Figure 15-13. **Normal lateral view of the rectum.** *Frequently, patients are unable to lie prone because of their physical condition (recent surgery, severe abdominal pain). These patients can turn on their left side and have a lateral view of the rectum exposed with a vertical beam to substitute for the prone radiograph. The lateral view of the rectum will usually demonstrate the presence or absence of air in the rectum or sigmoid (open black arrow).*

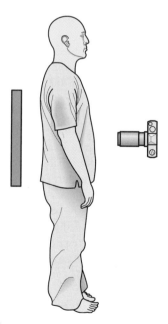

Figure 15-14. **Positioning of patient for an upright view of the abdomen.** *The patient stands or sits up and the x-ray beam is directed horizontally, parallel to the plane of the floor. The camera icon represents the x-ray tube, which would actually be positioned about 40 inches from the cassette, represented by the thick line.*

- **Substitute view**
  - Frequently, patients with the signs and symptoms of an acute abdomen cannot tolerate standing or sitting up for an upright view of their abdomen.
  - In such cases, a **left lateral decubitus view** of the abdomen is substituted for the upright radiograph.
    - For a left lateral decubitus view, the **patient lies on his or her left side on the x-ray table** (Fig. 15-15).
      - This is done so that any **"free air" will distribute itself at the highest part of the abdominal cavity,** which will be the patient's **right** side.
      - **Free air should be easily visible** over the **outside edge of the liver** where there is normally no bowel gas present (Fig. 15-16).

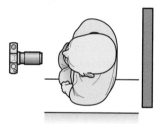

Figure 15-15. **Positioning of the patient for a left lateral decubitus view of the abdomen.** *Patients who cannot tolerate an upright view of their abdomen usually have a left lateral decubitus view as a substitute. The patient lies on their left side on the examining table, the x-ray tube is usually positioned anteriorly (camera icon) and the cassette (thick line) is placed in back of the patient. The x-ray beam is directed horizontally, parallel to the floor at a distance of about 40 inches from the patient.*

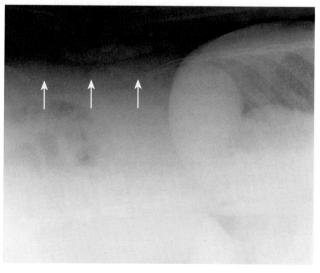

Figure 15-16. **Normal left lateral decubitus view of the abdomen.** *For a left lateral decubitus view, the patient lies on his or her left side on the examining table and an exposure is made with a horizontal x-ray beam (parallel to the floor). This is done so that any "free air" will distribute itself at the highest part of the abdominal cavity, which will be the patient's right side. If present, free air should be easily visible as a black crescent over the outside edge of the liver (closed white arrows), a location in which there is normally no bowel gas present. There is no free air in this patient.*

- If a right lateral decubitus view were obtained, any free air, if present, would rise to the left side of the abdomen.
- The left side of the abdomen is the normal location of the stomach bubble as well as gas in the splenic flexure of the colon, either of which could be confused for free air.
  - In order **to see** the **free air, the x-ray beam must be directed horizontally,** parallel to the floor, when a decubitus view is obtained.
- Box 15-2 summarizes the ingredients which must be present to be able to visualize air-fluid levels in the abdomen.

UPRIGHT VIEW OF THE CHEST

- **What it's good for**
  - Seeing **free air beneath the diaphragm**
  - Finding **pneumonia at the lung bases,** which might mimic the symptoms of an acute abdomen.
  - Finding **pleural effusions,** which could be secondary to an intra-abdominal process and help identify its presence.
    - **Pancreatitis,** for example, **may be associated with a left pleural effusion.**
    - Some **ovarian tumors** may occasionally be associated with **right-sided or bilateral pleural effusions.**
    - An abscess beneath the right hemidiaphragm (subphrenic abscess) **may be associated with a right pleural effusion.**
    - See Chapter 7 for more on the side-preference of selected diseases that cause pleural effusions.
- **How it's obtained**
  - The **patient stands or sits up** and an exposure of the thorax is made using a **horizontal x-ray beam** (Fig. 15-17).
- **Substitute view for an upright chest x-ray**
  - Frequently, patients with the signs and symptoms of an acute abdomen cannot tolerate standing for an upright view of their chest.
  - In those cases, **a supine view of the chest may be obtained** with the patient lying on the stretcher or x-ray table.
  - For a supine view, the x-ray beam is directed **vertically downward** and **free air, especially small amounts, may not be visible.**

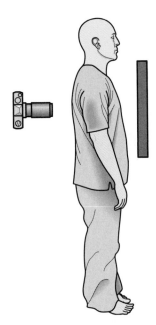

Figure 15-17. **Positioning of patient for an upright chest radiograph.** *The patient sits upright or stands with the anterior chest wall closest to the cassette. The camera icon represents the x-ray tube, which is actually about 72 inches from the cassette, represented by the thick line.*

Extraluminal Air

- Extraluminal air is discussed in Chapter 17, Recognizing Extraluminal Gas in the Abdomen.

Calcifications

- Abdominal calcifications are discussed in Chapter 18, Recognizing Abnormal Calcifications.
- Two abdominal calcifications should not be confused with pathologic calcifications:
  - **Phleboliths** are small, rounded calcifications that represent calcified venous thrombi that occur with increasing age, most often in the pelvic veins of women.
    - They classically have a lucent center (Fig. 15-18).
  - **Calcification of the rib cartilages** occurs with advancing age and, although not a true abdominal calcification, can sometimes be confused for renal or biliary calculi when it overlays the kidney or region of the gallbladder (Fig. 15-19).
    - Calcified cartilage tends to have an amorphous, speckled appearance, and the calcified cartilage will occur in an arc corresponding to that of the anterior rib cartilage as it sweeps back toward the sternum.

Organomegaly

- **Conventional radiographic evaluation of soft tissue structures in the abdomen** (e.g., the liver, spleen, kidneys, gallbladder, urinary bladder, or soft tissue masses such as tumors or abscesses) **is limited** because these structures are **soft tissue densities** and they are **surrounded by other soft tissues or fluid** of similar density.

Box 15-2

Requirements for Visualizing an Air-fluid Level on Conventional Radiograph
Air
Fluid
A horizontal x-ray beam (parallel to the plane of the floor)
Air-fluid interfaces cannot be visualized on conventional radiographs taken with a vertical x-ray beam

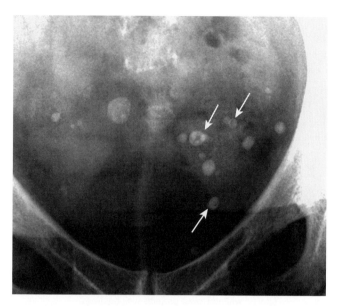

Figure 15-18. **Phleboliths.** *Phleboliths are small, rounded calcifications that represent calcified venous thrombi that occur with increasing age most often in the pelvic veins of women. They classically have a lucent center (closed white arrows). In the pelvic veins, they are considered incidental and nonpathologic calcifications.*

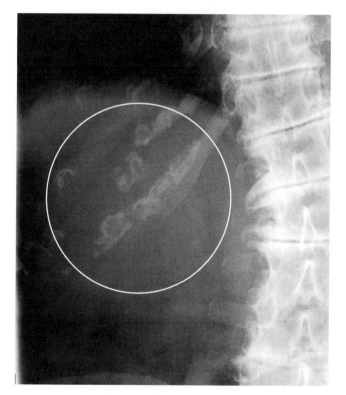

Figure 15-19. **Calcified rib cartilages.** *Calcification of the rib cartilages (white circle) occurs with advancing age and, although not a true abdominal calcification, can sometimes be confused for calculi when it overlays the kidney or region of the gallbladder. Calcified cartilage tends to have an amorphous, mottled appearance. Calcified rib cartilages will occur along an arc corresponding to the sweep of the anterior ribs as they turn back toward the sternum.*

- Only a **difference in density** between a particular structure and those surrounding it **will render that structure's outline visible** on conventional radiographs.
- Still, conventional radiographs are easy to obtain and frequently the first type of study ordered in a patient with abdominal symptoms.
- There are **two fundamental ways of recognizing the presence and estimating the size of soft tissue masses or organs** on conventional radiographs of the abdomen.
  - The first is by **direct visualization of the edges of the structure,** which can only occur if it surrounded by a tissue of a different radiographic density than soft tissue, like that of fat or free air.
  - The second is to recognize **indirect evidence of the mass** or enlarged visceral organ by **recognizing pathologic displacement of air-filled loops of bowel.**

LIVER

- **Normal**
  - The liver normally displaces all bowel gas from the right upper quadrant.
  - Occasionally, a **tongue-like projection of the right lobe** of the liver may extend to the iliac crest, **especially in females.**
    - This is called a *Riedel's lobe* and is normal (Fig. 15-20).
  - **Conventional radiographs are notoriously poor for estimating the size of the liver.**
- **Enlarged**
  - **An enlarged liver might be suggested** from conventional radiographs if there is displacement of all bowel from the right upper quadrant **down to the iliac crest** and **across the midline** (Fig. 15-21).
    - Imaging evaluation of liver size is best made using CT, MRI, or ultrasound.

SPLEEN

- **Normal**
  - The adult **spleen is about 12 cm in length and usually does not project below the 12th posterior rib.**
  - The **stomach bubble** (i.e., air in the gastric fundus) **usually nestles beneath the highest part of the left hemidiaphragm** about midway between the abdominal wall and the spine.
  - As a general rule, the **spleen is about as large as the left kidney.**
- **Enlarged**
  - If the spleen projects well below the 12th posterior rib or displaces the stomach bubble toward or across the midline, the spleen is probably enlarged (Fig. 15-22).

KIDNEYS

- **Normal**
  - Portions of the kidney outlines may be visible on conventional radiographs if there is an adequate amount of perirenal fat present.
  - The **kidney length is approximately the height of four lumbar vertebral bodies** or about **10 to 14 cm in an adult.**

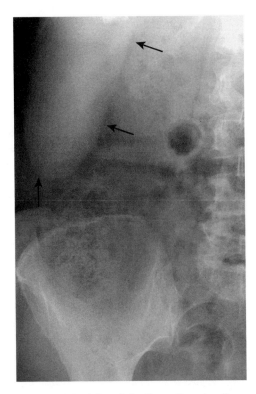

Figure 15-20. **Riedel's lobe of the liver.** *Occasionally, a tongue-like projection of the right lobe of the liver may extend to the iliac crest, especially in females. This is called a Riedel's lobe (closed black arrows) and is normal. Conventional radiographs are notoriously poor for estimating the size of the liver and CT, MRI, and ultrasound give a more accurate picture of liver size.*

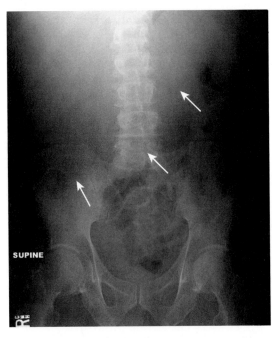

Figure 15-21. **Hepatomegaly.** *Sometimes, the liver can become so enlarged it will be obvious even on conventional radiographs. An enlarged liver might be suggested from conventional radiographs if there is displacement of all bowel loops from the right upper quadrant down to the iliac crest and across the midline (closed white arrows), such as in this patient with cirrhosis.*

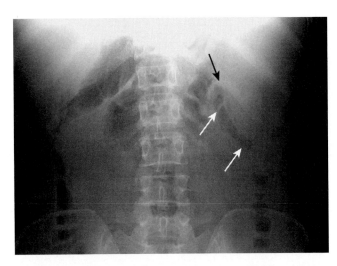

Figure 15-22. **Splenomegaly.** *The spleen is normally about 12 cm in length and usually does not project below the 12th posterior rib. If the spleen (closed white arrows) projects well below the 12th posterior rib (closed black arrow) or displaces the stomach bubble toward or across the midline, the spleen is probably enlarged, as it is in this patient with leukemia.*

- The liver depresses the right kidney so that the **right kidney is usually lower in the abdomen than the left kidney** (Fig. 15-23).
- The left **kidney is roughly the same length as the spleen.**
- Enlarged
  - Usually only extremely enlarged kidneys or large renal masses will be recognizable on conventional radiographs by displacement of bowel gas (Fig. 15-24).

URINARY BLADDER
- **Normal**
  - The bladder frequently is surrounded by **enough extravesical fat that at least the dome is visible** in most individuals as the top of an oval structure with its long axis parallel to the hips and the **base of the bladder just above the top of the symphysis pubis.**
  - When contracted, the urinary bladder is **about the size of a lemon;** it is about the size of a small cantaloupe when distended (Fig. 15-25).
- Enlarged
  - Bladder enlargement is usually recognized by displacement of bowel out of the pelvis by a large soft tissue mass.
    - Bladder outlet obstruction is much more common in men from enlargement of the prostate (Fig. 15-26A).

UTERUS
- **Normal**
  - The uterus usually sits atop the dome of the bladder.
  - There is frequently a lucency between the top of the bladder and the bottom the uterus.
  - The normal uterus is about 8 cm by 4 cm by 6 cm.
- **Enlarged**

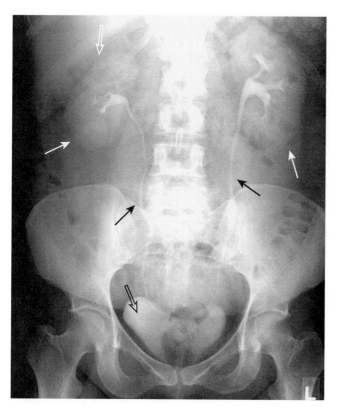

Figure 15-23. **Position of the kidneys.** *This image is from an* **intravenous urogram** *(aka* **intravenous pyelogram [IVP])** *in which the patient receives an intravenous injection of iodinated contrast material that is excreted by the kidneys. Both kidney outlines (closed white arrows), ureters (closed black arrows), and urinary bladder (open black arrow) can be seen. Other images of the kidneys, including oblique views, were often obtained to visualize the entire contour of the kidney. IVPs have largely been replaced by CT scans and CT urograms. The liver (open white arrow) depresses the right kidney more inferiorly than the left kidney.*

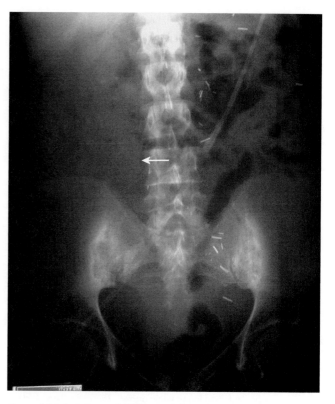

Figure 15-24. **Enlarged kidneys.** *Soft tissue masses or organomegaly can be diagnosed from a conventional radiograph either by visualizing the edge of the mass if there is fat or air surrounding it or by displacement of bowel, as in this case. Note that even though you don't see the outline of the right kidney, there is no bowel gas on the right side of the abdomen (closed white arrow), which should suggest that a soft tissue mass may be displacing the gas from this region. This patient's right kidney was markedly enlarged by multiple cysts. The sacroiliac joints are widened from secondary hyperparathoidism, a consequence of this patient's chronic renal disease.*

- **Ultrasound** is the **best** tool for **evaluating the size of the uterus and ovaries.**
- **Occasionally uterine enlargement,** when marked, **may be visible on conventional radiographs.**
  - The key to differentiating an enlarged uterus from a distended bladder is **identification of a lucency between the bladder and the uterus;** when the uterus is enlarged, the lucency will separate the uterus above from the flattened bladder below; when the soft tissue mass is a distended urinary bladder, the lucency will not be visible (Fig. 15-26B).

PSOAS MUSCLES

- One or both of these muscles may be visible if there is adequate extraperitoneal fat surrounding them.
- Inability to visualize one or both psoas muscles is not a reliable indicator of retroperitoneal disease (see Fig. 15-1).

WebLink

More information about the appearance of the normal abdomen on conventional radiographs is available to registered users on StudentConsult.com.

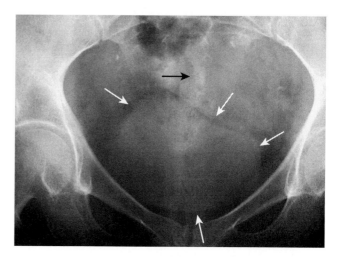

Figure 15-25. **Normal urinary bladder.** *Close-up of the pelvis demonstrates enough perivesical fat present to make the outline (closed white arrows) of the urinary bladder visible. In males, the sigmoid colon usually occupies the space just above the bladder (closed black arrow), but in females, this soft-tissue density may be the uterus or sigmoid colon.*

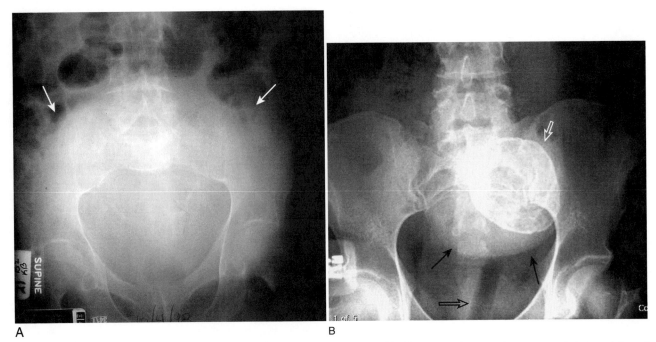

A   B

Figure 15-26. **Distended urinary bladder and enlarged uterus.** *The distended bladder* **(A)** *produces a soft tissue mass that ascends from the pelvis into the lower abdomen* (closed white arrows). *This was a 72-year-old man with bladder outlet obstruction from benign prostatic hypertrophy. The uterus enlarged by multiple leiomyomas* **(B)** *has a plane* (closed black arrows) *between it and the urinary bladder below it. One of the leiomyomas has calcified* (open white arrow). *This is a 60-year-old woman whose symptom of metrorrhagia could be suspected from the presence of a tampon* (open black arrow), *visible because there is air trapped between its fibers.*

🏠 TAKE-HOME POINTS: Recognizing the Normal Abdomen

Evaluation of the abdomen should focus on four main areas: the gas pattern, free air, soft tissue masses or organomegaly, and abnormal calcifications.

There is normally air present in the stomach and colon, especially the rectosigmoid, with a small amount of air (2–3 loops) normal in small bowel.

There is normally an air-fluid level in the stomach; there may be 2–3 air-fluid levels in nondilated small bowel and there is usually no fluid visible in the colon.

An acute abdominal series consists of a supine abdomen, prone abdomen (or its substitute, which is a lateral rectum view), upright abdomen (or its substitute, which is a left lateral decubitus view), and an upright chest (or its substitute, which is a supine chest).

The supine view of the abdomen is the general scout view to determine the bowel gas pattern, the presence of calcifications, and organomegaly or soft tissue masses.

The prone view allows air, if present, to be seen in the rectosigmoid, which is important in the evaluation of mechanical obstruction of the bowel.

The erect abdomen may demonstrate air-fluid levels in the bowel or free peritoneal air.

The erect chest may demonstrate free air beneath the diaphragm, pleural effusion (which may provide a clue as to the presence and nature of intra-abdominal disease), or pneumonia (which can mimic an acute abdomen).

CT, ultrasound, and MRI have essentially replaced conventional radiography in the assessment of organomegaly or soft tissue masses.

16 Recognizing Bowel Obstruction and Ileus

- In Chapter 15, we discussed how to recognize the normal intestinal gas pattern.
- In this chapter, you'll learn how to recognize and categorize four abnormal bowel gas patterns and their causes by **answering three key questions:**
  - **Is there air in the rectum or sigmoid?**
  - **Are there dilated loops of small bowel?**
  - **Are there dilated loops of large bowel?**

Abnormal Gas Patterns

- Abnormal intestinal gas patterns can be divided into two main categories, each of which can be subdivided into two subcategories (Box 16-1).
- *Functional ileus* is one main category in which it is presumed that **one or more loops of bowel lose their ability to propagate the peristaltic waves of the bowel,** usually due to some **local irritation or inflammation,** and hence **cause a functional type of "obstruction"** proximal to the affected loop(s).
- There are **two kinds** of **functional ileus:**
  - *Localized ileus (also called sentinel loops)* **affects only one or two loops** of (usually **small**) **bowel.**
  - *Generalized adynamic ileus* **affects all loops of large and small bowel,** and frequently the stomach.
- *Mechanical obstruction* is the other main category of abnormal bowel gas pattern.
- With mechanical obstruction, a **physical, organic obstructing lesion prevents the passage of intestinal content** past the point of either the small or large bowel blockage.
- There are **two kinds** of **mechanical obstruction:**
  - *Small bowel obstruction* (SBO)
  - *Large bowel obstruction* (LBO)

Laws of the Gut

- The bowel reacts to a mechanical obstruction in more or less predictable ways.
  - Loops **proximal** to the **obstruction** soon become **dilated with air and fluid.**
    - This can occur within 5 hours of a complete small bowel obstruction.
  - **Peristalsis will continue** (except in the loops of bowel involved in a functional ileus) in an attempt to propel intestinal contents through the bowel.
  - Loops **distal** to an **obstruction** will eventually become **decompressed or airless,** as their contents are evacuated.
  - In a mechanical obstruction, **the loop(s) that will become the most dilated** will either be:

- **The loop of bowel with the largest resting diameter before the onset of the obstruction** (e.g., **the cecum** in the large bowel), or
- The **loop(s) of bowel just proximal to the point of obstruction**
- Most patients with a mechanical obstruction will present with some form of **abdominal pain, abdominal distention,** and **constipation.**
  - Patients may present with **vomiting early** in the course of a **proximal small bowel obstruction** and later in the course of the illness with a **distal small bowel obstruction.**
- Let's look at each of the four abnormal bowel gas patterns in detail (Table 16-1).
  - For each of the four abnormalities, we'll look at their **pathophysiology, causes, key imaging features,** and **diagnostic pitfalls.**

Functional Ileus

LOCALIZED ILEUS—SENTINEL LOOPS

- **Pathophysiology**
  - **Focal irritation** of a loop or loops of bowel **occurs most often from inflammation of an adjacent visceral organ** (e.g., pancreatitis may affect bowel loops in the left upper quadrant, diverticulitis in the left lower quadrant).
    - The **loop(s) affected** are almost always loops of **small bowel,** and because they **herald the presence of underlying pathology,** they are called *sentinel loops.*
  - The **irritation causes these loops to lose their normal function and become aperistaltic,** which in turn leads to dilatation of these loops.
  - Because a **functional ileus does not produce the degree of obstruction that a mechanical obstruction does,** some gas continues to pass through the defunctionalized bowel past the point of the localized ileus.

Box 16-1

Abnormal Bowel Gas Patterns

| **Functional Ileus** |
| Localized ileus (sentinel loops) |
| Generalized adynamic ileus |
| **Mechanical Obstruction** |
| Small bowel obstruction (SBO) |
| Large bowel obstruction (LBO) |

Table 16-1

ABNORMAL GAS PATTERNS—SUMMARY

Condition	Air in Rectum or Sigmoid	Air in Small Bowel	Air in Large Bowel
Normal	Yes	Yes, 1–2 loops	Rectum and/or sigmoid
Localized ileus	Yes	2–3 dilated loops	Rectum and/or sigmoid
Generalized ileus	Yes	Multiple dilated loops	Yes, dilated
Small bowel obstruction	No	Multiple dilated loops	No
Large bowel obstruction	No	None unless ileocecal valve incompetent	Yes, dilated

- **Air** usually reaches and **is visible in the rectum or sigmoid.**
- **Causes of a localized ileus**
  - The **dilated loops of bowel tend to occur** in the **same anatomic area** as the **inflammatory or irritative process** of the adjacent abdominal organ, although this may not always be the case.
  - Table 16-2 summarizes **sites of a localized ileus and their most common cause.**
- **Key imaging features of a localized ileus**
  - There are **one or two** *persistently dilated* **loops of small bowel.**
    - *Persistently* means that these **same loops remain dilated** on **multiple views** of the abdomen (supine, prone, erect abdomen) or on **serial studies** done over the course of time.

Table 16-2

CAUSES OF A LOCALIZED ILEUS

Site of dilated loops	Cause(s)
Right upper quadrant	Cholecystitis
Left upper quadrant	Pancreatitis
Right lower quadrant	Appendicitis
Left lower quadrant	Diverticulitis
Mid-abdomen	Ulcer or kidney/ureteral calculus

- *Dilated* means the small bowel loops are **persistently larger than 2.5 cm.**
- Small bowel loops involved in a functional ileus **usually do not dilate as greatly as those which are mechanically obstructed.**
- In some instances the sentinel loop may be **large bowel,** rather than small bowel.
  - This can especially occur in the **cecum,** with diseases like appendicitis.
- **Frequently air-fluid levels** are seen in the **sentinel loops.**
- There is usually **gas in the rectum or sigmoid** in a localized ileus (Fig. 16-1).
- **Pitfalls: Differentiating a localized ileus from an early SBO**
  - A **localized ileus may resemble an** *early* **mechanical SBO,** i.e., there may be a few dilated loops of small bowel with air not yet expelled from the colon.
    - *Early* means the **patient has had symptoms for a day or two.**
    - Patients who have had obstructive symptoms for a week or more usually no longer demonstrate imaging findings of an early obstruction.
  - **Solution**
    - The **clinical findings** may help to **differentiate** localized ileus from small bowel obstruction in that the patient with a **localized ileus** will tend to **manifest the signs and symptoms** of the **underlying inflammatory process** rather than those of intestinal obstruction.
    - For example, elevated pancreatic enzymes may indicate that the dilated small bowel loops in the left upper quadrant are more likely to be sentinel loops from pancreatitis than from an early small bowel obstruction.

GENERALIZED ADYNAMIC ILEUS
- **Pathophysiology**
  - In a generalized adynamic ileus, the **entire bowel is aperistaltic or hypoperistaltic.**
  - Swallowed **air dilates, and fluid fills, all loops of both small and large bowel.**
  - A **generalized adynamic ileus is almost always the result of abdominal or pelvic surgery** in which the bowel is manipulated during the surgery.
- **Causes of a generalized adynamic ileus** are summarized in Table 16-3.
- **Key imaging features of a generalized adynamic ileus**
  - The **entire bowel is usually air-containing and dilated,** both large and small bowel.
    - Frequently the stomach is dilated as well.
  - The absence of peristalsis and the continued production of intestinal secretions usually produces **many long air-fluid levels in the bowel.**
  - Because this is not a mechanical obstruction, there is **usually gas in the rectum or sigmoid.**
  - **Bowel sounds are frequently absent or hypoactive** (Fig. 16-2).

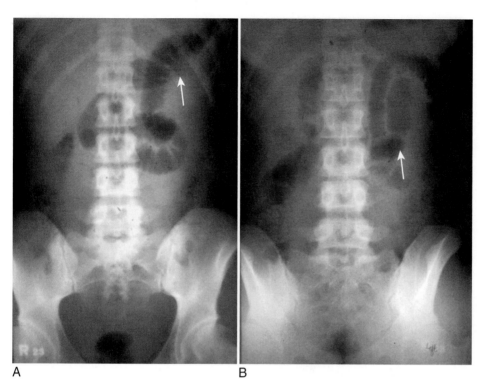

A   B

Figure 16-1. **Sentinel loops from pancreatitis.** *A single, persistently dilated loop of small bowel is seen in the left upper quadrant (closed white arrows) on both the supine **(A)** and prone **(B)** radiographs of the abdomen representing a sentinel loop or localized ileus. A localized ileus is called a **sentinel loop** because it often signals the presence of an adjacent irritative or inflammatory process. This patient had acute pancreatitis.*

Table 16-3

CAUSES OF A GENERALIZED ADYNAMIC ILEUS

Cause	Remarks
Postoperative	Usually abdominal surgery
Electrolyte imbalance	Especially diabetics in ketoacidosis

- **Pitfalls: Recognizing a generalized adynamic ileus**
  - Patients do not present to the emergency department with a generalized adynamic ileus unless they are 1 or 2 days postoperative (abdominal or gynecologic surgery) or they have a severe electrolyte imbalance (e.g., hypokalemia).
  - Many patients who have either **intestinal pseudo-obstruction** (see end of this chapter) **or aerophagia** (Chapter 15) are mistakenly identified as having a generalized ileus on abdominal radiographs.

Mechanical Obstruction

SMALL BOWEL OBSTRUCTION (SBO)

- We'll now shift away from functional ileus to mechanical obstruction of the bowel, starting with small bowel obstruction.
- **Pathophysiology**
  - A lesion either inside or outside the small bowel obstructs the lumen.

- Over time, **from the point of obstruction** *backward,* the **small bowel dilates** from continuously swallowed air and from intestinal fluid, which continues to be produced by the stomach, pancreas, biliary systems, and small bowel.
- **Peristalsis continues and may increase** in an effort to overcome the obstruction.
  - This can lead to **high-pitched, hyperactive bowel sounds.**
- Over time, **from the point of obstruction** *forward,* the **peristaltic waves empty the small bowel distal to the obstructing lesion and the colon of its contents.**
- If the obstruction is **complete** and if enough time has elapsed since the onset of symptoms, **there should be no air in the rectum or sigmoid.**
- **Causes of a mechanical small bowel obstruction** are summarized in Table 16-4.
- **Key imaging features of mechanical small bowel obstruction**
  - **Multiple dilated loops of small bowel** proximal to the point of the obstruction (>2.5 cm)
    - As they begin to dilate, **small bowel loops** *stack up on one another forming a* *step-ladder* appearance, usually beginning in the left upper quadrant and proceeding, depending on how distal the small bowel obstruction is, to the right lower quadrant (Fig. 16-3).
  - Generally speaking, **the more proximal the small bowel obstruction** (e.g., proximal jejunum), **the fewer dilated loops** there will be; the **more distal the**

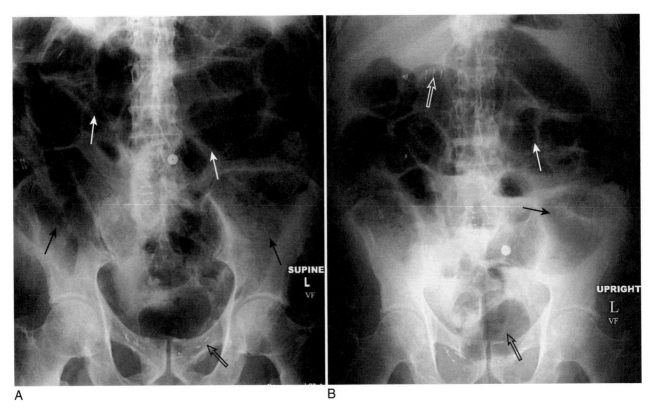

A   B

Figure 16-2. **Generalized adynamic ileus, supine (A) and erect (B) abdomen.** *Dilated loops of large* (closed black arrows) *and small bowel* (closed white arrows) *are seen down to and including the rectum* (open black arrows). *The upright image* **(B)** *shows surgical clips* (open white arrow) *just to the right of the upper lumbar spine. The patient had undergone abdominal surgery the day before.*

Table 16-4

CAUSES OF A MECHANICAL SMALL BOWEL OBSTRUCTION

Cause	Remarks
Postsurgical adhesions	Most frequent following appendectomy, colorectal surgery, and pelvic surgery
Malignancy	Primary malignancies of the small bowel are rare; secondary tumors (e.g., gastric and colonic carcinomas and ovarian cancers) may compromise the lumen of small bowel
Hernia	An inguinal hernia may be visible on conventional radiographs if air-containing loops of bowel are seen over the obturator foramen
Gallstone ileus	May be visible on conventional radiographs if air is seen in the biliary tree and (rarely) a gallstone in right lower quadrant (see Fig. 17-17)
Intussusception	Ileocolic intussusception is the most common form and produces small bowel obstruction
Inflammatory bowel disease	Thickening of the bowel wall may occur with compromise of the lumen in patients with Crohn's disease; this is most likely to occur in the terminal ileum

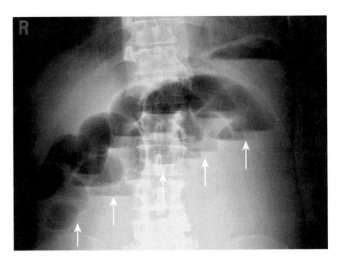

Figure 16-3. **Step-ladder appearance of obstructed small bowel.** *As they begin to dilate, small bowel loops stack up, forming a* **step-ladder** *appearance usually beginning in the left upper quadrant and proceeding, depending on how distal the small bowel obstruction is, to the right lower quadrant* (closed white arrows). *The more proximal the small bowel obstruction (e.g., proximal jejunum), the fewer dilated loops there will be; the more distal the obstruction (e.g., at the ileocecal valve), the greater the number of dilated small bowel loops. This was a distal small bowel obstruction caused by a carcinoma of the colon, which obstructed the ileocecal valve.*

obstruction (e.g., at the ileocecal valve), the **greater the number of dilated small bowel loops.**

- On erect or decubitus views, there will usually be **numerous air-fluid levels in the small bowel** proximal to the obstruction.
- If enough time has elapsed to decompress and empty the bowel distal to the point of obstruction, **there will be little or no gas in the colon, especially the rectum.**
- Remember, the key to recognizing a mechanical small bowel obstruction is to **recognize a disproportionate dilatation of small bowel compared to the large bowel** (Fig. 16-4).
- **Pitfalls: Differentiating a SBO from a functional (localized) adynamic ileus**
  - An early mechanical small bowel obstruction (patient will have had obstructive symptoms for a short time) **may resemble a localized functional ileus,** especially if the sentinel loops are located in the left upper quadrant.
  - An **intermittent** (also known as a *partial* or *incomplete*) mechanical small bowel obstruction allows some gas to pass the point of obstruction, at least at times, and can lead to a confusing picture because gas may pass into the colon and be visible long after the large bowel would be expected to be devoid of such gas (Fig. 16-5).
    - **Partial or incomplete small bowel obstruction** occurs **more often in patients** in whom **adhesions** are the cause.

- CT with oral contrast material or small bowel follow-through with either barium or iodinated, water-soluble contrast may be helpful in demonstrating a partial small bowel obstruction.
- For more about the CT findings of mechanical small bowel obstruction, see Chapter 19, Recognizing Tumors, Tics, and Ulcers.

LARGE BOWEL OBSTRUCTION (LBO)
- **Pathophysiology**
  - A lesion either inside or outside the colon causes obstruction to the lumen.
  - Over time, from the point of obstruction *backward,* the **large bowel dilates** with the **cecum frequently attaining the greatest diameter,** even if the obstruction is as far away as the sigmoid colon.
  - The large bowel normally functions to reabsorb water, so there are **usually few or no air-fluid levels in the obstructed colon.**
  - Over time, from the point of obstruction *forward,* continuing peristaltic waves **empty the colon distal to the point of obstruction,** especially the rectum.
  - There is **usually no air in the rectum in a mechanical large bowel obstruction.**
- **Causes of a mechanical large bowel obstruction** are summarized in Table 16-5.
- **Key imaging features of a mechanical large bowel obstruction**

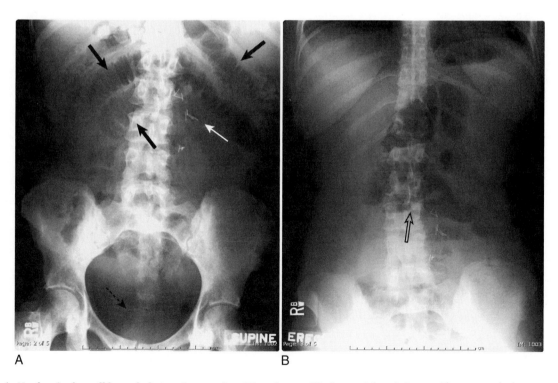

A   B

*Figure 16-4. **Mechanical small bowel obstruction, supine (A) and erect (B) views of the abdomen.** There are multiple air-containing and dilated loops of small bowel. On the supine image **(A),** there are dilated loops of small bowel (closed black arrows) and no gas is seen in the rectum (dotted black arrow). On the erect image **(B),** there are numerous dilated small bowel loops with air-fluid levels (open black arrow). Adhesions from prior surgery is the most likely cause of a mechanical small bowel obstruction, as it was in this patient (closed white arrow on image A points to surgical clips).*

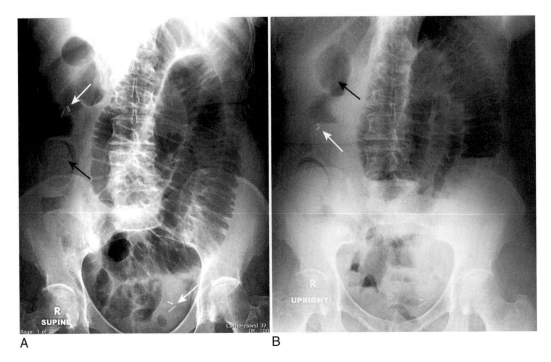

A   B

*Figure 16-5. **Partial small bowel obstruction, supine (A) and upright (B) views.** A partial or incomplete mechanical small bowel obstruction allows some gas to pass the point of obstruction, possibly on an intermittent basis. This can lead to a confusing picture because gas may pass into the colon (closed black arrows) and be visible long after the large bowel would be expected to be devoid of gas. The important observation is that the small bowel is disproportionately dilated compared to the large bowel, a finding suggestive of small bowel obstruction. Partial or incomplete small bowel obstructions occur more often in patients in whom adhesions are the cause. Notice the clips (closed white arrows) attesting to prior abdominal surgery.*

Table 16-5

CAUSES OF A MECHANICAL LARGE BOWEL OBSTRUCTION

Cause	Remarks
Tumor (carcinoma)	Most common cause of large bowel obstruction; more frequently obstructs when it involves the left colon
Hernia	May be visible on plain films if air is seen over the obturator foramen
Volvulus	Either the sigmoid or cecum may twist on its axis and obstruct the colon and/or small bowel (see Box 16-2)
Diverticulitis	Uncommon cause of colonic obstruction
Intussusception	Colo-colic intussusception usually occurs because of a tumor acting as a lead point

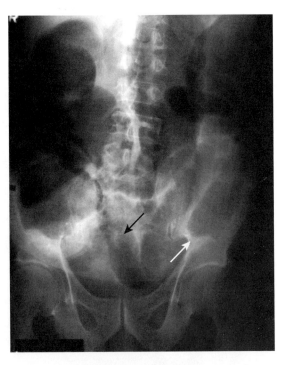

*Figure 16-6. **Mechanical large bowel obstruction.** The entire colon is dilated to a cut-off point in the distal descending colon (closed white arrow), the site of this patient's obstructing carcinoma of the colon. Some gas has passed backward through an incompetent ileocecal valve and outlines a dilated ileum (closed black arrow). Notice that the large bowel is disproportionately dilated compared to the small bowel, a finding of large bowel obstruction. This patient had an obstructing carcinoma at the sigmocolic junction.*

- The **colon is dilated to the point of obstruction.**
  - Because there are a limited number of large bowel loops, they tend not to overlap each other (as do the loops of small bowel), so **it is often possible to identify the site of obstruction** as the **last air-containing** segment of the colon (Fig. 16-6).

- Regardless of the point of obstruction, **the cecum is often the most dilated segment of the colon** (Fig. 16-7).
  - **When the cecum reaches a diameter above 12 to 15 cm, there is danger of cecal rupture.**
- The **small bowel is not dilated** unless the ileocecal valve becomes *incompetent* (see below).
- Because it is distal to the point of obstruction, **the rectum should contain little or no air.**
- Because the large bowel functions to reabsorb water, **there are usually no (or very few) air-fluid levels in the large bowel.**
- Pitfalls: How a LBO can mimic a SBO
  - **So long as the ileocecal valve** prevents gas from re-entering the small bowel in a retrograde direction (such an ileocecal valve is called **competent),** the colon will continue to dilate between the ileocecal valve and the point of colonic obstruction.
    - The **small bowel is not dilated.**
  - But if the intracolonic pressure rises high enough and the **ileocecal valve opens** (such a valve is called **incompetent), then gas from the dilated large bowel decompresses backward into the small bowel,** much like the air escaping from a balloon.

- This can produce a picture in which there is disproportionate dilatation of the small bowel compared to the decompressed large bowel.
  - This **picture mimics that of a mechanical small bowel obstruction** (Fig. 16-8).
- **Solution**
  - Ask for a barium enema or a CT scan of the abdomen; either should show the site of obstruction is in the colon and not the small bowel.
  - **Barium is not administered by mouth in a patient with a suspected large bowel obstruction** because water will be absorbed from the barium when it reaches the obstructed colon, increasing the viscosity of the barium and possibly leading to impaction.
- Volvulus of the colon is a particular kind of large bowel obstruction that produces a striking and characteristic picture that is summarized in Box 16-2 (Fig. 16-9).

Intestinal Pseudo-obstruction (Ogilvie's Syndrome)

- **Ogilvie's syndrome (acute intestinal pseudo-obstruction)** may occur in elderly individuals who are usually already hospitalized or at chronic bedrest.

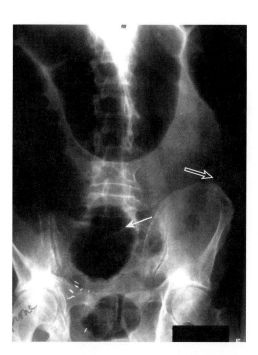

Figure 16-7. **Dilated cecum in large bowel obstruction of the descending colon.** *Although the point of this patient's large bowel obstruction is the mid-descending colon (open white arrow), notice that the cecum is the most dilated loop of colon (closed white arrow). With a mechanical obstruction, the loop(s) that will become the most dilated will be either the loop of bowel with the largest resting diameter before the onset of the obstruction (e.g., the cecum in the large bowel) or the loop(s) of bowel just proximal to the obstruction. This patient had an obstructing carcinoma of the mid-descending colon.*

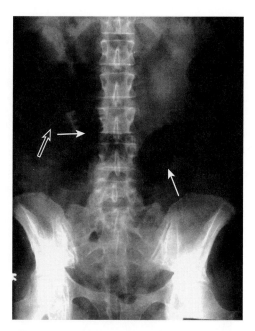

Figure 16-8. **Large bowel obstruction masquerading as a small bowel obstruction.** *There are air-filled and dilated loops of small bowel (closed white arrows) in this patient who actually had a mechanical large bowel obstruction from a carcinoma of the mid-descending colon. The pressure in the colon was sufficient to open the ileocecal valve, which then allowed much of the gas in the colon to decompress backward into the small bowel. The cecum still contains air (open white arrow) and is dilated, a clue that this is really a large bowel obstruction. Abdominal CT or a contrast enema can resolve the question of whether the large or small bowel is obstructed.*

Box 16-2

Volvulus—A Cause of Mechanical Large Bowel Obstruction

Most commonly, either the cecum or the sigmoid colon can twist upon itself, producing a mechanical obstruction known as a **volvulus**

Sigmoid volvulus is more common and tends to occur in older men

The volvulated sigmoid assumes a massive size rising up from the pelvis with the wall between the twisted loops of sigmoid forming a line that points from the left lower to the right upper quadrant

The appearance of the dilated sigmoid has been likened to a **coffee bean** (see Fig. 16-9)

When the cecum volvulates, it usually moves across the midline into the left upper quadrant producing dilated loops of bowel forming a line that characteristically points from the right lower to the left upper quadrant

A contrast enema can be both diagnostic (the obstructed sigmoid produces a **beak sign**) and therapeutic as the hydrostatic pressure of the enema can sometimes decompress the volvulus

- **Drugs with anticholinergic effects, such as antidepressants, phenothiazines, antiparkinsonian agents, and narcotics,** may cause or exacerbate the condition.
- The syndrome is characterized by a **loss of peristalsis,** resulting in sometimes **massive dilatation of the entire colon, resembling a large bowel obstruction** (Fig. 16-10).
  - Unlike a mechanical obstruction, **no obstructing lesion can be demonstrated** on CT or with barium enema.
  - Unlike a generalized ileus, **patients have more marked abdominal distention** and bowel sounds may be **normal or hyperactive** in almost half of patients with Ogilvie's syndrome.
  - The supine abdominal radiograph shows **marked bowel dilatation, almost always confined to the colon.**
  - Management is **pharmacologic stimulation of colonic contractions,** usually with neostigmine.

WebLink
More information on recognizing bowel obstruction and ileus is available to registered users on StudentConsult. com.

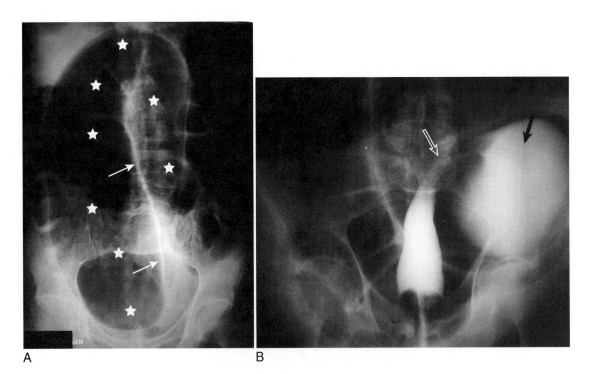

Figure 16-9. **Sigmoid volvulus.** *Supine abdominal film (A) shows a massively dilated sigmoid (white stars) with the wall between the twisted loops (closed white arrows) forming a line that points toward the right upper quadrant, findings characteristic of a sigmoid volvulus. B, One image from a barium enema shows a smoothly tapered segment of sigmoid colon likened to a bird's beak, a finding characteristic of a sigmoid volvulus (open white arrow). Some barium has entered the dilated volvulated sigmoid (closed black arrow).*

A   B

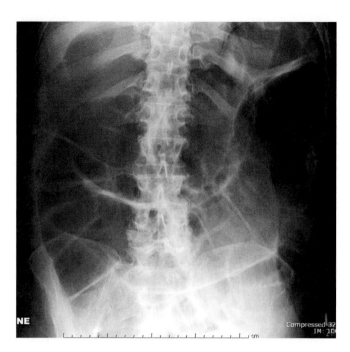

Figure 16-10. **Ogilvie's syndrome.** *Ogilvie's syndrome (acute intestinal pseudo-obstruction) may occur in elderly individuals who are usually already hospitalized or at chronic bedrest. Drugs with anticholinergic effects may cause or exacerbate the condition. The syndrome is characterized by a loss of peristalsis, resulting in sometimes massive dilatation of the entire colon, resembling a large bowel obstruction, as in this patient. Treatment is pharmacologic stimulation of the bowel.*

⊞ TAKE-HOME POINTS: Recognizing Bowel Obstruction and Ileus

Abnormal bowel gas patterns can be divided into two main groups: functional ileus and mechanical obstruction.

There are two varieties of functional ileus—localized ileus (sentinel loops) and generalized adynamic ileus—and there are two varieties of mechanical obstruction—small bowel obstruction (SBO) and large bowel obstruction (LBO).

In mechanical obstruction, the gut reacts in usually predictable ways: loops proximal to the obstruction become dilated, peristalsis attempts to propel intestinal contents through the bowel, and loops distal to the obstruction eventually are evacuated; the loop(s) that become the most dilated will either be the loop of bowel with the largest resting diameter or the loop(s) of bowel just proximal to the obstruction.

The key findings in a localized ileus (**sentinel loops**) are 2–3 dilated loops of small bowel with air in the rectosigmoid and an underlying irritative process that frequently is adjacent to the dilated loops.

Some causes of sentinel loops include pancreatitis (LUQ), cholecystitis (RUQ), diverticulitis (LLQ), and appendicitis (RLQ).

The key findings in a generalized adynamic ileus are dilated loops of large and small bowel with gas in the rectosigmoid and long air-fluid levels.

Postoperative patients develop generalized adynamic ileus, not patients presenting to the emergency room for abdominal pain.

The key imaging findings in a mechanical small bowel obstruction are disproportionately dilated and fluid-filled loops of small bowel with little or no gas in the rectosigmoid.

The most common cause of a SBO is adhesions; other causes include hernias, intussusception, gallstone ileus, malignancy, and inflammatory bowel disease (e.g., Crohn's disease).

An early SBO and sentinel loops may resemble each other, and partial SBO may present a somewhat confusing radiologic picture.

The key imaging findings in mechanical LBO include dilatation of the colon to the point of the obstruction and absence of gas in the rectum with no dilatation of the small bowel as long as the ileocecal valve remains competent.

Causes of mechanical LBO include malignancy, hernia, diverticulitis and intussusception.

If the ileocecal valve becomes incompetent, a LBO can present with a radiologic picture similar to a SBO; a CT scan or barium enema will usually be diagnostic.

Ogilvie's syndrome is characterized by a loss of peristalsis, resulting in sometimes massive dilatation of the entire colon resembling a large bowel obstruction but without a demonstrable point of obstruction; it can sometimes be confused for a generalized adynamic ileus.

17 Recognizing Extraluminal Air in the Abdomen

- Recognition of extraluminal gas is an important finding that can have an immediate effect on the course of treatment.
- Air is normally not present in the peritoneal or extraperitoneal spaces, bowel wall, or biliary system.
  - **Air outside the bowel** is called *extraluminal air.*
- **The four most common locations of extraluminal air:**
  - **Intraperitoneal (pneumoperitoneum)** (frequently called *free air)*
  - **Retroperitoneal air**
  - **Air in the bowel wall (pneumatosis intestinalis)**
  - **Air in the biliary system (pneumobilia)**

Signs of Free Intraperitoneal Air

- There are **three major signs of free intraperitoneal air,** arranged here in the order in which they are most commonly seen.
  - **A crescentic lucency beneath the diaphragm**
  - **Visualization of both sides of the bowel wall**
  - **Visualization of the falciform ligament**

AIR BENEATH THE DIAPHRAGM

- Air will rise to the highest part of the abdomen.
  - In the upright position, **free air will usually reveal itself under the diaphragm as a crescentic lucency that parallels the undersurface of the diaphragm** (Fig. 17-1).
  - The **size of the crescent** will be **roughly proportional to the amount of free air.**
    - The smaller the amount of free air, the thinner the crescent; the larger the amount of free air, the larger the crescent (Fig. 17-2).
- Although **free air is best demonstrated on CT scans of the abdomen** because of its greater sensitivity in detecting very small amounts of free air (Fig. 17-3), most surveys of the abdomen begin with conventional radiographs.
  - Conventional radiographs **serve as an important screening tool** for discovering many previously unsuspected cases of free air.
- On conventional radiographs, **free air is best demonstrated with the x-ray beam directed parallel to the floor** (i.e., a horizontal beam) (see Figs. 15-14 and 15-15).
  - **Small amounts of free air will not be visible on supine** radiographs in which the x-ray beam is directed vertically downward.
- Free air is **easier to recognize under the right hemidiaphragm** because that area is usually occupied by only the soft tissue density of the liver.

- Free air is **more difficult to recognize under the left hemidiaphragm** because air-containing structures such as the fundus of the stomach and the splenic flexure already reside in that location and may obscure accurate recognition of free air (Fig. 17-4).
- If the patient is unable to stand or sit upright, then a view of the abdomen with the patient lying on his or her left side (the right side pointing up) taken with a horizontal x-ray beam may show free air rising above the right edge of the liver.
  - This is the **left lateral decubitus view** of the abdomen (Fig. 17-5).
- **Pitfall: Chilaiditi's syndrome**
  - Occasionally, colon may be interposed between the dome of the liver and the right hemidiaphragm and, unless a **careful search** is made **for the presence of haustral folds** characteristic of the colon, it may be mistaken for free air (Fig. 17-6).
  - **Solution**
    - Obtain a left lateral decubitus view of the abdomen or, if necessary, a CT scan of the abdomen.

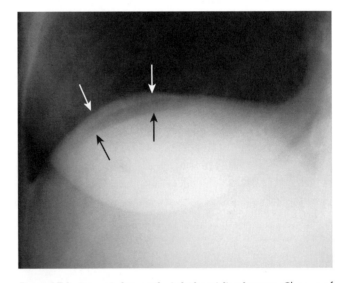

Figure 17-1. **Free air beneath right hemidiaphragm.** *Close-up of the right upper quadrant from an upright chest radiograph shows a thin crescent of air between the hemidiaphragm (closed white arrows) and the dome of the liver (closed black arrows) representing free intraperitoneal air. The patient had undergone abdominal surgery 5 days earlier. Free air can remain for up to 7 days after surgery in an adult, but serial studies should demonstrate a progressively decreasing amount of air.*

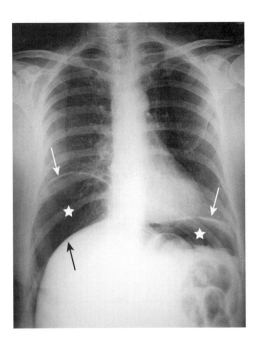

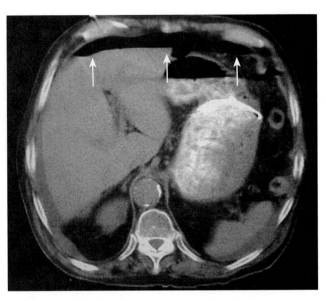

Figure 17-2. **Large amount of free air.** Upright view of the chest demonstrates a large amount of free air (white stars) beneath each hemidiaphragm (closed white arrows). The top of the liver (closed black arrow) is made visible by the air above it. The patient had a perforated gastric ulcer.

Figure 17-3. **Free air seen on CT scan of the abdomen.** Axial CT scan of the upper abdomen performed with the patient supine shows free air anteriorly (closed white arrows). The air is not contained within any bowel. Free intraperitoneal air will normally rise to the highest point of the abdomen which, in the supine position, is usually under the anterior abdominal wall.

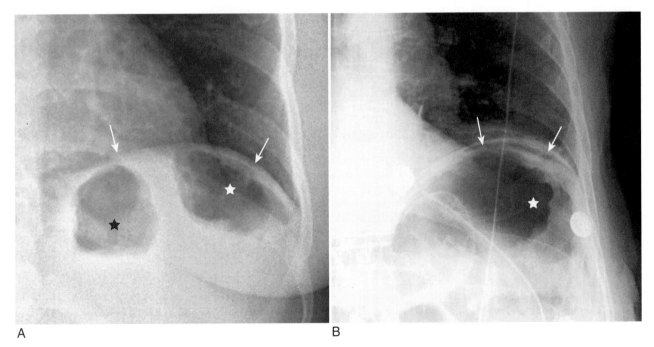

A   B

Figure 17-4. **Normal left hemidiaphragm (A) and free air under hemidiaphragm (B). A,** Close-up of the left upper quadrant demonstrates the difficulty in recognizing free air beneath the normal left hemidiaphragm (closed white arrows) because of the normal location of gas-containing structures such as the stomach (black star) and splenic flexure (white stars) in that location. **B,** A crescentic lucency beneath the left hemidiaphragm represents free air in another patient. It is easier to recognize free air beneath the right hemidiaphragm because there is usually no air interposed between the liver and the right hemidiaphragm.

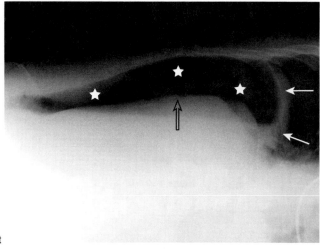

Feet   Head

Figure 17-5. ***Left lateral decubitus view showing free air.*** *Close-up of the right upper quadrant in a patient lying on their left side in the left lateral decubitus position shows a crescent of air (white stars) above the outer edge of the liver (open black arrow), beneath the right hemidiaphragm (closed white arrows). If the patient is unable to stand or sit for an upright view of the abdomen, a left lateral decubitus view can substitute. The x-ray beam must be directed horizontally.*

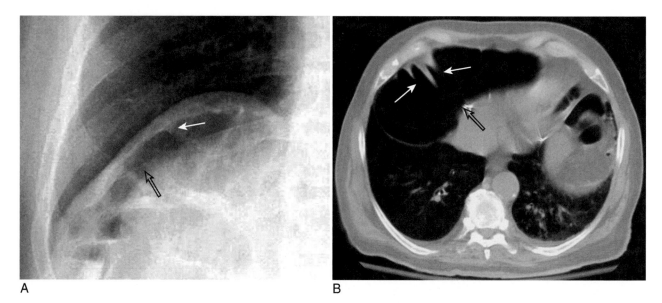

A   B

Figure 17-6. ***Chilaiditi's syndrome.*** *Close-up of the right hemidiaphragm on a conventional chest radiograph* ***(A)*** *and an axial CT scan at the level of the diaphragm* ***(B)*** *both demonstrate air beneath the diaphragm that could be mistaken for free air (open black arrows). Careful evaluation of this air demonstrates several haustral folds (closed white arrows) that traverse the air, indicating this is a loop of colon interposed between the liver and the diaphragm (Chilaiditi's syndrome) rather than free air. Most patients with this syndrome are completely asymptomatic, and it is only important as a potential diagnostic pitfall.*

VISUALIZATION OF BOTH SIDES OF THE BOWEL WALL

- In the **normal** abdomen, we visualize only the air **inside** the lumen of the bowel, **not the wall of the bowel itself.**
  - This is because the wall is soft tissue density and is surrounded by tissue of the same density.
- Introduction of **air into the peritoneal cavity enables us to visualize the wall of the bowel itself** because the wall is now surrounded on both the inside and outside by air.

- The **ability to see both sides of the bowel wall is a sign of free intraperitoneal air** called *Rigler's sign* (Fig. 17-7).
- It can be seen on supine, upright, or prone films of the abdomen so long as there is an adequate amount of free air present.
  - Rigler's sign usually requires large amounts of free air in order to be present.
- **Pitfall:** When dilated loops of small bowel overlap each other, they may occasionally produce the mistaken impression of seeing both sides of the bowel wall (Fig. 17-8).

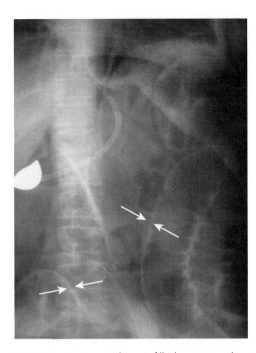

Figure 17-7. **Rigler's sign.** *When air fills the peritoneal cavity, both sides of the bowel wall will be outlined by air, making the wall of the bowel visible as a discrete line (closed white arrows). This is known as Rigler's sign and indicates the presence of a pneumoperitoneum.*

- **Solution:** Confirm the presence of free air with an upright view, left lateral decubitus view, or CT scan of the abdomen.

VISUALIZATION OF THE FALCIFORM LIGAMENT

- The **falciform ligament** courses over the **free edge of the liver anteriorly** just to the **right of the upper lumbar spine.**
  - It contains a remnant of the obliterated umbilical artery.
  - It is **normally invisible,** composed of soft tissue, and surrounded by tissue of similar density.
- When a (usually) large amount of free air is present and the **patient is in the supine position,** free air may rise over the anterior surface of the liver, **surround the falciform ligament,** and **render it visible.**
- Visualization of the falciform ligament is aptly called the *falciform ligament sign* (Fig. 17-9).
- The curvilinear appearance of the falciform ligament combined with the oval collection of air that collects beneath and distends the abdominal wall has been likened to the appearance a football with its laces, and is called the *football sign.*
- Table 17-1 summarizes the **three major signs of free air.**

Causes of Free Air

- The **most common cause of free intraperitoneal air** is **rupture of an air-containing loop of bowel,** either stomach, small intestine, or large intestine.

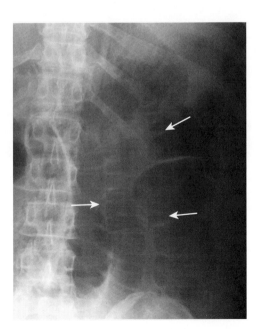

Figure 17-8. **Overlapping loops mimicking free air.** *Don't let overlapping loops of dilated small bowel (closed white arrows) fool you into thinking you are seeing both sides of the bowel wall because of free air. If there is doubt about the presence of free air, confirmation may be obtained through an upright or left lateral decubitus view of the abdomen or a CT scan of the abdomen.*

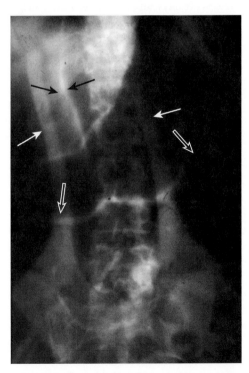

Figure 17-9. **Falciform ligament sign.** *Free intraperitoneal air may surround the normally invisible falciform ligament on the anterior edge of the liver causing that thin soft tissue structure to become visible (closed black arrows) just to the right of the upper lumbar spine. Notice also that both sides of the stomach wall are visible (Rigler's sign) (open white arrows) in this patient with a large pneumoperitoneum from a perforated gastric ulcer. The thick white bands (closed white arrows) represent folds of skin on the patient's back.*

Table 17-1

THREE SIGNS OF FREE AIR

Sign	Remarks
Air beneath diaphragm	Requires patient to be in the upright or left lateral decubitus position; a horizontal x-ray beam is used
Visualization of both sides of the bowel wall	Usually requires large amount of free air; will be visible in any position
Visualization of the falciform ligament	Usually requires large amounts of free air; patient is usually supine

- **Perforated peptic ulcer** is the most common cause of a perforated stomach or duodenum and is still the most common cause of free air.
- **Trauma,** whether accidental or iatrogenic, can also produce free air.
  - **Free air following penetrating trauma** usually **implies a perforation of the bowel,** not free air generated simply by penetration of the abdominal wall itself.
  - **For several days following abdominal surgery (about 5–7 days),** whether the surgery had been performed on the bowel or not, **it is normal to see free air** on postoperative studies.
    - The **amount** of free air following surgery **should diminish with each successive study.**
    - A complication of the surgery or of the original disease should be considered **if free air persists for longer than a week** or if the **amount increases on successive studies.**
- **Perforated diverticulitis and perforated appendicitis** usually produce walled-off abscess collections around the site of the perforation and rarely lead to significant amounts of free air.
- **Perforation of a carcinoma,** usually of the colon, is unusual but can also lead to free air.

Signs of Extraperitoneal Air (Retroperitoneal Air)

- Unlike the collections of free intraperitoneal air that outline loops of bowel and usually move freely in the abdomen, **extraperitoneal air can be recognized** by certain other characteristics:
  - **Streaky, linear appearance outlining extraperitoneal structures**
  - **Mottled, blotchy appearance** (anterior pararenal space, especially)
  - **Relatively fixed position, moving little,** if at all, **with changes in patient positioning**
- Extraperitoneal air may outline certain extraperitoneal structures:
  - **Psoas muscles**
  - **Kidneys, ureters, or urinary bladder**

- **Aorta or inferior vena cava** (Fig. 17-10)
- Inferior border of the diaphragm by collecting in the **subphrenic tissues**
- **Extraperitoneal air may extend through a diaphragmatic hiatus into the mediastinum** (and produce *pneumomediastinum*) or **may extend to the peritoneal cavity** through openings in the peritoneum (and produce *pneumoperitoneum).*
- Box 17-1 summarizes the signs of extraperitoneal air.

Causes of Extraperitoneal Air

- **Extraperitoneal air is most frequently the result of bowel perforation** secondary to either:
  - **Inflammatory disease (e.g., ruptured appendix),** or
  - **Ulcerative disease (e.g., Crohn's disease** of the ileum or colon)
- **Other causes of extraperitoneal air:**
  - **Blunt or penetrating trauma**
  - **Iatrogenic manipulation** (e.g., perforation of the bowel during sigmoidoscopy)
  - **Foreign body** (e.g., perforation of the extraperitoneal ascending colon by an ingested foreign body)

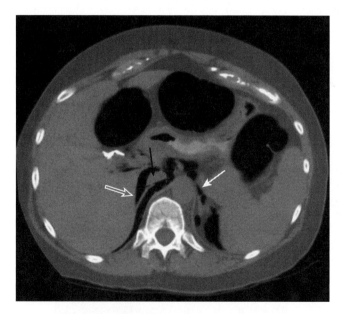

Figure 17-10. **Extraperitoneal air seen on CT.** *Air is seen in the retroperitoneum (open white arrow) on this axial CT scan of the upper abdomen. Air outlines the inferior vena cava (closed black arrow) and the aorta (closed white arrow). Unlike free air, extraperitoneal air is streaky, relatively fixed in position, and outlines extraperitoneal structures such as the vena cava, aorta, psoas muscles, and kidneys.*

Box 17-1

Signs of Extraperitoneal Air

Streaky, linear collections of air that outline extraperitoneal structures
Mottled, blotchy collections of air that remain in a fixed position

- **Gas-producing infection** originating in extraperitoneal organs (such as **perforated diverticulitis**).

Signs of Air in the Bowel Wall

- Air in the bowel wall is called *pneumatosis intestinales.*
- Air in the bowel wall is **most easily recognized when it is seen in profile** producing a **linear radiolucency (black line)** whose contour exactly parallels the bowel lumen (Fig. 17-11).
- **Air in the bowel wall seen *en face* is more difficult to recognize** but frequently has a **mottled appearance that resembles gas mixed with fecal material** (Fig. 17-12).
  - Clues to help differentiate pneumatosis from fecal material:
    - **Presence of such mottled gas in an area of the abdomen unlikely to contain colon**
    - **Lack of change** in the appearance of the mottled gas pattern over several images in **differing positions.**
- Table 17-2 summarizes the signs of air in the bowel wall.

Causes and Significance of Air in the Bowel Wall

- Pneumatosis intestinales can be divided into two major categories.
  - A **rare, primary form** called *pneumatosis cystoides intestinales* usually **affects the left colon,** producing **cyst-like collections of air in the submucosa or serosa** (Fig. 17-13).

- A **more common, secondary form** can occur in obstructive and necrotizing diseases:
  - **Chronic obstructive pulmonary disease,** presumably secondary to air from ruptured blebs dissecting through the mediastinum to the abdomen.
  - Diseases in which there is **necrosis of the bowel** wall (Fig. 17-14):

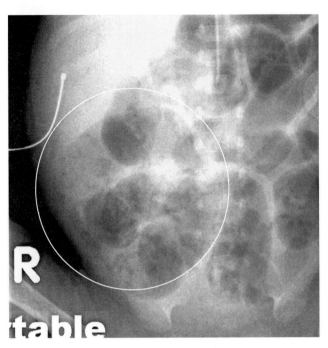

Figure 17-12. **Pneumatosis seen en face.** *Supine abdominal study of another infant shows multiple faint, mottled lucencies in the right lower quadrant (white circle), which is the appearance of pneumatosis intestinales when seen en face. The density has the same appearance as air mixed with stool, but can be distinguished from stool because it occurs in areas stool might not be expected and it does not change over time. This infant also had necrotizing enterocolitis.*

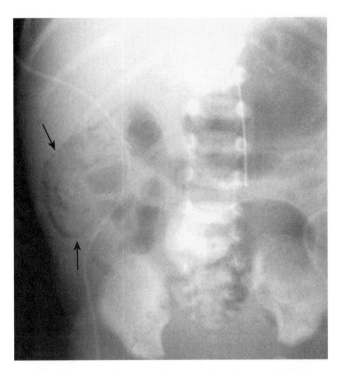

Figure 17-11. **Pneumatosis seen in profile.** *Close-up of the right lower quadrant in an infant demonstrates a thin curvilinear lucency that parallels the lumen of the adjacent bowel (closed black arrows), an appearance characteristic of gas in the bowel wall seen in profile. In infants, the most common cause for this finding is necrotizing enterocolitis, a disease found mostly in premature infants in which the terminal ileum is most affected. Pneumatosis intestinalis is pathognomonic for necrotizing enterocolitis in infants.*

Table 17-2

SIGNS OF AIR IN THE BOWEL WALL

Sign	Remarks
Linear radiolucency paralleling the contour of air in the adjacent bowel lumen	When seen in profile
Mottled appearance that resembles air mixed with fecal material	May occur in an area of the abdomen not expected for colon; doesn't change over time
Globular, cystlike collections of air that parallel the contour of the bowel	Unusual, benign condition affecting colon, usually left colon

- **Necrotizing enterocolitis** in infants
- **Ischemic bowel disease** in adults
- **Obstructing lesions of the bowel** that raise intraluminal pressure:

- **Hirschsprung's disease** or **pyloric stenosis** in children
- **Obstructing carcinomas** in adults
- Pneumatosis intestinales **associated with diseases that produce necrosis of bowel** is usually a **more ominous prognostic sign** than pneumatosis associated with **obstructing lesions of the bowel** or chronic obstructive pulmonary disease.
- **Complications of pneumatosis intestinales:**
  - **Rupture into the peritoneal cavity** leading to intraperitoneal free air (**pneumoperitoneum**)
  - Dissection of **air into the portal venous system** (Fig. 17-15)

Signs of Air in the Biliary System
- Air in the biliary system presents as **one or two tube-like, branching lucencies in the right upper quadrant overlying the central portion of the liver and conforming to the location and appearance of the major**

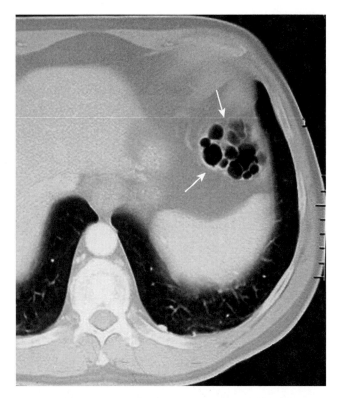

Figure 17-13. **Pneumatosis cystoides intestinalis.** Axial CT scan of the upper abdomen windowed for lung technique shows a cluster of air-containing cysts (closed white arrows) associated with the left colon, characteristic of **pneumatosis cystoides intestinales,** a rare but benign condition in which air-containing cysts form in the submucosa or serosa of the bowel.

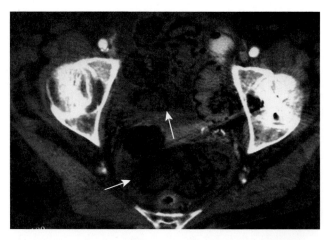

Figure 17-14. **Necrosis of bowel from mesenteric ischemia.** Axial CT image of the pelvis demonstrates multiple loops of bowel with punctate collections of air throughout their walls consistent with pneumatosis (closed white arrows). The patient had widespread ischemia of bowel from mesenteric vascular disease. Pneumatosis which results from bowel necrosis is an ominous sign.

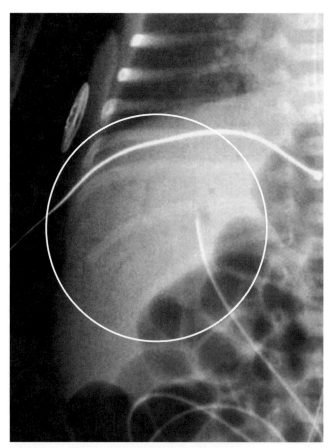

Figure 17-15. **Portal venous gas.** Numerous small black branching structures are visible over the periphery of the liver (white circle). This is air in the portal venous system, a finding most often associated with necrotizing enterocolitis in infants. Once thought to be an ominous prognostic sign, it now is considered less grave. Unlike air in the biliary system, this air is peripheral rather than central and has numerous branching structures rather than the few tubular structures seen with pneumobilia.

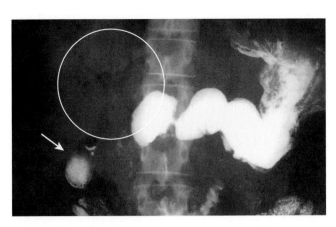

Figure 17-16. **Air in the biliary tree.** *Frontal view of the upper abdomen from an upper gastrointestinal series demonstrates several air-containing tubular structures over the central portion of the liver consistent with air in the biliary system (white circle). There is also barium in the gallbladder (closed white arrow). This patient had a history of a prior sphincterotomy for gallstones so that reflux of air and barium into the biliary system would be expected.*

bile ducts: the common duct, cystic duct, and the hepatic ducts (Fig. 17-16).

- Box 17-2 summarizes the **signs of air in the biliary system.**

Causes of Air in the Biliary System

- Gas in the biliary system **may be a "normal" finding** if the sphincter of Oddi, which guards the entrance of the common bile duct as it enters the duodenum, is open (said to be "incompetent").

- Prior **sphincterotomy,** such as might be done to allow gallstones to exit from the ductal system into the bowel, may be a cause.

- **Prior surgery** that results in the **reimplantation of the common bile duct** into another part of the bowel (i.e., choledocho-enterostomy) is frequently accompanied by gas in the biliary ductal system.

- Pathologic conditions that can produce pneumobilia include **uncommon causes:**

  - **Gallstone ileus** in which a **gallstone erodes through the wall of the gallbladder** into the **duodenum** (usually) producing a **fistula between the bowel and the biliary system.**
    - The **gallstone impacts in the small bowel,** usually in the narrower terminal ileum, and produces a mechanical obstruction (here called an "ileus") (Fig. 17-17).
  - **Gas-forming pyogenic cholangitis,** particularly from *Escherichia coli*

WebLink
More information on recognizing extraluminal air in the abdomen is available to registered users on StudentConsult.com.

Signs of Air in the Biliary Tract

Tube-like, branching lucencies in the right upper quadrant overlying the liver

Tubular structures are central in location and few in number compared to portal venous air, which is peripheral in location and fills innumerable vessels

Gas in the lumen of the gallbladder

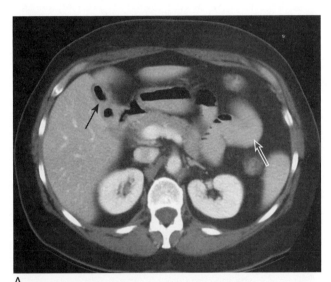

A

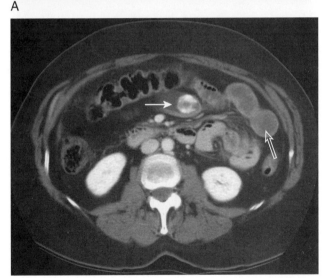

B

Figure 17-17. **Gallstone ileus.** *The three key findings of gallstone ileus are present on this study.* **A,** *Axial CT scan of the upper abdomen shows air in the lumen of the gallbladder (closed black arrow) and dilated small bowel (open white arrows) consistent with a mechanical small bowel obstruction. At a lower level, another axial CT scan of the abdomen* **(B)** *shows a large calcified gallstone inside the small bowel (closed white arrow). The gallstone had eroded through the wall of the gallbladder into the duodenum and then began a journey down the small bowel before becoming impacted and producing obstruction.*

TAKE-HOME POINTS: Recognizing Extraluminal Air in the Abdomen

Gas in the abdomen outside the normal confines of the bowel is called extraluminal air.

The four most common locations for extraluminal air are intraperitoneal air (**pneumoperitoneum**, frequently called **free air**), retroperitoneal air, air in the bowel wall (**pneumatosis**), and air in the biliary system (**pneumobilia**).

The three key signs of free air are air beneath the diaphragm, visualization of both sides of the bowel wall (**Rigler's sign**), and visualization of the falciform ligament.

The most common causes of free air are perforated peptic ulcer, trauma whether accidental or iatrogenic, perforated diverticulitis, and perforation of a carcinoma, usually of the colon.

The key signs of extraperitoneal (retroperitoneal) air are a streaky, linear appearance or a mottled, blotchy appearance outlining extraperitoneal structures and its relatively fixed position, moving little or at all with changes in patient positioning.

Extraperitoneal air outlines extraperitoneal structures (e.g., the psoas muscles, kidneys, aorta, or inferior vena cava).

Causes of extraperitoneal air include bowel perforation secondary to either inflammatory or ulcerative disease, blunt or penetrating trauma, iatrogenic manipulation, or foreign body ingestion.

The key signs of air in the bowel wall include linear radiolucencies paralleling the contour of air in the adjacent bowel lumen, a mottled appearance that resembles air mixed with fecal material, or uncommonly, globular, cystlike collections of air that parallel the contour of the bowel.

Causes of air in the bowel wall (pneumatosis intestinalis) include a rare primary form called **pneumatosis cystoides intestinales** and a more common secondary form that includes diseases in which there is necrosis of the bowel wall (e.g., necrotizing enterocolitis in infants and ischemic bowel disease in adults) as well as obstructing lesions of the bowel that raise intraluminal pressure (e.g., Hirschsprung's disease in children and obstructing carcinomas in adults).

Pneumatosis intestinales associated with diseases that produce necrosis of bowel is usually a more ominous prognostic sign than pneumatosis associated with obstructing lesions of the bowel or chronic obstructive pulmonary disease.

Signs of air in the biliary system include tube-like, branching lucencies in the right upper quadrant overlying the liver, which are central in location and few in number, and gas in the lumen of the gallbladder.

Causes of pneumobilia include incompetence of the sphincter of Oddi, prior sphincterotomy, prior surgery that results in the reimplantation of the common bile duct into another part of the bowel, and gallstone ileus.

The triad of findings in gallstone ileus are air in the biliary system, small bowel obstruction, and visualization of the gallstone itself.

18 Recognizing Abnormal Calcifications and Their Causes

- Soft tissue calcifications lend themselves to an intuitive approach that ties together a diverse group of diseases.
- Although this chapter focuses primarily on abdominal calcifications, the same approach applies to dystrophic calcification found anywhere in the body.
- Most soft tissue calcification occurs in tissue that is already abnormal.
  - Such calcification is called *dystrophic calcification.*
- The **nature of most calcifications can be determined by examining two of their characteristics:**
  - Their **pattern of calcification**
  - Their **anatomic location**

Patterns of Calcification

- Calcifications **tend to occur in one of four distinct patterns,** depending on the type of structure that has calcified.
- The patterns are named as follows:
  - **Rimlike**
  - **Linear or track-like**
  - **Lamellar (or laminar)**
  - **Cloudlike, amorphous, or popcorn**

RIMLIKE CALCIFICATION

- Rimlike calcifications imply **calcification that has occurred in the wall of a hollow viscus.**
- Examples of structures that manifest rimlike calcifications:
  - **Cysts**—calcification in any one of the following is relatively uncommon.
    - **Renal cysts**
    - **Splenic cysts**
    - **Extra-abdominal sites:**
      - Mediastinal cysts, such as pericardial and bronchial cysts (Fig. 18-1)
      - Popliteal cysts
  - **Aneurysms**
    - **Aortic aneurysm**
      - Most easily recognized on a lateral radiograph of the lumbar spine
      - The abdominal aorta should normally measure <3 cm in diameter, a measurement that requires both apposing walls be visible (Fig. 18-2).
    - **Splenic artery** or **renal artery** aneurysms
    - **Extra-abdominal sites:**
      - Femoral artery aneurysms
      - Cerebral aneurysms
  - **Saccular organs, such as the gallbladder or urinary bladder**
    - **Porcelain gallbladder**

- An uncommon entity (named after the gross appearance of the gallbladder which resembles porcelain) that occurs with chronic inflammation and stasis and is associated with gallstones and an increased incidence of carcinoma of the gallbladder (Fig. 18-3)
    - **Urinary bladder**
      - Uncommon occurrence in diseases such as **schistosomiasis, bladder cancer,** and **tuberculosis**
- Table 18-1 highlights key facts about rimlike calcifications.

LINEAR OR TRACK-LIKE CALCIFICATION

- Linear or track-like calcifications imply **calcification that has occurred in the walls of tubular structures** (Fig. 18-4).

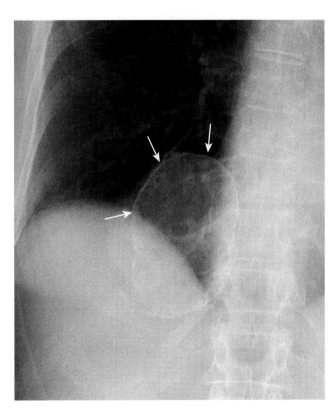

Figure 18-1. **Calcified pericardial cyst.** *A rimlike calcification (closed white arrows) identifies the structure containing the calcification as cystic or saccular. The calcification is in the right cardiophrenic angle, an ideal location for pericardial cysts. Pericardial cysts almost always occur on the right side and are most common at the cardiophrenic angle, as in this case. They are usually asymptomatic and discovered when a chest radiograph is obtained for another reason.*

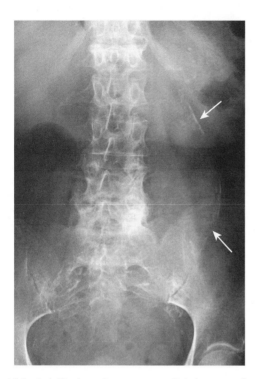

Figure 18-2. ***Calcified aortic aneurysm.*** *Calcification in the wall of the abdominal aorta is a common finding in atherosclerosis, especially in those with diabetes mellitus. In this patient, the aorta demonstrates a rimlike calcification (closed white arrows). The opposite wall is also calcified but overlaps the spine. When the diameter of the abdominal aorta exceeds its normal diameter by more than 50%, an aneurysm is present.*

- Examples of structures that have calcifications in the walls:
  - **Arteries**
    - **Common in atherosclerosis** and seen anywhere in the body
    - **Walls of veins do not calcify.**
      - In veins, **long, linear thrombi** or **small, focal thrombi** (the latter called *phleboliths*) may calcify (see Fig. 15-18).
  - **Tubular structures**
    - **Fallopian tubes and vas deferens**
      - Seen more often in diabetics (Fig. 18-5).
    - **Ureter**
      - Uncommon finding seen in schistosomiasis and even more rarely in tuberculosis (TB)
- Table 18-2 highlights key facts about linear or track-like calcifications.

Lamellar or Laminar Calcification

- **Lamellar** (or laminar) **calcifications imply calcification that forms around a nidus inside a hollow lumen** (Fig. 18-6).
  - A "hollow lumen" refers to a structure such as the gallbladder or urinary bladder.
  - **Calcification in concentric layers** begins with a central nidus around which alternating layers of calcified and noncalcified material form as a result of prolonged movement of the stone within the hollow viscus.

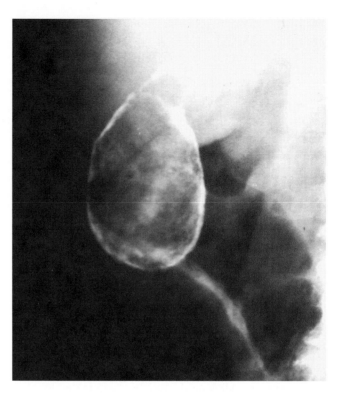

Figure 18-3. ***Calcified gallbladder wall.*** *A rimlike calcification is one that occurs in the wall of a cyst or saccular organ. This calcification is in the right upper quadrant, the location of the gallbladder. This is a* ***porcelain gallbladder,*** *an uncommon entity (so named because the gross appearance of the gallbladder resembles porcelain) that occurs with chronic inflammation and stasis and is associated with gallstones and an increased incidence of carcinoma of the gallbladder.*

Table 18-1

RIMLIKE CALCIFICATIONS

Organ of Origin	Remarks
Renal cyst	Thick and irregular calcifications, though uncommon, may indicate the presence of renal cell carcinoma
Splenic cysts	May be a manifestation of hydatid cyst, old trauma or prior infection
Aortic aneurysms	Occurs more often in diabetics with advanced atherosclerosis
Gallbladder	Associated with chronic stasis; called *porcelain gallbladder* for its gross appearance; higher incidence of carcinoma of the gallbladder

- Lamellar or laminated calcifications are usually called *stones* or *calculi* (singular: calculus) and include the following:
  - **Renal calculi**
    - CT is the study of choice.
    - Conventional radiographs are only about 50% to 60% sensitive for displaying renal calculi despite the fact that about 90% of renal calculi contain calcium (Fig. 18-7).

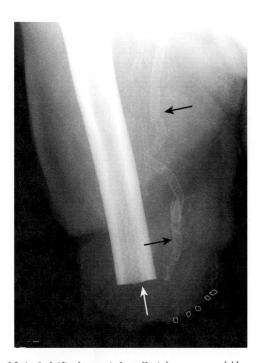

Figure 18-4. **Calcified arterial wall.** A linear or track-like calcification (closed black arrows) implies calcification that has occurred in the walls of tubular structures. This is calcification in the femoral artery. Such vessel wall calcification occurs in arteries, not veins, and is usually secondary to atherosclerosis, frequently associated with diabetes, or in patients with chronic renal disease. This patient obviously suffered one of the complications of diabetes and has had an above-the-knee amputation (closed white arrow) of a formerly gangrenous leg.

Table 18-2

LINEAR OR TRACK-LIKE CALCIFICATIONS

Organ of Origin	Remarks
Walls of smaller arteries	Mostly seen in atherosclerosis accelerated by diabetes and renal disease
Fallopian tubes or vas deferens	Usually accelerated by diabetes
Ureters	Uncommon occurrence described with schistosomiasis and, rarely, tuberculosis

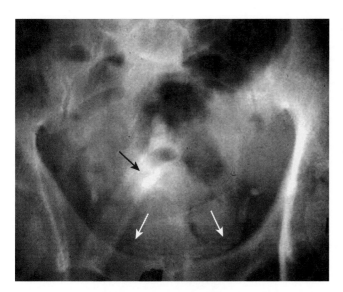

Figure 18-5. **Calcification of the vas deferens.** This male patient manifests two track-like calcifications (closed white arrows) symmetrically on each side of the urinary bladder that end in the urethra. The type of calcification identifies it as occurring in the wall of a tubular structure. The location identifies it as calcification in the walls of the vas deferens, which occurs more commonly and earlier in diabetics than in a natural degenerative process. There is another tube-like structure visible (closed black arrow) but it is synthetic: it represents a suprapubic cystostomy drainage tube, which had been inserted for a neurogenic bladder.

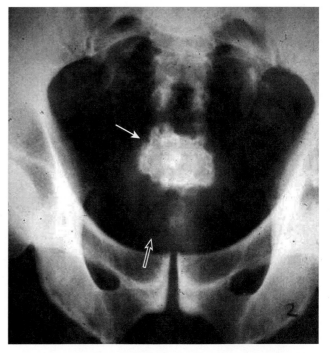

Figure 18-6. **"Jackstone" calculus of the urinary bladder.** A lamellated calcification is seen in the pelvis (closed white arrow). The lamination identifies it as a calculus that has formed in a hollow viscus. The anatomic location places it in the urinary bladder (open white arrow). This is called a "jackstone calculus" because of its irregular margin that resembles the playing piece used in the child's game. The irregularity results from the stone forming in a bladder with a heavily trabeculated inner surface, a consequence of chronic bladder outlet obstruction. The stone has not "fallen to the bottom of the bladder" because of its size and because the patient is supine.

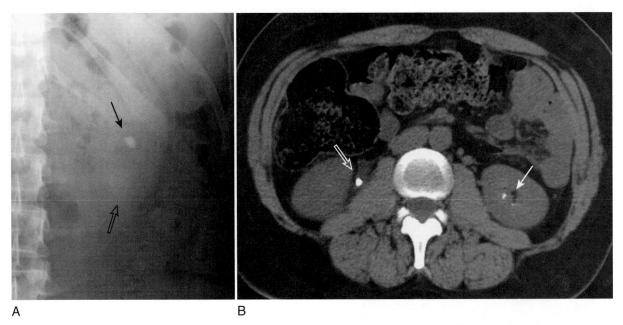

Figure 18-7. **Renal calculus, conventional radiograph (A) and axial CT scan (B). A,** *A small calcification* (closed black arrow) *overlies the shadow of the left kidney* (open black arrow)*. Although it is too small for lamination to be recognized, its location suggests a renal calculus.* **B,** *In a different patient, an image from an unenhanced axial CT scan, called a "stone search," reveals a large calcification in the proximal right ureter* (open white arrow) *and several smaller calcifications in the left intrarenal collecting system* (closed white arrow)*. Because of its greater sensitivity, a CT stone search has mostly replaced conventional radiography for the identification of renal and ureteral calculi.*

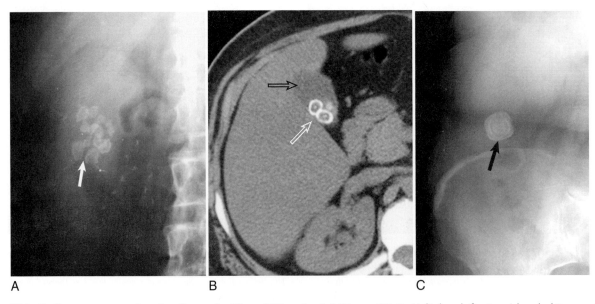

Figure 18-8. **Gallstones, conventional radiographs (A) and (C) and axial CT scan (B). A,** *Multiple calcifications* (closed white arrow) *have interlocking edges, suggesting that they all formed in a hollow viscus in proximity to each other. These calcifications are called* **faceted stones** *for their characteristic shapes.* **B,** *In a different patient, a close-up view of an unenhanced axial CT scan of the right upper quadrant shows several gallstones* (open white arrow)*, two of which clearly have a central nidus surrounded by laminated, concentric rings of noncalcified and calcified material. The gallbladder* (open black arrow) *contains bile fats and is less dense than the liver.* **C,** *A typical laminated gallstone* (closed black arrow) *is seen, the laminations implying that the stone has formed inside a hollow viscus, in this case the gallbladder.*

- **Gallstones**
  - Ultrasound is the study of choice.
  - Only about 10% to 15% of gallstones contain enough calcification to be visible on conventional radiographs (Fig. 18-8).
- **Bladder stones**
  - Usually secondary to chronic bladder outlet obstruction, they are very prone to develop lamination (Fig. 18-9).
- Table 18-3 highlights key facts about laminated or lamellar calcifications.

CLOUDLIKE, AMORPHOUS, OR "POPCORN" CALCIFICATION

- **Cloudlike, amorphous, or popcorn calcification is calcification that has formed inside a solid organ or tumor,** and examples include:

- **Body of the pancreas**
  - Pathognomonic for chronic pancreatitis (Fig. 18-10)
- **Leiomyomas of uterus**
  - Uterine fibroids or leiomyomas very commonly degenerate and calcify over time (Fig. 18-11).

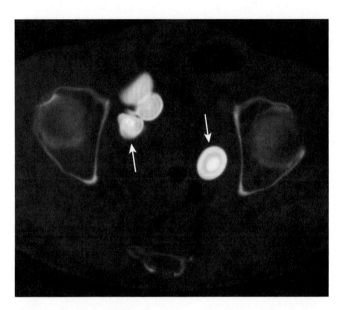

Figure 18-9. **Urinary bladder stones.** *Laminated calcifications (closed white arrows) are seen on this axial CT scan through the level of the pelvis and windowed to show the laminations better. The laminations imply that these calcifications have formed inside a hollow viscus. The anatomic location of these calculi places them in the urinary bladder.*

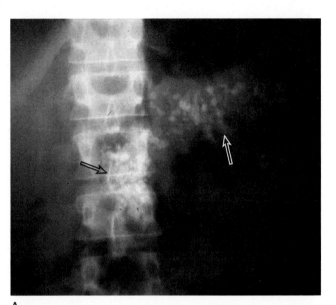

A

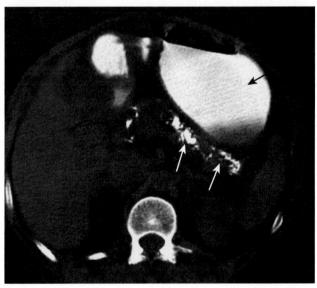

B

Figure 18-10. **Chronic calcific pancreatitis, conventional radiograph (A) and axial CT scan (B).** *A close-up view of the left upper quadrant of a conventional radiograph of the abdomen (A) shows amorphous calcifications (black and white open arrows) implying calcification in a solid organ or tumor. The anatomic distribution of the calcification corresponds to the location of the pancreas. In another patient (B), a nonenhanced image of the upper abdomen shows calcifications distributed along the course of the body and tail of the pancreas (closed white arrows). There is oral contrast material in the stomach (closed black arrow). These calcifications are pathognomonic of chronic pancreatitis, a chronic and irreversible disease occurring mostly secondary to alcoholism that leads to atrophy of the gland and diabetes.*

Table 18-3

LAMINAR OR LAMELLATED CALCIFICATIONS

Organ of Origin	Remarks
Kidney	Most calcified renal stones are composed of calcium oxalate crystals; most form due to stasis, infection
Gallbladder	Most calcified gallstones are calcium bilirubinate; form due to chronic infection and stasis
Urinary bladder	Most bladder calculi contain urate crystals; form most often from outlet obstruction

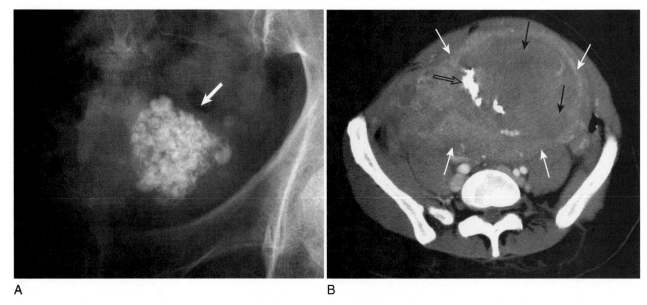

A   B

*Figure 18-11. **Calcified uterine leiomyoma (fibroid) on conventional radiograph and CT. A,** There is an amorphous (or popcorn, if you're hungry) calcification (closed white arrow) in the pelvis of this 48-year-old female. This type of calcification suggests formation in a solid organ or tumor. This is the anatomic location and the classical appearance of calcified uterine leiomyomas (fibroids). **B,** CT of another patient who has large uterine fibroids (closed white arrows), portions of which have necrosed (closed black arrows) and calcified (open black arrow). Ultrasound is the study of choice in diagnosing uterine fibroids.*

- **Pitfall**
  - Sometimes a **solid tumor will outgrow its blood supply and the center of the tumor will undergo necrosis,** leaving only a viable "outer shell."
  - The subsequent calcification will be **more rimlike than amorphous.**
    - Uterine fibroids are especially prone to this appearance (Fig. 18-12).
  - Solution
    - CT or US will reveal the true nature of the calcification.
- **Lymph nodes**
  - Can calcify anywhere in the body, mostly due to prior granulomatous infection, e.g., old tuberculosis.
- **Mucin-producing adenocarcinomas** of the stomach, ovary, and colon (Fig. 18-13).
- In structures outside the abdomen:
  - **Meningiomas** (see Fig. 25-20)
- Table 18-4 highlights key facts about amorphous, cloudlike, or popcorn calcifications.
- Table 18-5 summarizes the key findings of the four patterns of abnormal calcification.
- **No matter what its cause, the presence of calcification implies a process that is subacute or chronic.**

Location of Calcification

- Identifying the **pattern** of calcification helps in identifying its **type.**

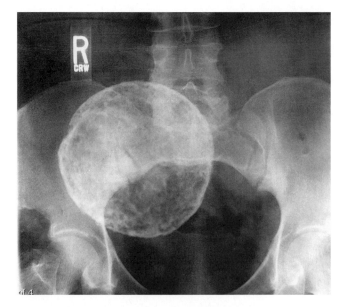

*Figure 18-12. **Calcified rim in uterine leiomyoma.** This is a rimlike calcification in the pelvis of a female patient, so it would be appropriate to consider that this calcification formed in the wall of a hollow viscus or saccular structure. In fact, this is a characteristic pattern of calcification in the outer wall of a degenerated uterine leiomyoma (fibroid). Cystic lesions of the ovary might produce this appearance, and ultrasound of the pelvis would be the study of choice to identify the organ of origin.*

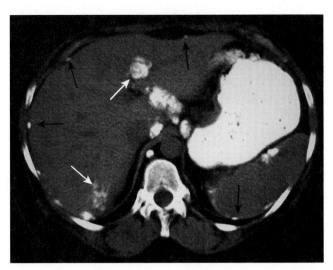

*Figure 18-13. **Calcified ovarian metastases.** An unenhanced axial CT scan of the upper abdomen shows multiple amorphous calcifications, some within the liver (closed white arrows) and others which stud the peritoneal surface of the abdomen (closed black arrows). This patient had a mucin-producing adenocarcinoma of the ovary which metastasized to the peritoneum and liver. Mucin-producing tumors of the stomach and colon can also produce calcified metastases, but ovarian malignancy is the most common to metastasize to the peritoneum.*

Table 18-4

AMORPHOUS, CLOUDLIKE, OR POPCORN CALCIFICATIONS

Organ of Origin	Remarks
Pancreas	Chronic pancreatitis, frequently secondary to alcoholism
Uterine fibroids (leiomyomas)	Degenerating fibroids calcify
Mucin-producing tumors	Mucin-producing tumors of the ovary, stomach, or colon may calcify as can their metastases
Meningioma	Benign, extra-axial brain tumor of older individuals that calcifies about 20% of the time

- Identifying the anatomic **location** of the calcification helps to identify its **organ or tissue of origin.**
  - Combining the **type** of calcification with its **anatomic location** should provide the key to the **cause** of most pathologic calcifications.
- Table 18-6 summarizes some of the possibilities for calcification in the abdomen.

WebLink
More information about recognizing abnormal calcifications is available to registered users on StduentConsult.com.

Table 18-5

IDENTIFYING THE FOUR TYPES OF ABNORMAL CALCIFICATION

Type of Calcification	Location	Examples
Rim-like	Formed in wall of hollow viscus	Calcification in cysts, aneurysms, gallbladder
Linear or track-like	Formed in walls of tubular structures	Calcification in ureters, arteries
Lamellar or laminar	Formed in stones	Renal, gallbladder, and bladder calculi
Amorphous, cloudlike, popcorn	Forms in a solid organ or tumor	Uterine fibroids, some mucin-producing tumors

Table 18-6

CALCIFICATION: LOCATION, LOCATION, LOCATION

Anatomic Quadrant in the Abdomen	Pattern of Calcification	Possible Organ of Origin	Cause
RUQ	Rim-like	Gallbladder wall	Chronic infection
	Track-like	Hepatic artery	Atherosclerosis
	Laminated	Gallbladder	Gallstones
	Amorphous	Head of pancreas	Chronic pancreatitis
LUQ	Rim-like	Splenic cyst	Amebic infection
	Track-like	Splenic artery	Atherosclerosis
	Laminated	Kidney	Renal stone
	Amorphous	Tail of pancreas	Chronic pancreatitis
RLQ	Rim-like	Iliac artery	Iliac artery aneurysm
	Track-like	Iliac artery	Atherosclerosis
	Laminated	Appendix	Appendicolith
	Amorphous	Uterus	Fibroids
LLQ	Rim-like	Iliac artery	Iliac artery aneurysm
	Track-like	Iliac artery	Atherosclerosis
	Laminated	NONE	
	Amorphous	Uterus or ovaries	Ovarian tumor

TAKE-HOME POINTS: Recognizing Abnormal Calcifications and Their Causes

Calcifications can be characterized by the pattern of their calcification and their anatomic location

There are four distinct patterns: rimlike, linear or track-like, lamellar (or laminar) and cloudlike, amorphous or popcorn

Rimlike calcifications imply calcification which has occurred in the wall of a hollow viscus

Examples of rimlike calcifications include cysts, aneurysms or saccular organs like the gallbladder

Linear or track-like calcifications imply calcification that has occurred in the walls of tubular structures

Examples of track-like calcifications include the walls of arteries and tubular structures such as the ureters, Fallopian tubes and vas deferens

Lamellar (or laminar) calcifications imply calcification that forms around a nidus inside a hollow lumen

Examples of lamellar calcifications include renal calculi, gallstones and bladder stones

Cloudlike, amorphous or popcorn calcification is calcification which has formed inside of a solid organ or tumor

Examples of amorphous or popcorn calcifications include pancreatitis, leiomyomas of the uterus, lymph nodes and mucin-producing adenocarcinomas

Combining the type of calcification with its anatomic location should provide the key to the cause of most pathologic calcifications

19 Recognizing Tumors, Tics, and Ulcers: Radiology of the Gastrointestinal Tract

Recognizing Abnormalities of the Gastrointestinal Tract from Top to Bottom

- In this chapter, you'll learn how to recognize some of the most common abnormalities of the gastrointestinal (GI) tract from the esophagus to the rectum.
- As you go through this chapter, you will probably want to refer to the two tables at the end of the chapter, one on **terminology** used in studies of the GI tract (see Table 19-3) and the other on **basic principles in GI radiology** (see Table 19-4), both of which will prove helpful in understanding the terms and concepts used here.
- In grossly oversimplified terms, there are **basically two major types of abnormality of the GI tract:** those that *stick in* and those that *stick out* (Table 19-1).
  - Lesions that **stick out** are **diverticula** and **ulcers**—each adds a **collection** of contrast agent that normally wouldn't be there.
  - Lesions that **stick in** are **benign and malignant tumors**, including **polyps** and **cancer**—each displaces contrast material and forms a **filling defect.**
- Fluoroscopic spot films and overhead films are usually obtained by the radiologist and radiologic technologist in several projections for each part of the GI tract being studied, depending in part on the **nature of the abnormality** and the **mobility of the patient.**
- CT, ultrasound, and MRI have essentially replaced conventional radiography and, in some instances, barium studies for the evaluation of the GI tract and the visceral abdominal organs (the latter in all cases).
- *Virtual endoscopy* is a technique made possible by newer, faster CT and MRI scanners and complex computer algorithms that allow for three-dimensional reconstruction of the appearance of the inside of the bowel lumen including time-of-flight (motion) displays without the use of an endoscope.

Esophagus

- Single or double contrast examination of the esophagus is performed with the patient drinking liquid barium either by itself (single contrast) or accompanied by a gas-producing agent that provides the "air" in a double contrast examination.
  - Because both the single and double contrast techniques have their own strengths, many esophagograms are routinely performed using both techniques, called a *biphasic examination.*
- *Video esophagography* (**video swallowing function**) is a study of the **swallowing mechanism,** usually performed with fluoroscopy and frequently captured in motion on videotape, digital video recorders, or film.
  - This is the study of choice for diagnosing and documenting **aspiration,** in which ingested substances pass into the trachea below the level of the vocal cords (Fig. 19-1).
- **Fluoroscopic observation** of the esophagus can also **reveal abnormalities in esophageal motility.**
  - *Tertiary waves* are a common but nonspecific abnormality of esophageal motility, representing disordered and nonpropulsive contractions of the esophagus.
    - They can be observed fluoroscopically and captured on spot films (Fig. 19-2).

ESOPHAGEAL DIVERTICULA

- Esophageal **diverticula occur in three locations:** the **neck, around the carina,** and just **above the diaphragm.**
- Diverticula of the GI tract, in general, are **usually produced when the mucosal and submucosal layers herniate through a defect in the muscular layer** of the bowel wall.
  - Wherever they occur in the GI tract, diverticula produce an **outpouching of barium** that projects well beyond the borders of the wall when viewed in profile (**stick-out lesions).**
  - They can **change in shape and size** during the course of a barium examination, a characteristic that **helps to differentiate a diverticulum from an ulcer,** another stick-out lesion that tends not to change in size or shape.

Table 19-1

"STICK-IN" AND "STICK-OUT" LESIONS OF THE GI TRACT

Part	Lesions That Stick In	Lesions That Stick Out
Esophagus	Leiomyoma, carcinoma	Diverticula
Stomach	Polyp, carcinoma/lymphoma	Ulcers
Duodenum	Polyp or carcinoma (rare)	Ulcers
Colon	Polyp, carcinoma	Diverticula

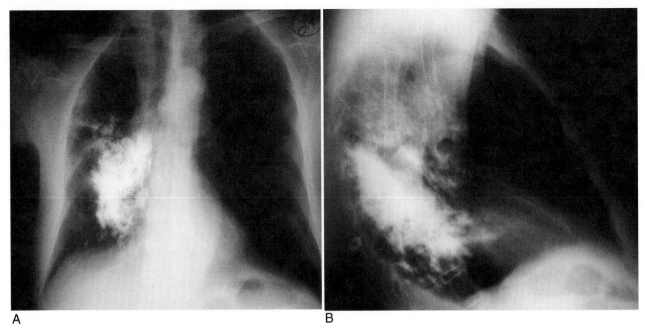

A   B

Figure 19-1. ***Aspiration, barium gone wild.*** *Frontal* ***(A)*** *and lateral* ***(B)*** *radiographs of the chest demonstrate a very high density material in the right lower lobe. The material is metal density and represents barium that was aspirated into the lung during an upper gastrointestinal series. Barium is inert and did not cause any additional symptoms the patient wasn't already experiencing from aspirating his own secretions. It will take some time, but most of this barium will be reabsorbed, most likely leaving only a small amount remaining.*

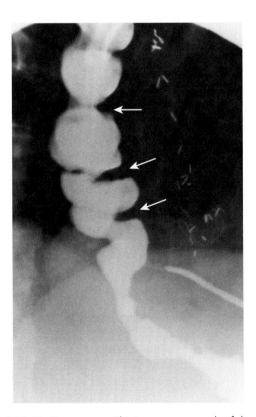

Figure 19-2. ***Tertiary waves.*** *This is a severe example of disordered and nonpropulsive waves of contraction in the esophagus called tertiary waves (closed white arrows). The term* ***corkscrew esophagus*** *is sometimes applied to this appearance. Tertiary waves are a nonspecific and very common abnormality that increases with advancing age.*

- In the neck, the diverticulum is posteriorly located and is called *Zenker's diverticulum* (Fig. 19-3A).
- Diverticula at the level of the carina may be due to extrinsic inflammatory disease such as tuberculosis *(traction diverticula)*; diverticula just above the esophagogastric junction are called *epiphrenic diverticula* (Fig. 19-3B and C).

ESOPHAGEAL CARCINOMA

- Esophageal carcinoma continues to be a disease with a very **poor prognosis**—more than **50% of patients will have metastases upon initial presentation.**
  - The **lack of an esophageal serosa** and a **rich supply of lymphatics** aid in the extension and dissemination of esophageal carcinoma.
- Esophageal malignancies are either **squamous cell carcinomas** or **adenocarcinomas,** the latter of which is **increasing in prevalence.**
  - **Adenocarcinomas** arise in esophageal epithelium that has undergone **metaplasia** from **squamous to columnar epithelium** (*Barrett's esophagus*), a process in which **gastroesophageal reflux plays a major role.**
- Barium esophagograms are **frequently the initial study** in patients with symptoms suggesting this diagnosis.
- Esophageal carcinomas may **appear in one or more of several forms:**
  - **Annular-constricting lesion** (Fig. 19-4A)
  - **Polypoid mass** (Fig. 19-4B)
  - **Superficial, infiltrating lesion**
  - **Ulceration and irregularity of the wall** (Fig. 19-4C)

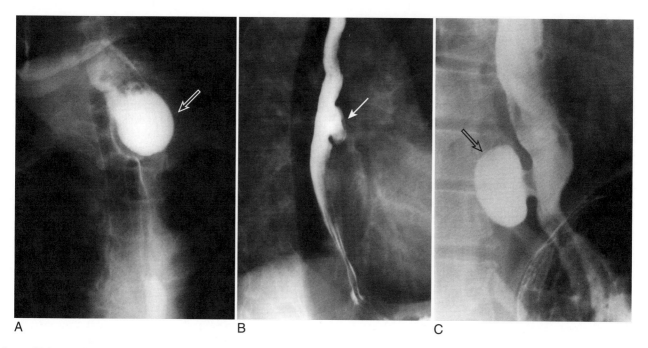

Figure 19-3. **Esophageal diverticula.** *Esophageal diverticula characteristically occur in the neck* **(A)** *from a localized weakness in the posterior wall of the hypopharynx* **(Zenker's diverticulum)** *(open white arrow); in the midesophagus* **(B)** *from extrinsic disease (e.g., TB) that causes fibrosis, which pulls the esophagus, forming a* **traction diverticulum** *(closed white arrow); or just above the diaphragm in the distal esophagus* **(C) (epiphrenic diverticulum)** *(open black arrow). Only the traction diverticulum is a* **true** *diverticulum in that it contains all layers of the esophagus; Zenker's and epiphrenic diverticula are* **false** *or pseudodiverticula in that the mucosa and submucosa herniate through a defect in the muscular layer. Zenker's diverticulum is the only one of the three that produces symptoms.*

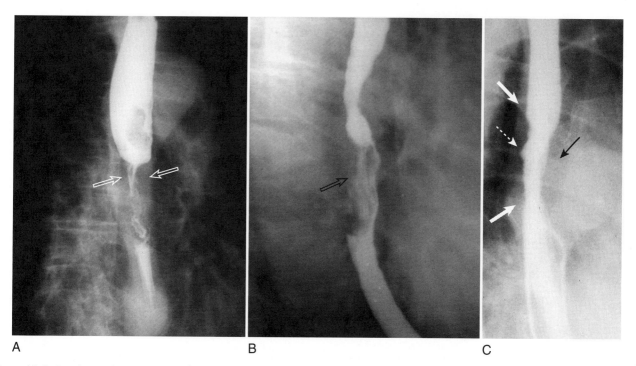

Figure 19-4. **Esophageal carcinomas.** *Three patients are shown with different appearances of esophageal carcinoma.* **A,** *An* **annular constricting** *lesion is seen in the midesophagus (open white arrows). The tumor encircles the normal lumen and obstructs it in this case.* **B,** *A* **polypoid mass** *arises from the right lateral wall of the esophagus and displaces the barium around it (open black arrow).* **C,** *The wall is irregular and rigid (closed white arrows) and contains a small* **ulceration** *(dotted white arrow); the aortic knob is producing a normal indentation on the opposite wall of the esophagus (closed black arrow).*

Hiatal Hernia and Gastroesophageal Reflux Disease

- **Hiatal hernias** are a **common** abnormality that increase in incidence with age and in which the esophagogastric (EG) junction is usually above the level of the diaphragm.
- Hiatal hernias are divided into the **sliding type** (almost all) in which the **esophagogastric junction lies above the diaphragm** or the **paraesophageal type (1%)** in which a **portion of the stomach herniates through the esophageal hiatus but the EG junction remains below the diaphragm.**
- **Most hiatal hernias are asymptomatic,** but there is an association between the presence of some hiatal hernias and clinically significant *gastroesophageal reflux disease (GERD).*
  - **Gastroesophageal reflux also occurs in patients without** any visible **hiatal hernia,** usually due to some dysfunction of the lower esophageal sphincter, which normally acts to prevent gastric acid from repeatedly refluxing into the esophagus.
- The **radiologic findings of hiatal hernia**
  - **Failure of the esophagus to narrow** on multiple images **as it passes through the esophageal hiatus**
  - **Extension of multiple gastric mucosal folds above the diaphragm** (Fig. 19-5)
  - Sometimes, a thin, circumferential filling defect in the distal esophagus called *Schatzki's ring* may be visible.

- Schatzki's ring **marks the position of the esophagogastric junction** so that its visualization above the diaphragm defines a sliding hiatal hernia (Fig. 19-6).
- Some limit use of the term Schatzki's ring to esophageal rings associated with **dysphagia.**
- **Gastroesophageal reflux may be evident during fluoroscopy** when barium is seen to move from the stomach backward into the esophagus, but reflux is intermittent so that it may not occur during the course of the examination.
  - Demonstration of reflux **does not indicate the patient has the complications of GERD, i.e., esophagitis, stricture, and Barrett's esophagus.**
  - Each of those complications can be visible (but may not be) on an esophagogram.
  - Lack of demonstration of reflux during the course of the examination **does not exclude reflux.**

Stomach and Duodenum

- Today, the lumen of the stomach is often studied by upper endoscopy, and the wall thickness and structures outside the stomach are studied by CT examination of the abdomen with oral contrast agent.
- Nevertheless, biphasic upper gastrointestinal (UGI) examinations, which include study of the esophagus, stomach, and duodenum, remain a sensitive, cost-effective, readily available, and noninvasive examination.

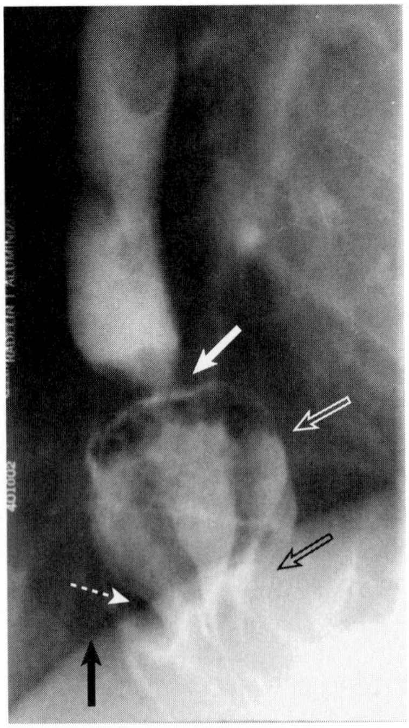

*Figure 19-5. **Hiatal hernia.** A bulbous collection of contrast material (open white arrow) represents the stomach herniated above the diaphragm (closed black arrow). Gastric folds in the hernia identify it as part of the stomach (dotted white arrow). Notice that the esophagus does not narrow as it does normally when passing through the esophageal hiatus (open black arrow). The narrowing seen above the hernia (closed white arrow) is the level of the esophagogastric junction.*

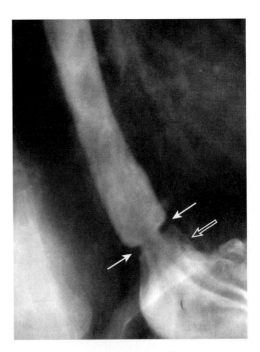

*Figure 19-6. **Hiatal hernia with Schatzki's ring.** A hiatal hernia (open white arrow) is identified by the multiple gastric folds and the lack of narrowing as the esophagus passes through the diaphragmatic hiatus. Just above the hernia is a thin, weblike filling defect characteristic of a Schatzki's ring (closed white arrows). The Schatzki's ring marks the level of the esophagogastric junction.*

GASTRIC ULCERS

- In the United States, the **incidence of gastric ulcer disease has been declining.**
- In adults, infection with *Helicobacter pylori* accounts for almost three fourths of the cases of gastric ulcer disease.
  - **Nonsteroidal anti-inflammatory agents account for most of the rest.**
- The **radiologic findings of gastric ulcers** are similar to those for ulcers anywhere in the GI tract:
  - **Peristent collection of barium**
    - An ulcer provides a receptacle for the retention of barium and it will be present on multiple images of the same area (persistence).
  - The **collection extends outward from the lumen** beyond the normal contours of the stomach (when seen in profile) ("*stick-out lesion*") (Fig. 19-7).
    - In the stomach, most ulcers occur on the **lesser curvature** or **posterior wall** in the region of the **body or antrum.**
  - **Radiating folds typically extend to the ulcer margin** (Fig. 19-8).
  - A **surrounding margin of edema** of varying size presents as a **lucency at the base of the ulcer** when seen in profile.
- About **95% of all gastric ulcers are benign.**
  - Only 5% will represent ulcerations in gastric malignancies.

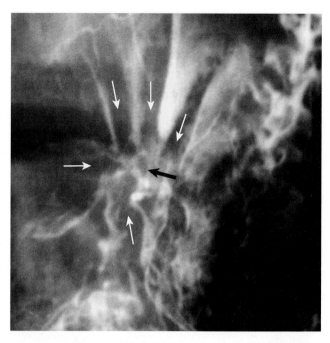

Figure 19-8. ***Benign gastric ulcer.*** *Numerous gastric folds (closed white arrows) all radiate to a central lesion (closed black arrow) that represents a gastric ulcer. On double contrast examinations, ulcers that are on the nondependent surface of the stomach at the time of the exposure will be etched with barium rather than fill in as a collection of barium. In this case, the ulcer is represented by the oval density to which the black arrow is pointing. This was a benign gastric ulcer.*

- Although determination of the benign or malignant nature of a gastric ulcer can be suggested using radiographic criteria, that differentiation now relies less on radiographic findings than it does on endoscopic biopsy.

GASTRIC CARCINOMA

- There has been a dramatic **decline in the incidence of gastric carcinoma in the United States.**
  - The **mortality rate, however, remains quite high,** because they are frequently not diagnosed until after they have spread.
- Most gastric carcinomas (actually, they are adenocarcinomas) **occur in the distal third of the stomach** on the **lesser curvature.**
- Double contrast upper gastrointestinal series can demonstrate gastric carcinoma in the following forms:
  - **Polypoid**
  - **Infiltrating** = *linitis plastica*
  - **Ulcerative**
- The **key findings in gastric carcinoma**
  - A **mass that protrudes into the lumen** and produces a filling defect, displacing barium (***stick-in lesion***) (Fig. 19-9)
  - **Rigidity of the wall and nondistensibility of the lumen** (Fig. 19-10)
  - **Eccentric, irregular ulceration in a mass** (see Fig. 19-9)
  - **Thickened, irregular gastric folds** (>1 cm), especially localized to one area of the stomach

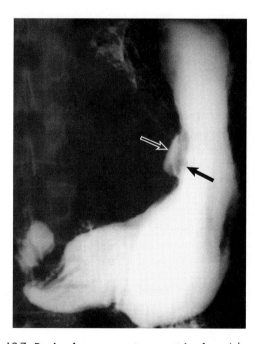

Figure 19-7. ***Benign lesser curvature gastric ulcer.*** *A large collection of barium protrudes beyond the expected contour of the normal stomach (stick-out lesion) representing a gastric ulcer (open white arrow). A mound of edematous tissue surrounds the ulcer and is seen in profile in this example as a lucent zone at the base of the ulcer called an* ***ulcer collar*** *(closed black arrow).*

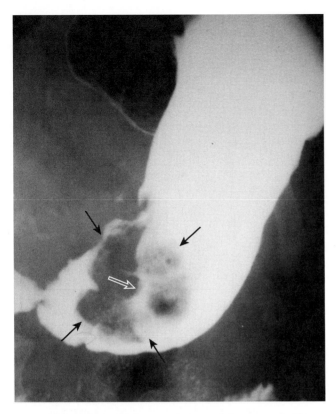

Figure 19-9. **Polypoid adenocarcinoma of the stomach.** *This large, polypoid filling defect in the antrum of the stomach (stick-in lesion) displaces the barium around it (closed black arrows). Contained within the mass and seen en face is an irregularly shaped, linear collection that represents an ulceration in the mass and that fills in with barium (open white arrow). Differential possibilities for such a lesion might include an ulcerating adenocarcinoma of the stomach, a leiomyoma (leiomyomas frequently ulcerate) or lymphoma. This was an adenocarcinoma of the stomach.*

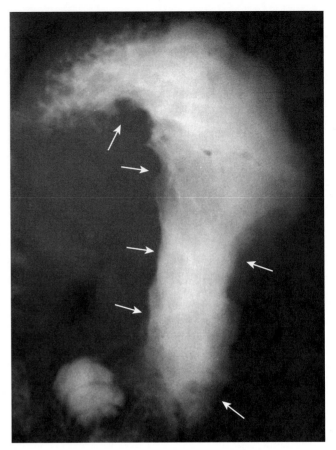

Figure 19-10. **Linitis plastica.** *The entire body of the stomach displays a lack of distensibility, losing the normal tendency to balloon outward that every portion of the GI tract demonstrates when filled with enough barium or air. Instead, the walls of the stomach are concave inward (closed white arrows) and rigid. This stomach would have the same appearance on all images. This is the typical appearance of **linitis plastica,** caused by an infiltrating adenocarcinoma of the stomach.*

- Other mass lesions may resemble gastric carcinoma, including *leiomyomas,* a wall lesion that characteristically ulcerates, and *lymphoma,* which may produce diffusely thickened folds or localized masses in the stomach.

DUODENAL ULCER

- **Duodenal ulcers are two to three times more common than gastric ulcers.**
    - Almost all duodenal ulcers occur in the **bulb,** the majority on the **anterior wall** of the bulb.
- They are **overwhelmingly caused by *H. pylori* infection** (85–95%).
- Complications include **obstruction, perforation** (into the peritoneal cavity), **penetration** (such as into the pancreas), and **hemorrhage.**
- Double contrast upper GI series has a sensitivity that exceeds 90% in detecting duodenal ulcers.

- The **radiologic findings of duodenal ulcers**
    - **A persistent collection of contrast material,** more often seen *en face* than in profile, in the duodenal bulb (Fig. 19-11)
        - It is unusual, therefore, to see a duodenal ulcer as a *stick-out lesion.*

- Frequently, **surrounding spasm and edema**
- **Healing of duodenal ulcers produces predictable deformities** of the bulb, among which is the *clover-leaf deformity,* which occurs from scarring following an ulcer that was located in the central portion of the bulb (Fig. 19-12).

DUODENAL DIVERTICULA

- They **occur in about 5% of people** and are **almost always asymptomatic** because they contain fluid and do not usually become obstructed and perforate, as do colonic diverticula.
- Most occur on the **medial wall of the second portion of the duodenum** at or near the site of the insertion of the common bile duct and **resemble a "mushroom" when seen in profile** *(stick-out lesion)* (Fig. 19-13).

Small Bowel

OBSTRUCTION

- For the findings of mechanical small bowel obstruction on conventional radiographs, see Chapter 16, "Recognizing Bowel Obstruction and Ileus".

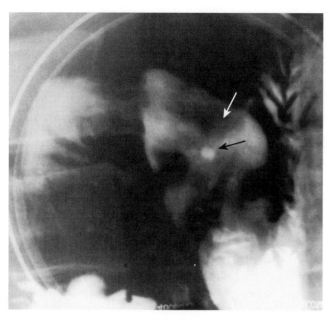

Figure 19-11. Acute duodenal ulcer. *Contained within the duodenal bulb on its anterior wall is a collection of barium (closed black arrow) surrounded by a zone of edema (closed white arrow) that displaces the barium from around the ulcer. This collection was persistent on multiple images of the bulb and is characteristic of an acute duodenal ulcer. When this centrally located ulcer heals, it is likely to produce the clover-leaf deformity, seen in Figure 19-12.*

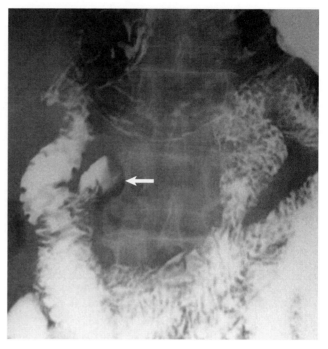

Figure 19-13. Duodenal diverticulum. *This collection of barium (stick-out lesion) protrudes from the medial border of the second portion of the duodenum in a characteristic location for a duodenal diverticulum (closed white arrow). The lesion typically has a "mushroom" shape and arises at or near the ampulla of Vater. Typically, these lesions produce no symptoms and are found serendipitously on examinations performed for other reasons.*

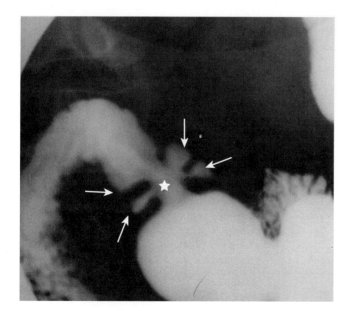

Figure 19-12. Clover-leaf deformity of chronic duodenal ulcer disease. *The duodenal bulb is deformed by scarring that has occurred from an ulcer previously located in the center of the bulb (white star). The scarring puckers the walls in such a way as to leave three or four projections of the unaffected normal bulb (closed white arrows). This pattern was once thought to resemble a clover leaf and is called a* **clover-leaf deformity.**

- The **most common cause of a mechanical small bowel obstruction is adhesions** from previous surgery.
  - Other causes include **hernias, intussusception, and gallstone ileus.**
- **CT is the most sensitive study** for diagnosing mechanical small bowel obstruction.
  - Ingestion of contrast material (containing either barium or iodine) helps in **identifying dilated loops** of bowel and in finding the *transition point* between the **proximal dilated** bowel and the **distal collapsed** bowel.
- The **CT findings of a small bowel obstruction**
  - **Fluid-filled and dilated loops of small bowel** (>2.5 cm in diameter) proximal to the point of obstruction
  - Identification of a *transition point,* which is where the **bowel changes caliber** from dilated to normal, indicating the site of the obstruction
    - In the absence of identifying a mass or hernia at the transition point, the cause is almost certainly adhesions.
  - **Collapsed small bowel or colon distal to the point of obstruction** (Fig. 19-14)

CROHN'S DISEASE

- Crohn's disease is a **chronic, relapsing, granulomatous inflammation of the small bowel and colon,** usually involving the **terminal ileum,** resulting in ulceration, obstruction, and fistula formation.
- Crohn's disease **typically involves the ileum and right colon,** presents with *skip areas* (abnormal bowel

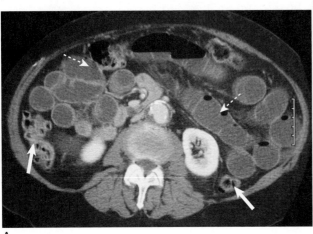

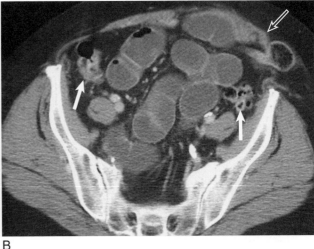

A   B

Figure 19-14. **Mechanical small bowel obstruction, CT.** These two patients have distal mechanical small bowel obstructions demonstrated on CT studies. **A,** There are multiple dilated loops of small bowel (dotted white arrows). The colon (closed white arrows) is collapsed. Therefore, there is a small bowel obstruction. **B,** There is a rent in the musculature of the left lateral abdominal wall called a **Spigelian hernia** through which a loop of small bowel has herniated (open white arrow) and obstructed. The colon (closed white arrows) is collapsed.

interposed between normal bowel), is prone to **fistula formation,** and has a **propensity for recurring** following surgical resection and reanastomosis in whatever loop becomes the new terminal ileum.

- Crohn's disease may be demonstrated by either a barium **small bowel follow-through** series or **CT of the abdomen and pelvis.**

- The **imaging findings in Crohn's disease**
  - **Narrowing, irregularity, and ulceration of the terminal ileum** frequently with proximal small bowel dilatation
  - **Separation of the loops of bowel** due to fatty infiltration of the mesentery surrounding the ileum making the affected loop(s) stand apart from the surrounding loops of small bowel (*proud loop*) (Fig. 19-15)
  - The *string-sign*—narrowing of the terminal ileum into a near slit-like opening by spasm and fibrosis
  - Fistulae—especially between the ileum and colon but also to the skin, vagina, and urinary bladder. (Fig. 19-16A)
    - **Streaky collections of barium** may emanate from the abnormal loop and join another luminal structure (e.g., the colon) or end blindly as a *sinus tract.*
    - **On CT, thickening of the wall and infiltration of the surrounding fat** by streaky or hazy densities indicate surrounding inflammatory changes (Fig. 19-16B).

Large Bowel

- The intraluminal surface of the colon is most often studied with endoscopy or double contrast barium enema examination.
  - Virtual colonoscopy utilizing either CT or MRI can provide information on the intraluminal anatomy of the colon while, at the same time, allowing for visualization of the other abdominal structures outside the colon.

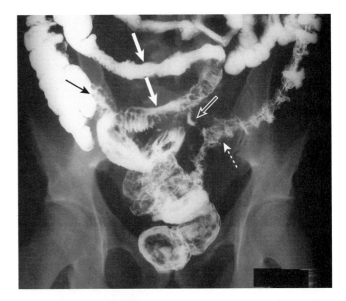

Figure 19-15. **Crohn's disease.** Several loops of abnormal small bowel (closed white arrows) all show narrowing, rigidity, and ulcerations. The terminal ileum (closed black arrow) is also abnormal, as is characteristic of this disease. The small bowel loops are widely separated from each other, in large part because of the increased amount of mesenteric fat present in patients with this disease **(proud loops).** A streak of barium (open white arrow) connects the small bowel to the sigmoid colon (dotted white arrow) and represents an **enterocolic fistula,** a common complication of this disease.

DIVERTICULOSIS

- **Colonic diverticula,** like most diverticula of the GI tract, represent herniation of the mucosa and submucosa through a defect in the muscular layer *(false diverticula).*
- They occur more frequently with increasing age and may be due, at least in part, to increase in intraluminal pressure and weakening of the colonic wall.

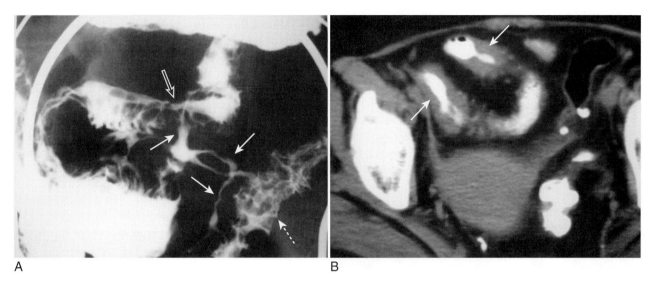

A   B

*Figure 19-16. **Crohn's disease, small bowel series and CT.** These two patients have Crohn's disease. **A,** A single close-up image of the right lower quadrant from a small bowel follow-through study shows multiple streaks of barium (closed white arrows) representing multiple fistulae originating from an abnormal loop of small bowel (open white arrow) and connecting with each other and the large bowel (dotted white arrow). **B,** An image of the pelvis from a CT scan shows an abnormal loop of small bowel in the right lower quadrant with a thickened wall (closed white arrows). Normal small bowel wall thickness is 3 mm or less with the loop distended, which means that a bowel loop opacified with contrast agent has essentially no visible wall when normal. In patients with Crohn's disease, the wall may be up to a 10 mm thick. Notice how the loop is surrounded by extra fat in the mesentery.*

- They are **usually multiple *(diverticulosis),*** are almost always **asymptomatic** (about 90% of the time), but **can become inflamed or bleed.**
  - **Diverticulosis is the most common cause of massive lower GI bleeding.**
  - When they bleed, the right-sided diverticula seem to bleed more than those on the left.

- They occur most often in the sigmoid colon and are readily **identified on either barium enema or CT examination as small spikes or smoothly domed outpouchings of air or contrast material** (Fig. 19-17).

DIVERTICULITIS
- Diverticula can become inflamed and perforate *(**diverticulitis**),* most likely secondary to mechanical irritation or obstruction.

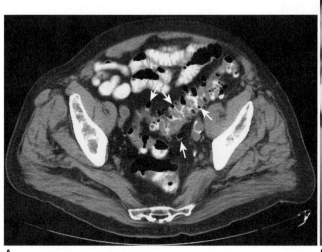

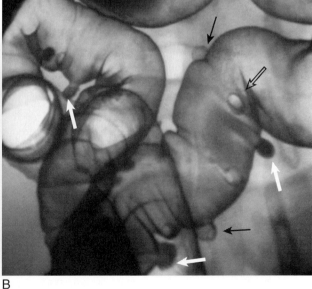

A   B

*Figure 19-17. **Diverticulosis. A,** In this CT scan of the pelvis, diverticula contain mostly air and appear as small, usually round outpouchings in the region of the sigmoid colon especially (closed white arrows). **B,** Numerous outpouchings of barium (stick-out lesions) are seen in the sigmoid colon of this double-contrast barium enema examination. Some diverticula contain barium (closed white arrows) but others contain air and are outlined with barium (closed black arrows). Where a diverticulum is seen en face, it produces a circular density (open black arrow), which can sometimes produce an appearance that can be similar to a polyp on double-contrast examinations.*

- **CT is the modality of choice** for the **diagnosis of diverticulitis** because the pericolonic soft tissues can be visualized using CT, which is impossible with either barium enema or endoscopy.
- The **CT findings of acute diverticulitis**
  - **Presence of diverticula**
  - **Pericolonic inflammation**—hazy areas of increased attenuation or streaky and disorganized linear and amorphous densities in the pericolonic fat (Fig. 19-18)
  - **Thickening of the adjacent colonic wall** (>4 mm) (see Fig. 19-18)

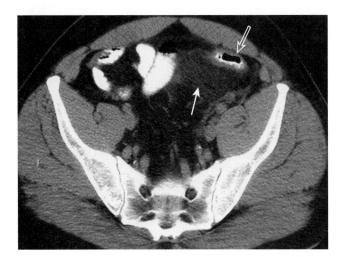

Figure 19-18. **Diverticulitis, CT.** Infiltration of the pericolonic fat is demonstrated by a hazy increase in attenuation (closed white arrow) surrounding an abnormally thickened wall in a loop of large bowel (open white arrow). Focal infiltration of fat is a common characteristic of inflammatory diseases.

- **Abscess formation**—multiple small bubbles of air or pockets of fluid contained within a pericolonic soft tissue masslike density (Fig. 19-19A)
- **Perforation of the colon**—extraluminal air or contrast either around the site of the perforation or, less likely, free in the peritoneal cavity (Fig. 19-19B)

COLONIC POLYPS

- The **incidence of polyps increases with age** and the **incidence of malignancy increases with the size** of the polyp.
  - Patients with polyposis syndromes in which multiple adenomatous polyps are present have a much higher risk of developing a colonic malignancy.
- Most colonic polyps are **hyperplastic polyps** that have **no malignant potential.**
- **Adenomatous polyps carry** a low **potential for malignancy that increases with the size of the polyp** so that those **larger than 1.5 cm** have about a **10% chance of being malignant.**
- Therefore, the early detection and removal of adenomatous polyps will decrease the chances of malignant transformation.
- The **imaging findings of colonic polyps on barium enema examination**
  - A **persistent filling defect in the colon**—barium is displaced by the polyp *(stick-in lesion)* (Fig. 19-20A).
  - The polyp may have a stalk *(pedunculated polyp)* or be attached to the wall *(sessile polyp)* (Fig. 19-20B).
  - The polyp **may contain numerous fronds** that produce an irregular, wormlike surface with numerous crypts that may contain barium *(villous polyp)* (Fig. 19-21).

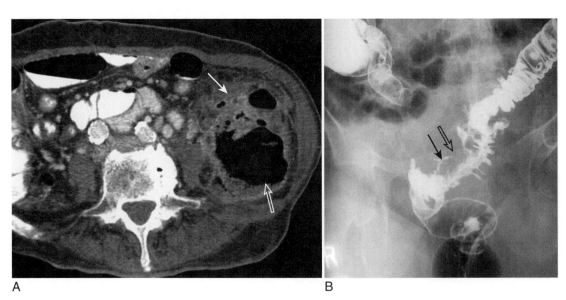

A   B

Figure 19-19. **Diverticulitis, CT and barium enema.** A large abscess cavity (open white arrow) is seen in the left lower quadrant in this close-up of a CT scan of the lower abdomen **(A)**. There are adjacent small bubbles of gas that are not contained within bowel (closed white arrow). These findings are secondary to a confined perforation with abscess formation from perforated diverticulitis. **B,** A barium enema examination from a different patient is shown. The two major findings of diverticulitis on barium enema are extraluminal barium (closed black arrow) and mass effect on the colon (open black arrow).

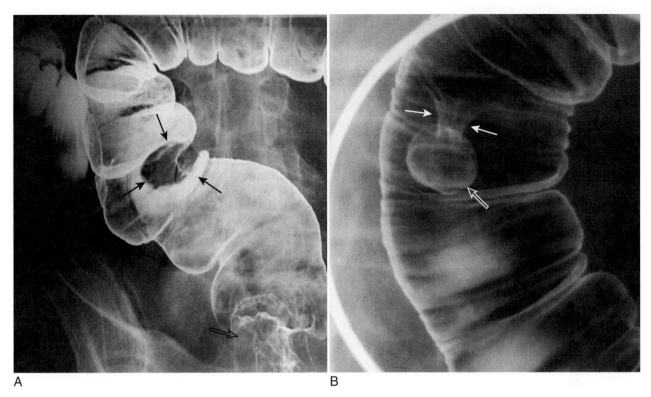

Figure 19-20. **Sessile and pedunculated polyps of the colon. A,** *A sessile filling defect (attaches directly to wall) is seen in the pool of barium along the medial wall of the sigmoid colon (closed black arrows). The size of the lesion should raise concern for malignancy. This is the same patient shown in Figure 19-23 with an annular constricting carcinoma of the rectosigmoid (open black arrow).* **B,** *A double contrast barium enema was performed on another patient with a filling defect in the sigmoid colon etched by barium (open white arrow). In this patient, the polyp is attached to the wall of the colon by a stalk (closed white arrows). Polyps on a stalk are called* **pedunculated polyps.**

- Villous polyps tend to be larger and have more of a malignant potential than other adenomatous polyps.
- Occasionally, a polyp may serve as a *lead point* for an *intussusception,* in which the polyp drags and prolapses one part of the bowel into the lumen of the bowel immediately ahead of it.

- The bowel proximal to the intussusception is usually obstructed and dilated.
- Intussusception may produce a characteristic *coiled-spring* appearance on barium enema or CT (Fig. 19-22).

COLONIC CARCINOMA

- **Colon cancer is the most common cancer of the GI tract.**

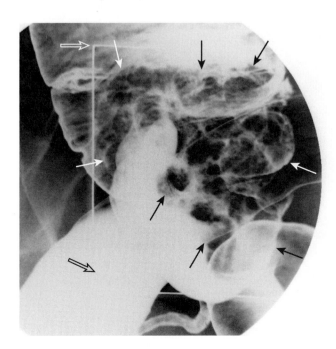

Figure 19-21. **Villous tumor of cecum.** *Contained within this large, polypoid mass in the cecum (outlined by black and white closed arrows) is an interlacing network of white lines representing barium that is trapped within the interstices of the frondlike projections from this tumor. This is a characteristic appearance for a villous adenomatous tumor. The rectosigmoid (open black arrow) is superimposed on the cecum in this projection. The white square (open white arrow) is part of a fluoroscopic device used to compress the abdomen to reduce the amount of soft tissue the x-ray beam must traverse.*

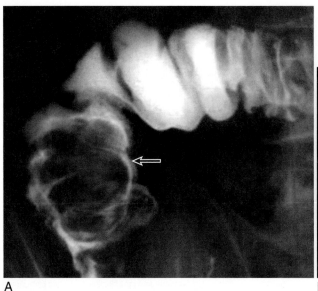
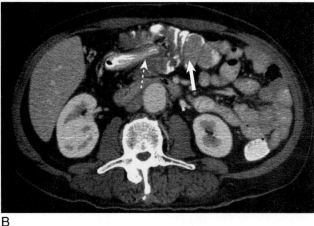

A   B

*Figure 19-22. **Intussusception, barium enema and CT scan. A,** When one loop of bowel prolapses inside the loop immediately distal to it, the resultant obstruction produces a **coiled-spring** appearance on barium enema examination since two loops of bowel are superimposed on one another (open white arrow). **B,** In another patient with an intussusception, a loop of large bowel (dotted white arrow) is seen prolapsing into the loop distal to it (closed white arrow), producing a filling defect.*

- Most cancers occur in the rectosigmoid region and take years to develop.
- Risk factors include adenomatous polyps, family history of colonic polyps or colon cancer, ulcerative colitis and Crohn's disease, polyposis syndromes, and prior pelvic irradiation.
- The **imaging findings of carcinoma of the colon**
  - A **persistent, large, polypoid filling defect**
  - **Annular constriction** of the colonic lumen producing an *apple-core lesion* (Fig. 19-23)
  - **Frank or micro-perforation**—infiltration of the pericolonic fat with streaky or hazy densities of increased attenuation with or without the presence of extraluminal air
  - **Large bowel obstruction**—either antegrade obstruction and/or retrograde obstruction demonstrated by the inability of rectally administered barium to pass the point of the colon cancer (see Fig. 16-6)
  - **Metastases,** especially to the liver and the lungs

LARGE BOWEL OBSTRUCTION

- Large bowel obstruction is most often caused by a carcinoma of the colon, typically involving the left colon, followed by inflammatory disease, volvulus, and hernia (see Chapter 16).
- In most cases, the diagnosis can be made on the basis of clinical history and conventional radiographs.
  - The location and cause of the obstruction can frequently be determined by either barium enema examination or lower endoscopy.
- CT is obtained to confirm the diagnosis, identify the level and possible cause of the obstruction, assess for free intraperitoneal air, and identify associated lesions, such as metastases.
- **Recognizing a large bowel obstruction on CT** (Fig. 19-24)

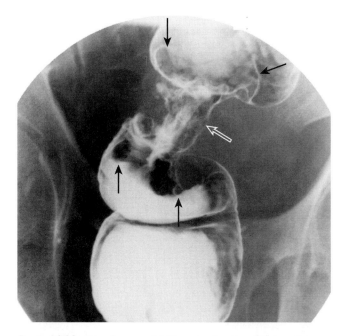

*Figure 19-23. **Annular constricting carcinoma of the rectum.** This characteristic **apple-core** lesion of the rectum is caused by circumferential growth of a colonic carcinoma. The margins of the lesion (closed black arrows) demonstrate what is called an **overhanging edge** where tumor tissue projects into the normal lumen, typical of this type of lesion. The "core" of the "apple" (open white arrow) is composed of tumor tissue—all the normal colonic mucosa has been replaced. Identification of such a lesion is pathognomonic for carcinoma.*

- The large bowel is **dilated to the point of obstruction,** then normal in caliber distal to the obstructing lesion.

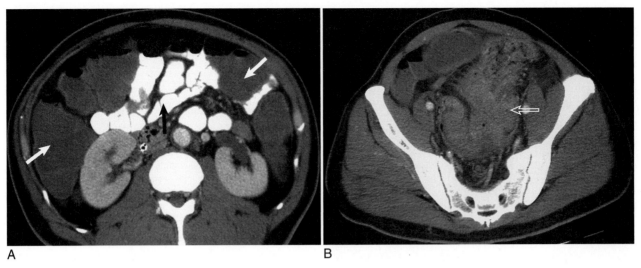

A   B

Figure 19-24. **Large bowel obstruction, CT.** *Two CT images from the same patient demonstrate dilated and fluid-filled loops of large bowel (closed white arrows) and nondilated loops of small bowel (closed black arrow)* **(A). B,** *A large soft tissue mass in the sigmoid (open white arrow) represents the patient's carcinoma of the sigmoid colon and the cause of the large bowel obstruction.*

- The point of obstruction, frequently a carcinoma, can usually be located on CT and identified as a **soft tissue mass.**
- So long as the ileocecal valve remains competent, the **small bowel is not dilated.**

APPENDICITIS

- Pathophysiologically, the development of appendicitis is invariably preceded by obstruction of the appendiceal lumen.
- An **appendicolith is a calcified concretion found in the appendix** of about 15% of all people.
  - The combination of **abdominal pain** and the **presence of an appendicolith is** associated with **appendicitis about 90% of the time** and indicates a higher probability for **perforation.**
  - CT is now the modality of choice for diagnosing appendicitis.
  - The **key CT findings in acute appendicitis**
    - Identification of a **dilated appendix** (>6 mm), which does **not** fill with oral contrast
    - **Periappendiceal inflammation,** which is evidenced by streaky, disorganized linear high attenuation densities in the surrounding fat (Fig. 19-25)
    - **Increased enhancement of the wall of the appendix** with intravenous contrast material due to inflammation
    - **Identification of** a calcification in about one fourth of cases, usually in the lumen of the appendix, which represents an *appendicolith* (Fig. 19-26)
    - **Perforation,** which occurs in up to 30% of cases and is **recognized by small quantities of periappendiceal extraluminal air or a periappendiceal abscess**
  - Because obstruction of the appendiceal lumen is a prerequisite for appendicitis, the presence of free

intraperitoneal air should point to another diagnosis.
- Table 19-2 indicates the study of **first choice** for several **different clinical scenarios** relating to **abdominal pain.**

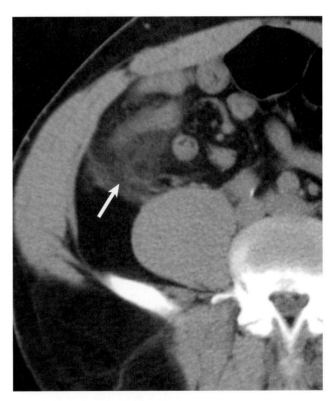

Figure 19-25. **Appendicitis, CT.** *Infiltration of the periappendiceal fat in the right lower quadrant is manifested by the increased attenuation in the mesenteric fat demonstrated on this CT scan (closed white arrow). Focal infiltration of fat is a common characteristic of inflammatory diseases and helps in their localization.*

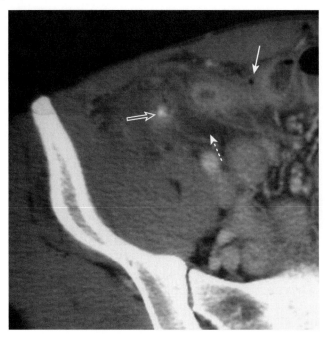

Figure 19-26. **Appendicolith in appendicitis, CT.** *Contained within the lumen of the appendix is a small calcification (open white arrow) or* **appendicolith.** *Inflammatory infiltration of the surrounding fat produces increased attenuation (dotted white arrow). A very small amount of air is present outside the appendiceal lumen from a confined perforation (closed white arrow). An appendicolith can be found in about one fourth of the cases of acute appendicitis. The combination of an appendicolith and acute appendicitis is a strong predictor of a perforated appendix.*

Terminology

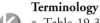

- Table 19-3 defines the terminology used in studies of the GI tract.

Table 19-2

INITIAL IMAGING STUDY OF CHOICE BY SITE OF PAIN

Site of Pain	Imaging Study	Likely Cause of Pain
Right upper quadrant	Ultrasound	Cholecystitis
Right lower quadrant	CT	Appenddicitis
Upper midline	Upper GI series	Ulcer
Pelvis	Ultrasound (female), CT (male)	Pelvic inflammatory disease; diverticulitis
Left upper quadrant	CT	Pancreatitis
Left lower quadrant	CT	Diverticulitis

Table 19-3

TERMINOLOGY FOR GI TRACT STUDIES

Term	Definition
Fluoroscopy	The special use of x-ray imaging to observe in real time the dynamic movement of the bowel and to optimally position the patient so as to obtain diagnostic images frequently referred to as "spot films."
Barium enema	Barium sulfate in suspension (an inert, radiopaque material prepared in liquid form) used to study the intraluminal anatomy of the GI tract and administered by tube via the rectum
Single contrast	A (full column) GI imaging procedure in which only barium is employed as the contrast agent
Double contrast (air contrast study)	A study of the GI tract using both thicker barium and air in a way that barium coats the mucosa and air distends the lumen
Biphasic examination	A study of the upper GI tract that utilizes an initial double contrast study followed by a single contrast agent to optimize the study
Filling defect	A lesion, usually of soft tissue density, that protrudes into the lumen *(sticks in)* and displaces the intraluminal contrast (e.g., a polyp is a filling defect)
Ulcer	A peristent collection of contrast that projects outward *(sticks out)* from the contrast-filled lumen and originates either through a break in the mucosal lining (as in gastric ulcer) or indside a GI mass (as in an ulcerating malignancy)
Diverticulum	A persistent collection of contrast material that projects outward *(sticks out)* from the contrast-filled lumen of the GI tract; it may appear like an ulcer but can change in shape, unlike an ulcer; many diverticula of the GI tract occur in anatomically predictable locations and are lined by mucosa and submucosa
Spot films	Static images obtained by the radiologist during fluoroscopy to position the patient for the optimum image
Overhead films	Additional images obtained by the radiologic technologist to complement fluoroscopic spot films using an x-ray tube mounted on the ceiling of the radiographic room (thus, the term "overhead")
Intraluminal (luminal)	Lesions generally arising from the mucosa, (e.g., polyps and carcinomas)
Intramural (mural)	Lesions arising from the wall of, in this case, the GI tract (e.g., leiomyomas and lipomas)
Extrinsic	Lesions arising outside the GI tract (e.g., serosal metastases or endometriosis implants)
En face and in profile	When you look at a lesion directly "head-on," you are seeing it *en face*; a lesion seen tangentially (from the side) is seen in profile; except for those that are perfect spheres, lesions will have a different appearance when viewed *en face* and in profile

Common Principles for All Gastrointestinal Barium Studies

- Table 19-4 explains the basic principles of barium studies.

WebLink
More information on radiology of the gastrointestinal tract is available to registered users on StudentConsult.com.

Table 19-4

PRINCIPLES COMMON TO ALL BARIUM STUDIES

Term	Definition
Fully distended vs. collapsed	Only loops that are fully distended by contrast can be accurately evaluated, no matter what part of the GI tract is being studied or whether the images are obtained using fluoroscopy or CT; evaluating certain criteria (such as wall thickness) by examining collapsed loops may introduce errors of diagnosis.
Change and distensibility	Over time (usually measured in seconds), the walls of all the GI luminal structures, from esophagus to rectum, change in contour, distending and ballooning outward with increasing volumes of barium or air. Change and distensibility are normal.
Rigid, stiff, fixed, nondistensible	If the wall of bowel is infiltrated by tumor, blood, edema, or fibrous tissue, to name a few, the bowel may lose its ability to change and distend; terms applied to this lack of distensibility are **rigid, stiff, fixed, nondistensible**. This is abnormal.
Irregularity	Except for the normal marginal indentations caused by the folds in the stomach, small bowel, and colon, the walls of the entire GI tract appear relatively smooth and regular; diseases can produce ulceration, infiltration and nodularity with resultant irregularity of the wall.
Persistence	Almost without exception, an apparent abnormality must be seen on more than one image to be considered a pathologic finding; transient changes in the GI tract caused by peristalsis, ingested food, the presence of stool, or incompletely distended loops of bowel will disappear over time, but true abnormalities will remain constant and persistent.

TAKE-HOME POINTS: Recognizing Tumors, Tics and Ulcers

In grossly oversimplified terms, there are basically two major types of abnormality of the GI tract: those that *stick in* and produce filling defects, like polyps and cancer, and those that *stick out* and are collections, like diverticula and ulcers.

Single contrast (barium only), double contrast (air and barium) and biphasic (combination of single and double contrast) examinations of the gastrointestinal tract are utilized with fluoroscopic spot films and overhead films usually obtained by the radiologist and radiologic technologist in several projections for whatever the part being studied.

Esophageal diverticula occur in the neck (Zenker's), around the carina (traction) and just above the diaphragm (epiphrenic); only the Zenker's diverticulum tends to produce symptoms.

Esophageal carcinoma continues to have a poor prognosis with an increasing incidence of adenocarcinomas forming in Barrett's esophagus, a condition in which GERD plays a major role in stimulating metaplasia of the squamous to columnar epithelium.

Esophageal carcinomas appear in one or more of several forms including an annular-constricting lesion, a polypoid mass and a superficial, infiltrating type lesion.

Hiatal hernias are a common abnormality that may be associated with GERD, although GERD can occur even in the absence of a demonstrable hernia; they are usually of the sliding variety in which the EG junction lies above the diaphragm.

A Schatzki's ring is a thin, circumferential ring that marks the position of the EG junction; some limit the use of that term to only those rings with associated dysphagia while others apply it to any such ring in the distal esophagus.

The radiologic findings of gastric ulcer include a persitent collection of barium that extends outward from the lumen beyond the normal contours of the stomach usually along the lesser curvature or posterior wall in the region of the body or antrum; the ulcer usually has radiating folds which typically extend to the ulcer margin and a surrounding margin of edema that varies in size.

The key findings in gastric carcinoma are a mass that protrudes into the lumen and produces a filling defect, displacing barium; they are associated with rigidity of the wall and non-distensibility of the lumen and sometimes eccentric, irregular ulceration or thickening and irregularity of the gastric folds (>1 cm), especially localized to one area of the stomach.

The radiologic findings of duodenal ulcers include a persistent collection of contrast, more often seen *en face* than in profile with surrounding spasm and edema.

Healing of duodenal ulcers produces predictable deformities of the bulb, amongst which is the clover-leaf deformity which occurs from scarring following an ulcer that was located in the central portion of the bulb.

Duodenal diverticula are relatively common lesions that occur on the medial wall of the second portion of the duodenum at or near the site of the insertion of the common bile duct and resemble a "mushroom" when seen in profile; they usually produce no symptoms.

(Continued)

TAKE-HOME POINTS: Recognizing Tumors, Tics and Ulcers—cont'd

The most common cause of a mechanical small bowel obstruction is adhesions caused by previous surgery.

CT is the most sensitive study for diagnosing small bowel obstruction and the findings include fluid-filled and dilated loops of small bowel (>2.5 cm in diameter) proximal to the point of obstruction, frequent identification of a transition point, which is where the bowel changes caliber from dilated to normal, and collapsed small bowel and/or colon distal to the point of obstruction.

Crohn's disease is a chronic, relapsing, granulomatous inflammation of the small bowel and colon, usually involving the terminal ileum, resulting in ulceration, obstruction and fistula formation; it may have skip areas, is prone to fistula formation and has a propensity for recurring following surgical removal of an involved segment.

The imaging findings in Crohn's disease include narrowing, irregularity and ulceration of the terminal ileum frequently with proximal small bowel dilatation; separation of the loops of bowel (proud loop), the string-sign, fistulae—especially between the ileum and colon, as well as thickening of the wall and infiltration of the surrounding fat on CT.

Colonic diverticulosis increases in incidence with increasing age, most often involves the sigmoid colon and is almost always asymptomatic, although it can lead to diverticulitis or massive GI bleeding, especially from right-sided diverticula.

CT is the study of choice for imaging diverticulitis and the findings include pericolonic inflammation, thickening of the adjacent colonic wall (> 4 mm), abscess formation and/or perforation of the colon.

On barium enema examinations, the direct radiologic signs of diverticulitis are extraluminal contrast and mass effect; spasm may be seen secondarily.

Most colonic polyps are hyperplastic and have no malignant potential; adenomatous polyps carry a malignant potential that is related, in part, to their size.

Double contrast barium enema examinations and now virtual colonoscopy are the imaging studies of choice for diagnosing colonic polyps and the signs include a persistent filling defect in the colon with or without a stalk; some larger, villous adenomatous polyps have a higher malignant potential and may contain barium within the interstices of their fronds.

The imaging findings of colonic carcinoma are a persistent, large, polypoid or annular constricting filling defect of the colon with or without frank or micro-perforation or large bowel obstruction and metastases, especially to the liver and the lungs.

Large bowel obstruction is most often caused by carcinoma of the left colon, can usually be diagnosed with conventional radiographs or barium enema and may be further defined by CT, which can evaluate extra-colonic extension or metastases.

CT is the study of choice in diagnosing appendicitis with findings including a dilated appendix (>6 mm) which does not fill with oral contrast, periappendiceal inflammation, increased enhancement of the wall of the appendix with intravenous contrast and sometimes identification of an appendicolith, a finding frequently associated with perforation of the appendix.

20 Recognizing the Basics on CT of the Abdomen

General Considerations

- Conventional radiography, ultrasonography, CT, and MRI are all utilized in the imaging evaluation of abdominal abnormalities.
- Each has advantages and disadvantages inherent to its own particular technology, and the choice of modality is frequently based on the patient's clinical condition (Table 20-1).
- History and physical examination continue to be an essential part of evaluating abdominal abnormalities not only to suggest a cause but also in helping to determine which, if any, imaging study (or studies) will provide the best yield in establishing the correct diagnosis.

ABDOMINAL TRAUMA

- The role of advanced imaging techniques deserves special mention in abdominal trauma.
- Radiology has made a significant impact on the lives of traumatized patients by distinguishing those patients who can be managed conservatively from those who need surgical or other interventions and by helping to direct the most appropriate intervention for those who need it.

Table 20-1

IMAGING OF THE ABDOMEN AND PELVIS

Modality	Uses	Advantages	Disadvantages
Conventional radiography	Primarily used for screening in abdominal pain	Availability	Lower sensitivity
		Cost	Ionizing radiation
		Patients tolerate procedure well	
Ultrasonography	Primary imaging mode for gallbladder and biliary tree	Availability	Operator dependent
	Screening for aortic aneurysm	Cost	More difficult to interpret
	Identification of vascular abnormalities and flow	No ionizing radiation	
	Detection of ascites	Patients tolerate procedure well	
	Primary imaging mode for the female pelvis		
CT	Diagnostic modality of choice for most abdominal abnormalities including trauma	Availability	Cost
		Cost	Ionizing radiation
		High spatial resolution and image reconstruction	Contrast reactions
		Evaluates multiple organ systems simultaneously	Inability to use IV contrast in renal insufficiency
MRI	Problem solving for difficult diagnoses	Soft tissue contrast	Cost
	Extension of known disease into surrounding soft tissues (staging)	No ionizing radiation	Availability
	Vascular anatomy	No iodinated contrast	Longer scan times
		Image reconstruction	Claustrophobia
			Monitoring issues in acutely ill

- **CT is the study of choice in abdominal trauma.**
  - **Intravenous contrast CT is always used** to identify devascularized areas, hematomas, active extravasation of blood, and extraluminal urine (after contrast material has passed through the kidneys).
    - If **head CT is to be done,** it should be **done first** before contrast material is injected for the abdomen.
- **Oral contrast** is usually not administered for abdominal trauma.
- **Rectal contrast** is occasionally administered in penetrating trauma to search for a bowel laceration.
- It is always best to consult with the radiologist so as to tailor the best study to fit the patient's needs.
- The **most commonly affected solid organs in blunt abdominal trauma** (in order of decreasing frequency) are the **spleen, liver, kidney, and urinary bladder.**
  - If penetrating lesions are also considered, the liver is most frequently traumatized.
  - Traumatic injuries to each of them will be discussed under each organ.

Liver

GENERAL CONSIDERATIONS

- The liver receives its **blood supply** from both **hepatic arteries** and **portal veins** and **drains** to the inferior vena cava via the **hepatic veins.**

- For practical purposes, the **vascular distribution of the liver defines its anatomy** because the vascular anatomy is what directs the surgical approach to liver lesions.
  - The liver is divided into **right, left, and caudate lobes** by its vessels.
    - The **right lobe** is subdivided into **two segments**—the **anterior and posterior**—and the **left lobe** is subdivided into **two segments**—the **medial and lateral.**
    - A prominent, fat-filled fissure that contains the **falciform ligament** and **ligamentum teres** (formerly the umbilical vein) separates the **medial and lateral segments** of the **left lobe** of the liver.
- Evaluation of **liver masses** is usually done with a **combination** of scans obtained **before and after intravenous contrast** injection.
  - **Postcontrast** scans are obtained in **two phases:** one is done quickly **(hepatic arterial phase)** and then a second is done about a minute later **(portal venous phase);** the combination helps to best define and characterize liver masses.
  - This combination of three separate scans done **without contrast** and then during the **arterial phase** followed by the **venous phase** is called a *triple phase scan* (Fig. 20-1).

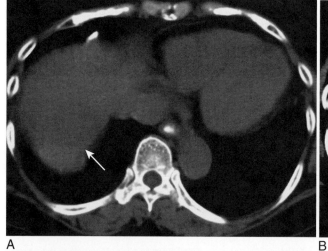

A

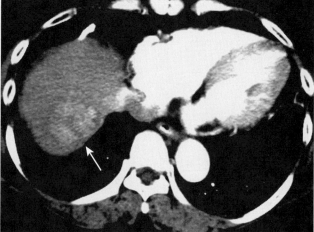

B

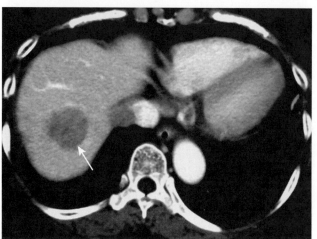

C

Figure 20-1. **Hepatocellular carcinoma, triple-phase CT scan of the liver.** *Evaluation of liver masses is usually done with a combination of scans including an unenhanced scan (**A**) and then two postcontrast scans: one quickly (hepatic arterial phase) (**B**) and a second done slightly later (portal venous phase) (**C**). The combination of these three scans is called a **triple phase scan.** This case shows the typical findings of a focal hepatocellular carcinoma. Most are low density (hypodense) or the same density as normal liver (isodense) without contrast (closed white arrow in **A**), enhance on the arterial phase with IV contrast (hyperdense) (closed white arrow in **B**), and then return to hypodense or isodense on the venous phase (closed white arrow in **C**).*

FATTY INFILTRATION

- Fatty infiltration of the liver is a **very common** abnormality in which there is fat accumulation in the hepatocytes in such diseases as alcohol ingestion, obesity, diabetes, hepatitis, and cirrhosis.
- Most patients with a fatty liver are **asymptomatic.**
- The **fatty infiltration** may be **diffuse** or **focal.**
  - Focal lesions may be **solitary** or **multiple.**
- **Recognizing fatty infiltration of the liver on CT**
  - When diffuse, the **liver is usually slightly enlarged.**
  - The **blood vessels stand out prominently** but are usually **neither obstructed nor displaced.**
  - The **spleen is denser than the liver** with or without intravenous contrast (Fig. 20-2A).
    - Normally, the **liver is equal to or greater than the density of the spleen.**
  - **Focal** fatty infiltration can produce an appearance that **mimics tumor,** but fatty infiltration usually produces **no mass effect** and the lesions have the ability to **appear and disappear** in a matter of weeks, quite unlike tumor masses (Fig. 20-2B).

CIRRHOSIS

- Cirrhosis is a chronic, irreversible disease of the liver that features destruction of normal liver cells and diffuse fibrosis and appears to be the final common pathway of many abnormalities including **hepatitis C** and **B, alcoholism, nonalcoholic fatty infiltration of the liver,** and miscellaneous diseases, e.g., **hemochromatosis** and **Wilson's disease.**
- Complications of cirrhosis include **portal hypertension, ascites, renal dysfunction, hepatocellular carcinoma, hepatic failure,** and **death.**
- **Recognizing cirrhosis of the liver on CT**

- **Early** in the disease, the liver may demonstrate **diffuse fatty infiltration.**
- As the disease progresses, the liver **contour becomes lobulated.**
- The **liver shrinks in volume** with the **right lobe** characteristically becoming **smaller** while the **caudate lobe and left lobe become disproportionately larger.**
  - This is especially so in alcoholic cirrhosis (Fig. 20-3).
- There is a **mottled, inhomogeneous** appearance to the liver parenchyma following intravenous contrast enhancement due to a mixture of regenerating nodules, focal fatty infiltration, and fibrosis.
- **Portal hypertension** may develop and can lead to **dilated vessels** around the stomach, splenic hilum, and esophagus representing **varices.**
- **Splenomegaly** may develop (Fig. 20-4).
- **Ascites** may be present.
  - Patients may have a combination of ascites and pleural effusion for a number of reasons, including cirrhosis, ovarian tumors, metastatic disease, hypoproteinemia, and congestive heart failure.
  - Sometimes it can be difficult to differentiate between ascites and pleural effusion on CT examinations (Table 20-2).
  - Both ascitic fluid and pleural fluid at the lung base may appear posterior to the liver (Fig. 20-5).

SPACE-OCCUPYING LESIONS OF THE LIVER

- CT studies are best at demonstrating liver masses when performed both with and without contrast, as either study alone may fail to reveal an *isodense* mass, i.e., one that has the identical attenuation as the surrounding normal tissue.

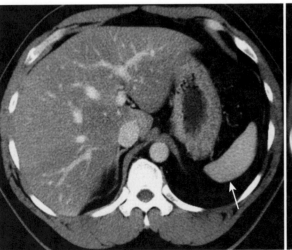
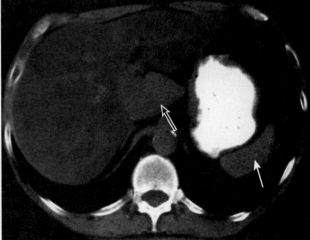

A   B

*Figure 20-2. **Diffuse and focal fatty infiltration of the liver.** Fatty infiltration of the liver is a very common abnormality. The fatty infiltration may be diffuse (**A**) or focal (**B**). The blood vessels stand out prominently but are usually neither obstructed nor displaced. **A,** Contrast-enhanced CT demonstrates diffuse fatty infiltration of the liver. The liver is less dense than the spleen (closed white arrow). **B,** A nonenhanced CT of another patient with fatty infiltration of the liver that spares the caudate lobe (open white arrow). The remainder of the liver is less dense than the spleen (closed white arrow).*

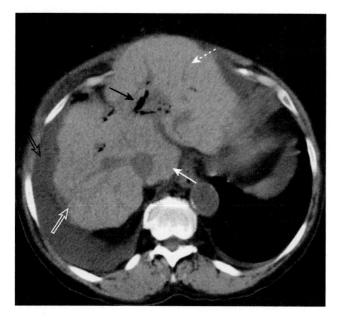

Figure 20-3. **Cirrhosis.** *As cirrhosis progresses, the liver contour becomes lobulated. The liver shrinks in volume with the right lobe (open white arrow) characteristically becoming smaller, while the caudate lobe (closed white arrow) and left lobe (dotted white arrow) become disproportionately larger. This is especially so in alcoholic cirrhosis. This patient has air in the ductal system (closed black arrow) from a stent that was placed from the distal common bile duct to the duodenum as a drain. The stent allows air to enter the biliary system from the bowel. There is also ascites present (open black arrow).*

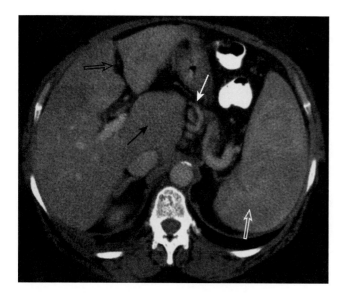

Figure 20-4. **Splenomegaly and varices from portal hypertension.** *Portal hypertension can lead to dilated vessels around the stomach, splenic hilum (closed white arrow), and esophagus representing varices. Splenomegaly may develop (open white arrow). There is characteristic enlargement of the caudate lobe (closed black arrow). The open black arrow points to the falciform ligament.*

Table 20-2

DIFFERENTIATING ASCITES FROM PLEURAL EFFUSION*		
Factor	**Ascites**	**Pleural Effusion**
Positioning relative to the hemidiaphragm	**Ascitic fluid** will appear **anterior to the hemidiaphragm** in the axial plane	**Pleural effusion** will be located **posterior to the hemidiaphragm**
Contact with the liver	Ascitic fluid **will not contact the "bare" area of the liver posteriorly,** where there is no peritoneal lining	Pleural fluid may appear to contact the posterior border of the liver; **fluid that seems to contact the posterior bare area is pleural in location**

*See Figure 20-5

- One of the primary aims of imaging studies, no matter what part of the body is being studied, is to accurately differentiate between benign and malignant processes using techniques that do not place the patient in danger or subject them to unnecessary pain.
  - This is the central goal in evaluating liver masses as well.
- **Metastases**
  - Metastases are the **most common malignant hepatic masses.**
  - Although **most are multiple,** metastases also represent the **most common cause** of a **solitary malignant mass** in the liver.
- **Most originate in the gastrointestinal tract,** in particular the **colon,** and almost all reach the liver via the bloodstream.
  - Other primary sites of metastatic spread to the liver include stomach, pancreas, esophagus, lung, melanoma, and breast.
- **Recognizing liver metastases on CT**
  - They are usually **multiple, low attenuation masses** (Fig. 20-6).
  - **Larger metastases** may demonstrate areas of necrosis that can be recognized as mottled areas of low attenuation within the mass.
  - **Mucin-producing carcinomas,** such as might originate in the stomach, colon, or ovary, can **calcify** both the primary tumor and the metastases (see Fig. 18-13).
- **Hepatocellular carcinoma (hepatoma)**
  - Hepatocellular carcinoma is the **most common primary malignancy** of the liver.
  - Virtually all arise in livers with preexisting abnormalities such as **cirrhosis** and **hepatitis.**
  - **Most are solitary,** but up to 20% can be multiple, mimicking metastases.

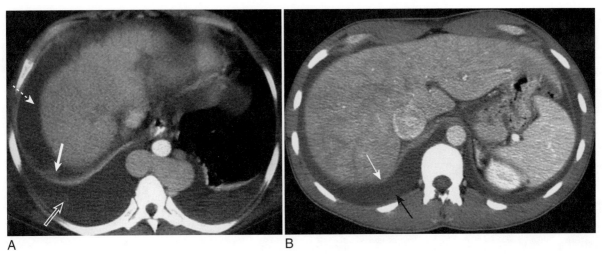

Figure 20-5. ***Differentiating pleural effusion from ascites.*** **A,** *Patients may have a combination of ascites* (dotted white arrow) *and pleural effusions* (open white arrow) *for a number of reasons, cirrhosis being one of them. Ascitic fluid will appear anterior to the hemidiaphragm* (closed white arrow) *in the axial plane. Pleural effusion will be located posterior to the hemidiaphragm.* **B,** *Ascites will never completely encircle the entire liver because of the "bare area"* (closed white arrow), *not covered by peritoneum. Fluid posterior to the bare area* (closed black arrow) *must be in the pleural space.*

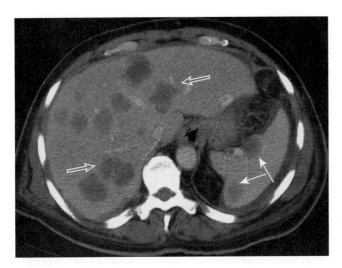

Figure 20-6. ***Metastases to the liver and spleen.*** *Metastases usually appear as multiple, low attenuation masses* (open white arrows). *There are also low attenuation lesions in the spleen* (closed white arrows) *in this patient with primary adenocarcinoma of the colon.*

- **Vascular invasion is common,** particularly of the portal system.
- **Recognizing hepatocellular carcinoma on CT.**
  - There are **three patterns** of appearance for hepatocellular carcinoma:
    - **Solitary mass,** frequently large (see Fig. 20-1)
    - **Multiple** nodules
    - **Diffuse infiltration** throughout a segment, lobe, or entire liver (Fig. 20-7)
  - Most are **low density (hypodense)** or the same density as normal liver **(isodense) without contrast,**

enhance on the **arterial phase** with IV contrast **(hyperdense),** and then return to **hypodense** or **isodense** on the **venous phase** (see Fig. 20-1).
- Low attenuation areas from **necrosis** are common.
- **Calcification** occurs relatively frequently.

- **Cavernous hemangiomas**
  - Cavernous hemangiomas are the **most common primary liver tumor** and **second in frequency to metastases for localized liver masses.**
  - They are more common in **women,** are usually **solitary,** and are almost always **asymptomatic.**
  - They are complex structures composed of multiple, large vascular channels lined by a single layer of endothelial cells.
- **Recognizing cavernous hemangiomas of the liver on CT**
  - **Usually hypodense lesions on unenhanced scans,** hemangiomas have a characteristic nodular enhancement **from the periphery** inward following injection of intravenous contrast and **become isodense** in the venous phase.
  - Contrast tends to be retained within the numerous vascular spaces of the lesion so that it characteristically appears **denser than the rest of the liver on delayed** (10-minute) **scans** (Fig. 20-8).
- **Cysts**
  - Believed to be **congenital** in origin, they are easily identified as **sharply marginated,** spherical lesions of **low attenuation (fluid density)** compared to the remainder of the liver, on both unenhanced and enhanced scans.
  - They are usually **solitary** and are **homogeneous** in density (Fig. 20-9).

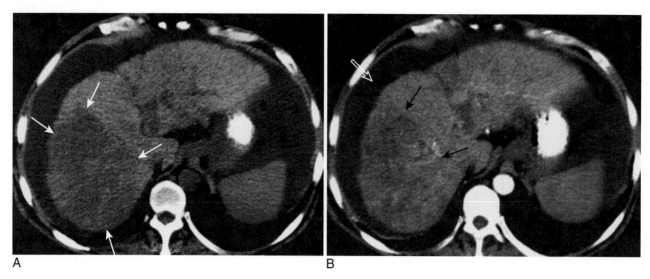

Figure 20-7. **Diffuse hepatocellular carcinoma of the liver.** *There are three patterns of appearance for hepatocellular carcinoma: solitary mass (see Fig. 20-1), multiple nodules, and diffuse infiltration throughout a segment, lobe (as in this case) or entire liver.* **A,** *A typical low attenuation lesion is seen on the nonenhanced scan (closed white arrows).* **B,** *The arterial phase demonstrates patchy enhancement (closed black arrows) indicating the probability of tumor necrosis in the low attenuation areas. Ascites is present (open white arrow). The overall volume of the liver is decreased and the contour is lobulated from underlying cirrhosis.*

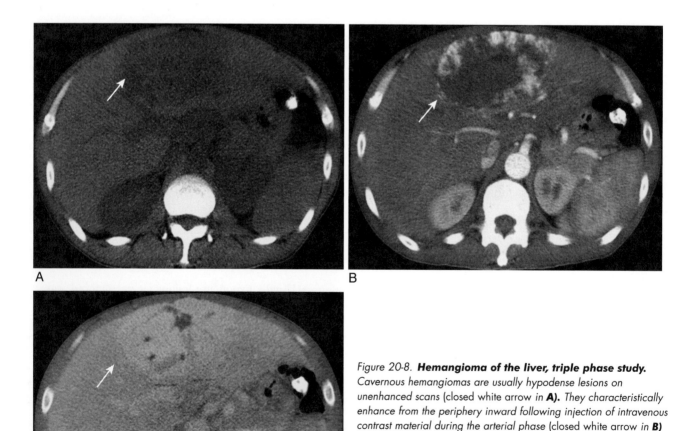

Figure 20-8. **Hemangioma of the liver, triple phase study.** *Cavernous hemangiomas are usually hypodense lesions on unenhanced scans (closed white arrow in **A).** They characteristically enhance from the periphery inward following injection of intravenous contrast material during the arterial phase (closed white arrow in **B)** and become isodense in the venous phase. Contrast tends to be retained within the numerous vascular spaces of the lesion so that they characteristically appear denser than the rest of the liver on delayed scans (closed white arrow in **C).***

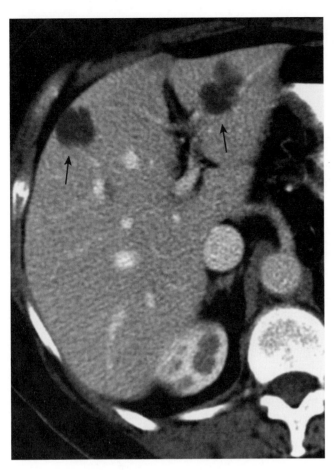

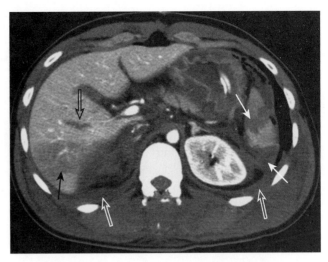

Figure 20-10. **Hepatic and splenic lacerations, hepatic contusion.** *Contrast-enhanced CT demonstrates a hepatic laceration (open black arrow). There is also a contusion of the liver (closed black arrow). This patient also has splenic lacerations (closed white arrows) and retroperitoneal blood (open white arrows). The patient had been struck by an automobile.*

Figure 20-9. **Hepatic cysts.** *Believed to be congenital in origin, hepatic cysts are easily identified as sharply marginated, spherical lesions of low attenuation (fluid density) compared to the remainder of the liver on both unenhanced and enhanced scans (closed black arrows). They are homogeneous in density.*

LIVER TRAUMA

- If both penetrating and blunt trauma are included, the liver would be the most frequently injured organ.
- Injury to the liver accounts for the **majority of deaths from abdominal trauma.**
- **Contrast-enhanced CT is the study of choice,** and because of its ability to demonstrate both the nature and extent of the trauma, the overwhelming majority of patients with liver trauma are now managed conservatively and do not require surgery.
- **CT findings in hepatic trauma**
  - **Lacerations**—irregularly marginated, low attenuation branching defects (Fig. 20-10)
  - **Hematomas**—focal, high attenuation lesions first caused by blood; may progress to low attenuation mass-like lesions filled with serous fluid
  - **Subcapsular hematomas**—lenticular fluid collections that conform to the shape of the outer contour of the liver but which frequently flatten the adjacent liver parenchyma
  - **Wedge-shaped defects** of devascularized liver parenchyma

- **Pseudoaneurysms and acute hemorrhages**—collections of contrast that often require angiography with embolization and/or surgery

Biliary System

GENERAL CONSIDERATIONS

- **Ultrasound is the study of first choice** for abnormalities of the biliary system.
- CT may be helpful in cases with difficult or unusual anatomy, for detecting masses or in determining the extent of disease already diagnosed.

ACUTE CHOLECYSTITIS AND GALLSTONES

- Ultrasound is the study of first choice, but CT may be helpful if the **ultrasound is equivocal or complicated.**
  - Because gallstones may be the same density as the surrounding bile, **CT is less sensitive than ultrasound in detecting stones** (see Fig. 18-8B).
- CT findings in acute cholecystitis include **thickening and enhancement** of the **gallbladder wall (>3 mm)** and **pericholecystic fluid or air in the wall or lumen of the gallbladder** *(emphysematous cholecystitis)* (Fig. 20-11).
- Radionuclide scans **(HIDA scans)** are used in the **diagnosis of acute cholecystitis.**
  - Hepatoiminodiacetic acid (HIDA) is tagged with a radioactive tracer (technetium-99m, or ^{99m}Tc), injected intravenously, and imaged with a special camera after it has been excreted by the liver into the bile and emptied into the small intestine.
  - In patients with **obstruction of the cystic duct,** the tracer will not appear in the **gallbladder,** and in patients with **obstruction of the common duct,** the tracer will **not appear in the small intestine,** both of which are usually caused by an obstructing gallstone.

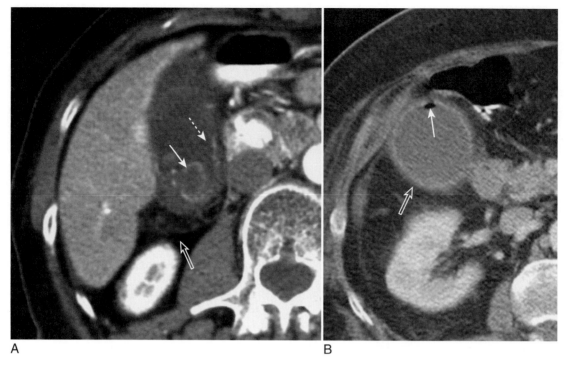

A   B

Figure 20-11. **Acute cholecystitis.** *These are two different patients with acute cholecystitis.* **A,** *A gallstone is visible (closed white arrow) in a distended gallbladder that demonstrates pericholecystic infiltration of the surrounding fat (open white arrow). Enhancement of gallbladder wall (dotted white arrow) is also seen.* **B,** *A small dot of air is in the lumen of gallbladder (closed white arrow), a sign of emphysematous cholecystitis. There is enhancement and thickening of the wall (open white arrow).*

Spleen

GENERAL CONSIDERATIONS

- The **liver should always be denser than or equal to the density of the spleen.**
- On early contrast-enhanced scans, the spleen may be inhomogeneous in its attenuation, a finding that should disappear over the course of the next several minutes.
- Most focal lesions in the spleen are not malignant.
- The spleen is usually **about 12 cm long, does not project** substantially below the margin of the **12th rib,** and is about the **same size as the left kidney.**

SPLENIC INFARCTION

- Splenic infarctions are **best seen on contrast-enhanced scans** in patients with such abnormalities as sickle cell disease, emboli originating on the left side of the heart in patients following acute myocardial infarction, polycythemia, lymphoma, and leukemia.
- Classically, a splenic infarct appears as a **low attenuation, wedge-shaped lesion at the periphery of the spleen that causes no mass effect** (Fig. 20-12).

SPLENIC TRAUMA

- Splenic trauma is usually caused by **deceleration injuries** in unrestrained occupants of motor vehicle collisions, by a fall, or by being struck by a motor vehicle as a pedestrian.

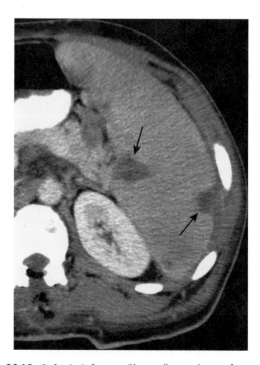

Figure 20-12. **Splenic infarcts.** *Classically, a splenic infarct appears as a low attenuation, wedge-shaped lesion at the periphery of the spleen that causes no mass effect (closed black arrows). This patient had lymphoma, and there was associated splenomegaly.*

- Because the **spleen is a highly vascular organ,** hemorrhage represents the most serious complication of trauma.
  - Despite its vascular nature, **most splenic trauma is treated conservatively** (nonsurgically).
- **CT findings in splenic trauma**
  - **Contusion**— alterations in the normal homogeneous appearance of the spleen including mottled areas of low attenuation
  - **Hematoma**—intrasplenic, rounded area of low attenuation (Fig. 20-13)
  - **Laceration**—irregular, low attenuation defect that usually transects the spleen
  - **Subcapsular hematoma**—crescent-shaped collection of fluid in the subcapsular space that frequently compresses the normal splenic parenchyma
  - **Intraperitoneal fluid or blood**—including small amounts of blood in the pelvis

Kidneys

GENERAL CONSIDERATIONS

- The kidneys are retroperitoneal organs, encircled by varying amounts of fat and enclosed within a fibrous capsule.
  - They are surrounded by the ***perirenal space,*** which, in turn, is delimited by the **anterior and posterior renal fasciae.**
  - Certain fascial attachments, muscles, and other organs define a series of spaces that produce predictable patterns of abnormality when those spaces are filled with fluid, pus, blood, or air.

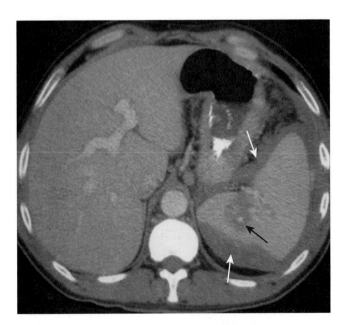

Figure 20-13. ***Intrasplenic and perisplenic hematomas.***
Because the spleen is a highly vascular organ, hemorrhage represents the most serious sequela of trauma. This patient has both an intrasplenic hematoma (closed black arrow), seen as a rounded area of low attenuation, and a perisplenic hematoma (closed white arrows), seen as crescent-shaped collections of fluid in the perisplenic space.

- So long as they are functioning properly, the **kidneys are the route** through which intravenously injected, iodinated **contrast** material is **excreted from the body.**
  - They should therefore **enhance** whenever intravenous contrast is administered.
  - If the kidneys are not functioning properly, contrast is excreted though alternative pathways (bile, bowel), a process called ***vicarious excretion*** of contrast.

URINARY TRACT CALCULI

- Unenhanced, multislice spiral CT scans have replaced conventional radiography in the search for renal and ureteral calculi and their complications.
  - A **negative stone search study has a negative predictive value of 98%.**
  - Besides urinary tract calculi, CT scans detect **symptomatic lesions in other organ systems** in almost one third of patients in whom a stone search study is conducted.
- **Recognizing a calculus on a stone search study** (all signs discussed are on the symptomatic side)
  - The **direct finding** is a calcific density in the ureter, at the ureterovesical junction, or in the bladder (Fig. 20-14A).
  - **Indirect findings**
    - Signs of **obstruction—dilatation of the ureter** or **intrarenal collecting system** or overall **enlargement of the kidney** (Fig. 20-14B).
    - Signs of **inflammation—perinephric stranding** (Figs. 20-14C).

ACUTE PYELONEPHRITIS

- Acute pyelonephritis is a **clinical diagnosis.**
  - Radiologic imaging is used to evaluate underlying disease and to detect any complications (e.g., abscess or emphysematous pyelonephritis).
- Pyelonephritis is an **inflammation of the renal parenchyma** and renal pelvis due to an infectious source.
  - Most often, it is secondary to an ascending lower urinary tract infection from gram-negative bacteria.
- Patients can have **flank pain, pyuria, and elevated white blood cell count.**
- **Recognizing acute pyelonephritis on CT**
  - **Enlarged kidney(s)**
  - **Wedge-shaped areas of low attenuation** secondary to decreased perfusion (Fig. 20-15)
  - **Perinephric stranding**
  - **Hydronephrosis**

SPACE-OCCUPYING LESIONS

- **Renal cysts**
  - Simple renal cysts are a **very common** finding on CT scans of the abdomen occurring in more than half of the population over 55 years of age.
  - Simple cysts are **benign, fluid-filled** structures that are frequently **multiple** and **bilateral.**
  - **Recognizing simple cysts of the kidney on CT**
    - They tend to have a **sharp margin** where they meet the normal renal parenchyma.

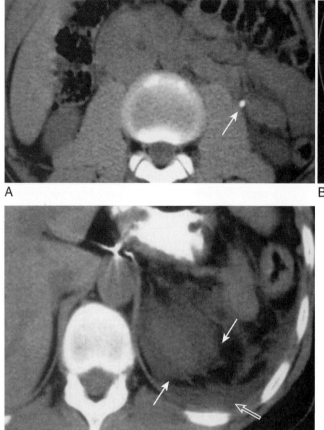

A

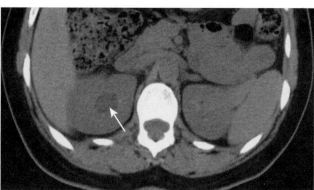

B

C

Figure 20-14. **Imaging findings of ureteral calculi, three different patients. A,** A calcified stone is visible in the left ureter (closed white arrow). **B,** There is hydronephrosis on the right with enlargement of the right kidney (closed white arrow). **C,** There is considerable perinephric stranding (closed white arrows) and retroperitoneal fluid most likely from a rupture of one of the renal fornices (open white arrow).

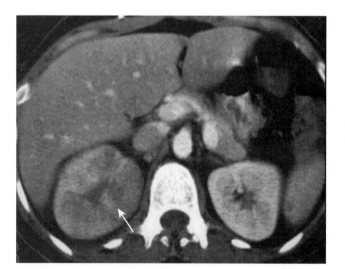

Figure 20-15. **Acute pyelonephritis.** The right kidney is larger than the left and has numerous wedge-shaped areas of low attenuation (closed white arrow) secondary to decreased perfusion, findings seen with acute pyelonephritis. Acute pyelonephritis is a clinical diagnosis.

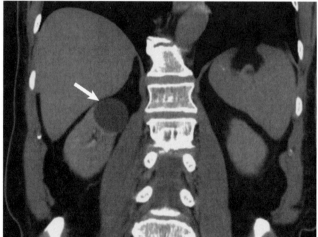

Figure 20-16. **Renal cyst on CT urogram.** This image from a CT urogram demonstrates a low attenuation mass (closed white arrow) in the upper pole of the right kidney which is homogeneous in density and sharply marginated. These findings are characteristic of a simple cyst.

- They have density measurements (Hounsfield numbers) of **water density** (−10 to +20).
- They **do not contrast-enhance** (Fig. 20-16).
- **Other lesions can resemble simple cysts:**

- **Complex cysts** into which hemorrhage has occurred or which become infected have higher attenuation numbers (whiter) and can be symptomatic (pain).

- **Renal abscesses** are thick-walled and may contain gas and pus.
- **Adult polycystic kidney disease** is an autosomal dominant disorder in which there are characteristically **innumerable cysts in the kidneys, liver, and pancreas** (Fig. 20-17).

- **Renal cell carcinoma (hypernephroma)**
  - Renal cell carcinoma is the **most common primary renal malignancy** in **adults.**
  - Solid masses in the kidneys of adults are usually renal cell carcinomas.
  - They have a propensity for **extending into the renal veins,** up the **inferior vena cava,** and producing **nodules in the lung.**
  - When they metastasize to bone, they are **purely lytic** and **often expansile.**
  - **Recognizing renal cell carcinoma on CT**
    - Ranging from **completely solid** to **completely cystic,** they are **usually solid lesions with low attenuation areas of necrosis.**
    - Even though renal cell carcinomas **enhance with intravenous contrast,** they still tend to remain **lower in density than the surrounding normal kidney.**
    - **Renal vein invasion occurs in up to one third of patients with renal cell carcinoma** and may appear as filling defects in the lumen of the renal veins (Fig. 20-18).

RENAL TRAUMA

- Motor vehicle accidents are the most common cause of blunt abdominal trauma to the kidneys in the United States.
- Almost all patients with renal trauma will have **hematuria.**

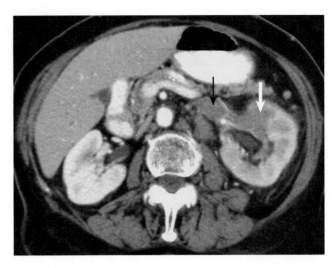

Figure 20-18. ***Renal cell carcinoma.*** *There is a low-density tumor involving the anterior portion of the left kidney (closed white arrow). The tumor is seen to extend directly into the left renal vein (closed black arrow), which renal cell carcinomas have a propensity for doing.*

- **CT findings in renal trauma**
  - **Contusion**—patchy, low attenuation areas in the contrast-enhanced kidney
  - **Laceration**—low attenuation linear defects (Fig. 20-19A)
  - **Fracture**—a laceration through the hilum
  - **Subcapsular hematoma**—low attenuation crescentic density that compresses the underlying renal parenchyma
  - **Vascular injuries**—if arterial, there may be no flow to the kidney and hence, no contrast enhancement
  - **Injuries to the collecting system**—extraluminal contrast (Fig. 20-19B)

Pancreas

GENERAL CONSIDERATIONS

- The pancreas is a retroperitoneal organ oriented obliquely so that the entire organ is not seen on any one axial image of the upper abdomen.
  - The **tail** is usually **most superior,** lying in the hilum of the spleen.
  - Proceeding inferiorly, the **body of the pancreas** crosses the midline and rests anterior to the **superior mesenteric artery** (Fig. 20-20A).
  - The **head of the pancreas** is nestled in the duodenal loop (Fig. 20-20B).
  - The **uncinate process** is part of the head and curves around the **superior mesenteric vein.**
- The **splenic vein** courses along the posterior border of the pancreas to the **superior mesenteric vein** and the **splenic artery** runs along the superior border of the pancreas from the **celiac axis** to the spleen.
- The main pancreatic duct empties into the duodenum as the **duct of Wirsung** and sometimes through an **accessory duct of Santorini.**

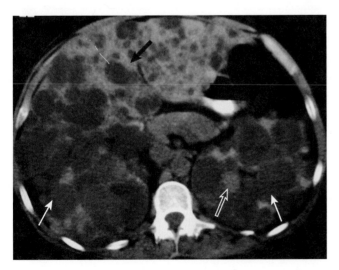

Figure 20-17. ***Adult polycystic kidney disease.*** *Bilaterally huge kidneys are almost completely filled with innumerable cysts (closed white arrows). There are also cysts in the liver (closed black arrow). This is adult polycystic kidney disease. There may occasionally be hemorrhage into a cyst (open white arrow), which causes it to appear denser than the other, fluid-filled cysts.*

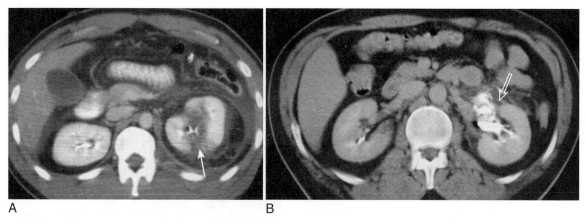

Figure 20-19. **Renal laceration and hematoma and perforation of the ureter. A,** A laceration of the left kidney is manifested by the low attenuation linear defect (closed white arrow). **B,** A tear of the ureter at the level of the ureteropelvic junction is visible by identifying extraluminal contrast representing contrast-containing urine that is leaking from the collecting system (open white arrow).

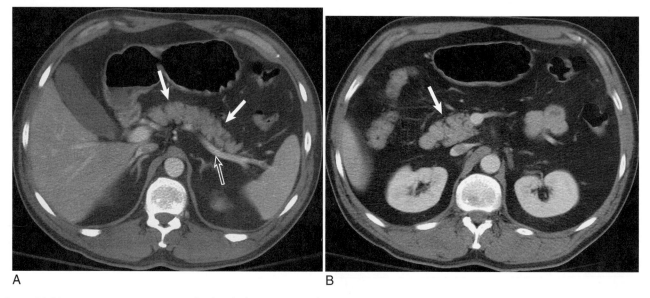

Figure 20-20. **Normal pancreas. A,** Body (closed white arrows). Splenic artery (open white arrow). **B,** Normal head (closed white arrow). The pancreas is a retroperitoneal organ oriented obliquely so that the entire organ is not seen on any one axial image of the upper abdomen. The tail is most superior, and the body and then head are usually visualized on successively more inferior slices.

PANCREATITIS

- The two most common causes of pancreatitis are **alcoholism** and **gallstones.**
- Inflammation of pancreatic tissue leading to disruption of the ducts and spillage of pancreatic juices occurs readily because of the lack of a capsule surrounding the pancreas.
- Pancreatitis is a **clinical diagnosis** with CT serving to document either a **cause** (e.g., gallstones) or **complication** (e.g., pseudocyst formation).
- **Recognizing acute pancreatitis on CT**
  - **Enlargement** of all or part of the pancreas (normal measurements for the pancreas: head 3 cm; body 2.5 cm; and tail 2 cm)

- **Peripancreatic stranding** or **fluid collections** (Fig. 20-21)
- **Low attenuation** lesions in the pancreas from **necrosis** (areas of nonviable pancreas; usually develops **early** in the course of the disease)
  - Requires IV contrast administration and is important in predicting prognosis
- **Pseudocyst formation**—fibrous tissue encapsulates a walled-off collection of pancreatic juices released from the inflamed pancreas (Fig. 20-22)
  - The **wall of a pseudocyst is usually visible by CT** and **may contrast-enhance.**
- **Chronic pancreatitis**

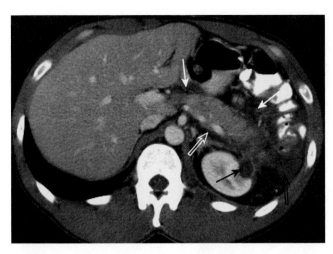

Figure 20-21. ***Acute pancreatitis.*** *There is a diffusely enlarged pancreas (open white arrow). There is infiltration of the peripancreatic fat (closed white arrows) and a peripancreatic effusion (open black arrow). All these findings are consistent with acute pancreatitis in the proper clinical setting. This patient had markedly elevated amylase and lipase levels. There is an incidental cyst of the left kidney present (closed black arrow).*

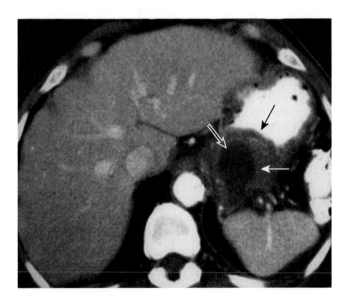

Figure 20-22. ***Pancreatic pseudocyst.*** *Pseudocysts of the pancreas (open white arrow) occur when fibrous tissue encapsulates a walled-off collection of pancreatic juices released from the inflamed pancreas. They may have an enhancing wall (closed white arrow). The cyst is indenting a loop of adjacent bowel (in this case, the posterior wall of the stomach, closed black arrow) which is called a* ***pad sign.***

- Chronic pancreatitis is a continuous and irreversible disease of the pancreas most often secondary to **alcohol abuse** leading to **fibrosis, atrophy of the gland, ductal dilatation,** and frequently **diabetes.**
- The **hallmarks** of the disease are **multiple, amorphous calcifications** that form within the **dilated ducts** of the **atrophied gland** (see Fig. 18-10B).

PANCREATIC ADENOCARCINOMA
- Risk factors include **alcoholism, cigarette smoking, chronic pancreatitis,** and **diabetes.**
- Pancreatic adenocarcinoma has an **exceedingly poor prognosis:** most tumors are unresectable and incurable at the time of diagnosis.
- Most of the time (75%), the tumor is located in the head of the pancreas; about 10% occur in the body and 5% in the tail.
- About half of the patients present with **jaundice,** and most of the time, there is **associated pain.**
  - Ultrasound is the study of first choice in the workup of the jaundiced patient.
- **Recognizing pancreatic adenocarcinoma on CT**
  - **Focal pancreatic mass,** usually **hypodense** to the remainder the gland (Fig. 20-23)
  - **Ductal dilatation**
    - Usually involving **both** the **pancreatic and biliary ducts**
    - The normal **pancreatic duct** measures **less than 4 mm** in the head and tapers to the tail; the **common duct** should be **less than 7 mm** in diameter.
  - Spread to contiguous organs, enlarged lymph nodes, and ascites

Small and Large Bowel
GENERAL CONSIDERATIONS
- Opacification and distention of the bowel lumen is necessary for proper evaluation of the bowel wall no matter what modality is used.
- **Pitfall: Collapsed or unopacified loops of bowel can introduce errors of diagnosis** related to our inability to first visualize and then to differentiate real from artifactual findings or to accurately characterize the abnormality even if recognized.
- On CT scans of the abdomen and pelvis, unopacified loops of bowel may mimic masses or adenopathy and wall thickness is difficult to assess if the bowel is not distended.
- Therefore, orally administered contrast, frequently given in temporally divided doses to allow earlier contrast to reach the colon while later contrast opacifies the stomach, is routinely utilized for most abdominal CT scans except those performed for **trauma,** the *stone search study,* and studies specifically directed toward evaluating vascular structures (e.g., the **aorta).**
  - Oral contrast material used for CT examinations is either a dilute solution containing barium or iodinated contrast.
- Several common and important findings can affect any part of the bowel and are key to the diagnosis of bowel abnormalities by CT.
- The **key bowel findings on CT**
  - **Thickening of the bowel wall**
    - The normal **small bowel** does not exceed about 2.5 cm in diameter and the wall is usually **no thicker than 3 mm.**

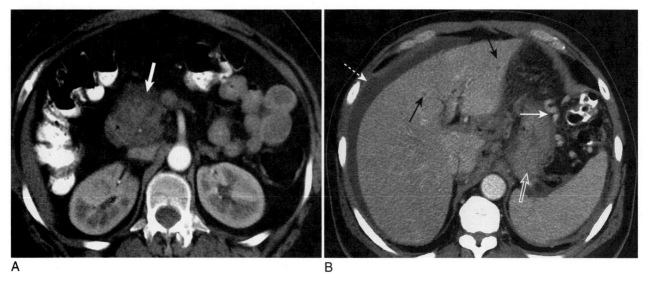

A   B

*Figure 20-23. **Pancreatic adenocarcinoma, two different patients. A,** There is focal enlargement of the head of the pancreas (closed white arrow). **B,** There are two small, ring-enhancing metastases to the liver (closed black arrows) and ascites (dotted white arrow). Gastric varices are visible as dilated and enlarged vessels (closed white arrow) at the periphery of the stomach (open white arrow).*

- The **colonic wall does not exceed 3 mm** with the lumen distended.
- **Submucosal edema or hemorrhage**
  - Submucosal infiltration produces varying degrees of *thumbprinting,* nodular indentations into the bowel lumen representing focal areas of submucosal infiltration by edema, hemorrhage, inflammatory cells, tumor (lymphoma), or amyloid.
- **Hazy or strandlike infiltration of the surrounding fat**
  - Extension of inflammatory reaction outside the bowel into the adjacent fat is a sentinel finding that heralds associated disease.
- **Extraluminal contrast or extraluminal air** (Fig. 20-24)
  - Indicates the presence of a bowel perforation

COLITIS
- Colitis is inflammation of the wall of the large bowel.
  - The numerous causes of colitis include infectious, ulcerative and granulomatous, ischemic, radiation-induced, and antibiotic-associated.
- Many forms of colitis appear similar radiographically, so once again, clinical history is of paramount importance.

- **Recognizing colitis on CT scans**
  - Segmental **thickening** of the bowel wall
  - Irregular narrowing of the bowel lumen due to edema: *thumbprinting* (Fig. 20-25)
  - **Infiltration** of the surrounding fat
  - **Mesenteric ischemia** due to diminished blood flow from either occlusion of vessels (thrombus) or from slow flow, as in congestive heart failure, may differ in appearance from some of the other colitides because there may be no bowel wall enhancement with contrast and there can be intramural or portal venous gas.

SHOCK BOWEL
- Shock bowel usually occurs with **blunt abdominal trauma** in which there is **severe hypovolemia and profound hypotension,** with complete reversibility of these findings following resuscitation (Fig. 20-26).
- **Recognizing shock bowel on CT**
  - **Diffuse thickening** of the **small bowel** wall with **increased enhancement.**
  - **Fluid-filled** and **dilated loops of bowel**
  - Other findings include **small IVC** (<1 cm) and **aorta** (<6 mm) and decreased perfusion of the spleen.

DIVERTICULOSIS AND DIVERTICULITIS
- Diverticulosis and diverticulitis are discussed in Chapter 19.

APPENDICITIS
- Appendicitis is discussed in Chapter 19.

Female Pelvis

GENERAL CONSIDERATIONS
- **Ultrasound is the study of first choice in evaluation of suspected abnormalities of the female pelvis.**
- MRI has assumed an increasingly important role in defining the anatomy of the uterus and ovaries and in clarifying questions in patients in whom ultrasound findings are confusing.
  - MRI is also used in surgical planning.

UTERINE LEIOMYOMAS (FIBROIDS)
- Leiomyomas are **benign smooth muscle tumors** of the uterus that occur in up to 50% of women over the age of 30.
- Although most women with fibroids are **asymptomatic,** they can cause **pain, infertility, menorrhagia,** and urinary or bowel symptoms if they grow large enough.

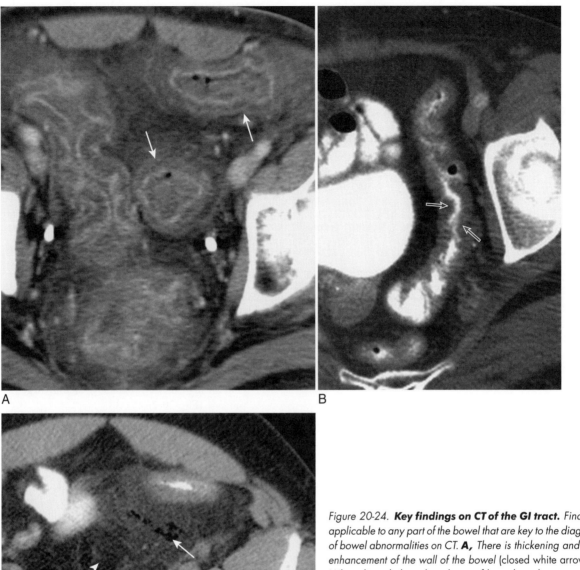

A

B

C

Figure 20-24. **Key findings on CT of the GI tract.** *Findings applicable to any part of the bowel that are key to the diagnosis of bowel abnormalities on CT.* **A,** *There is thickening and enhancement of the wall of the bowel (closed white arrows). When distended, as these loops of large bowel are, the bowel wall is normally very thin.* **B,** *There is submucosal infiltration of the wall (thumbprinting) (open white arrows). In this case of ischemic colitis, it most likely represents edema with some hemorrhage.* **C,** *There is infiltration of the surrounding fat (dotted white arrow), a sentinel finding that usually heralds adjacent inflammation. There is also extraluminal air (closed white arrow), a sign of bowel perforation. This patient had diverticulitis.*

- **Ultrasound and MRI are the imaging studies of first choice** in evaluating uterine fibroids.
  - Nevertheless, fibroids are frequently visualized on CT scans of the pelvis performed for other reasons.
- **Recognizing uterine leiomyomas on CT**

- Characteristically, they are **lobulated soft tissue masses** that **frequently calcify** with **amorphous or popcorn calcification** and **undergo central necrosis with low attenuation areas** when they grow large enough (see Fig. 18-11B).

- The **myometrium** is very vascular and **enhances greatly** on contrast-enhanced CT scans of the pelvis.
- The viable portions of uterine myomas also enhance dramatically following injection of intravenous contrast.

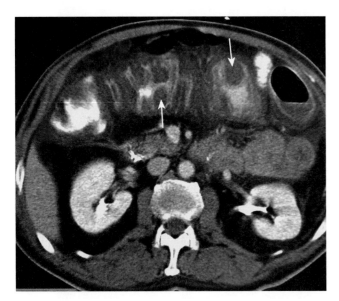

Figure 20-25. **Colitis.** *The colon demonstrates* **thumbprinting** *(closed white arrows) and a pattern that is called the* **accordion sign.** *This patient had C. difficile colitis, formerly called pseudomembranous colitis, and now known to be caused almost exclusively by toxins produced by Clostridium difficile. The colitis frequently follows antibiotic therapy. The diagnosis is usually made clinically by visualization of the pseudomembrane on endoscopy. The* **accordion sign** *represents contrast material that is trapped between enlarged folds and indicates the presence of marked edema or inflammation, but it is not specific for C. difficile colitis.*

OVARIAN TUMORS, CYSTS, AND PELVIC INFLAMMATORY DISEASE

- **Normal findings**
  - **Ultrasound is the imaging study of choice for evaluating the ovaries.**
  - Normal-sized ovaries are usually visualized on contrast-enhanced CT studies in premenopausal women.
  - In premenopausal women, the ovaries are approximately 2 cm × 3 cm × 4 cm in size.
  - They frequently contain cystic follicles.
- **Ovarian tumors**
  - Primary tumors of the ovary are **usually cystic in nature** with **thick and irregular walls** and **internal septations.**
  - Primary route of spread is throughout **peritoneal cavity.**
  - *Omental cake* is the term that applies to metastatic implants in the omentum and on the peritoneal surface, frequently producing an elongated nodular mass.
    - An omental cake is usually caused by ovarian, stomach, and colon metastases (Fig. 20-27).
  - **Ascites** usually indicates peritoneal spread.
- **Ovarian cysts**
  - Common entities which are **usually incidental findings on CT** done for some other reason.
  - Characteristically, they are **well-defined, thin-walled with homogeneous internal fluid density** but may contain high-density material if hemorrhage occurs into the cyst (Fig. 20-28).
- **Pelvic inflammatory disease (PID)**
  - This term is used to collectively describe a **group of infectious diseases affecting the uterus, Fallopian tubes, and ovaries.**
  - Most cases of PID **begin as a transient endometritis** and ascend to infection of the tubes and ovaries.
  - Patients can have pain, vaginal discharge, adnexal tenderness, and elevated white blood cell count.

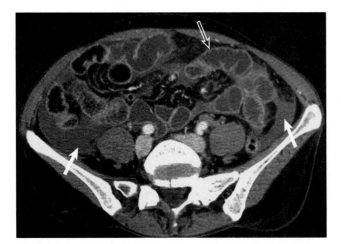

Figure 20-26. **Shock bowel.** *There is marked enhancement of the bowel wall with multiple dilated and fluid-filled loops (open white arrow). Retroperitoneal fluid is also present (closed white arrows). Shock bowel usually occurs in severe hypovolemia and profound hypotension.*

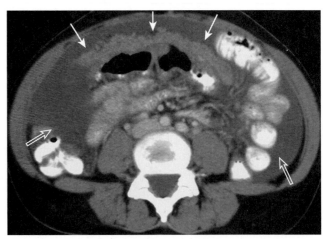

Figure 20-27. **Omental metastases, omental cake. Omental cake** *is the term that applies to metastatic implants in the omentum and the peritoneal surface, frequently producing an elongated nodular mass (closed white arrows). Ascites is also present in this patient with known ovarian carcinoma (open white arrows).*

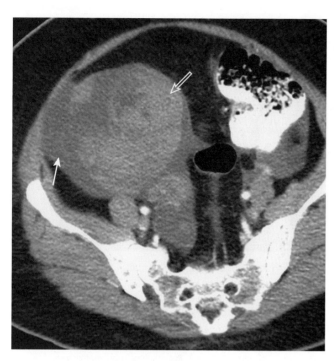

Figure 20-28. **Hemorrhagic ovarian cyst.** *Ovarian cysts can become painful if they undergo torsion or if there is hemorrhage into the cysts, as in this case. The hemorrhage (open white arrow) appears denser than the fluid in the remainder of the cyst (closed white arrow).*

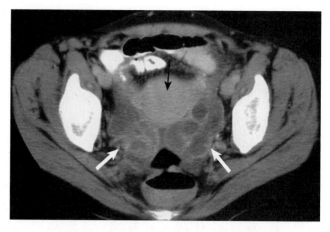

Figure 20-29. **Bilateral pyosalpinges in pelvic inflammatory disease.** *There are dilated, serpiginous, and fluid-filled tubular structures bilaterally (closed white arrows) representing pyosalpingitis of both fallopian tubes. The closed black arrow points to the uterus.*

- Complications include **infertility** or **ectopic pregnancy.**
- The **female pelvis is typically imaged initially using ultrasound,** but ultrasound can be insensitive for mild abnormalities and nonspecific for other findings.
  - CT is used for complicated PID or for those in whom the history may not have pointed to that diagnosis.
- **Recognizing PID on CT**
  - **Haziness of pelvic fat**
  - **Thickened tubes** may be folded upon themselves and appear as a fluid-filled multicystic mass (Fig. 20-29).
  - **Ovaries may be enlarged** and enhance with contrast.
  - **Enlarged uterus** with increased endometrial enhancement and fluid
  - **Pyosalpinx**—purulent infection of a dilated tube
  - **Tubo-ovarian abscess**—adnexal mass with focal areas of hypodensity
  - **Pelvic ascites**

Urinary Bladder

GENERAL CONSIDERATIONS

- The bladder is an **extraperitoneal organ,** the extraperitoneal space being continuous with the retroperitoneum.
  - The **dome of the bladder** is covered by the **inferior reflection of the peritoneum.**
- The **bladder wall measures 5 mm or less** with the bladder distended.
- The bladder is **best evaluated when distended** with either urine or urine containing contrast.

- The **bladder wall is usually visible** whether or not intravenous contrast has been administered.

BLADDER TUMORS

- Most malignant bladder tumors are **transitional cell tumors.**
  - Transitional cell tumors may occur simultaneously anywhere along the uroepithelium from the bladder to the ureter to the kidney.
- The **primary tumor** appears as **focal thickening of the bladder wall** and produces a **filling defect in the contrast-filled bladder** (Fig. 20-30).

RUPTURE OF THE URINARY BLADDER

- About **70% of bladder ruptures occur with pelvic fractures** and about **10% of patients with pelvic fractures have an associated rupture of the bladder.**
- They are best demonstrated by a **CT cystogram** in which contrast is infused under gravity through a Foley catheter into the bladder, but they can also be well demonstrated by **antegrade filling of the bladder** from renal excretion of intravenously injected contrast.
- **Two major types of bladder rupture**
  - **Extraperitoneal**—more common (Fig. 20-31)
    - Usually the **result of a pelvic fracture** with **direct puncture** of the bladder.
    - Extraluminal contrast **remains around bladder,** especially the retropubic space.
  - **Intraperitoneal rupture**—less common
    - Usually the **result of a forceful blow to the pelvis with a distended bladder**
    - Rupture usually occurs at the **dome** of the bladder adjacent to the peritoneal cavity.
    - Contrast flows freely through the **peritoneal cavity, surrounds bowel, and extends into the paracolic gutters.**

Abdominal Aortic Aneurysms

GENERAL CONSIDERATIONS

- The **abdominal aorta measures up to 3 cm in diameter.**

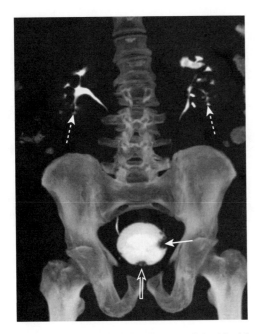

Figure 20-30. **Transitional cell carcinoma of the bladder, CT urogram.** There is a filling-defect in the left lateral wall of the contrast-filled bladder (closed white arrow). The defect at the base of the bladder is caused by the prostate gland (open white arrow). The calyceal collecting systems are both normal (dotted white arrows).

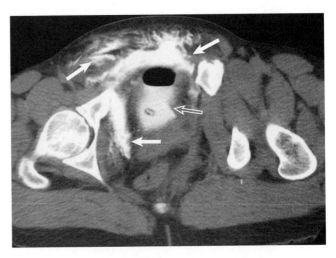

Figure 20-31. **Extraperitoneal bladder rupture.**
An extraperitoneal bladder rupture is demonstrated by contrast-containing urine (closed white arrows) that has leaked into the extraperitoneal spaces after being instilled in the bladder. Contrast, a Foley catheter, and air are seen inside a partially filled urinary bladder (open white arrow). Extraperitoneal ruptures are more common than intraperitoneal and are usually the result of a pelvic fracture. This patient did have several pelvic fractures.

- It divides into the right and left iliac arteries at the level of L4.
- Most aortic aneurysms occur in the abdominal aorta.

ANEURYSMS

- An aneurysm is defined as a localized dilation of an artery by at least **50% over its normal size.**

- Most abdominal aortic aneurysms (AAAs) begin **inferior to the origin of the renal arteries,** but they **frequently extend into one or both iliac arteries.**
- The **diameter of an aneurysm** is directly **related to its risk of rupture.**
  - For aneurysms **less than 4 cm,** there is a **less than 10%** chance of rupture.
  - For aneurysms **4 to 5 cm** in diameter, the risk of rupture increases to **almost 25%.**

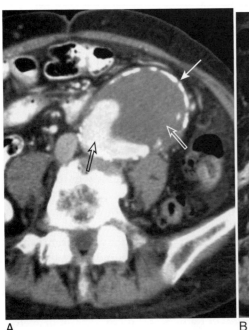
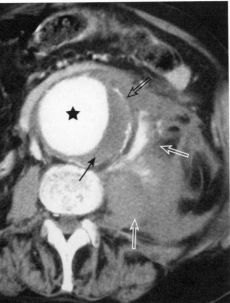

Figure 20-32. **Abdominal aortic aneurysms. A,** Contrast material is seen in the lumen (open black arrow) along with a large clot (open white arrow). Calcification is seen in the wall of the aorta (closed white arrow). **B,** This aneurysm has ruptured. Contrast is seen in the lumen (black star) along with a crescentic clot (closed black arrow). Calcification is present in the wall (open black arrow). The more critical finding is active extravasation of contrast-containing blood (open white arrows).

A   B

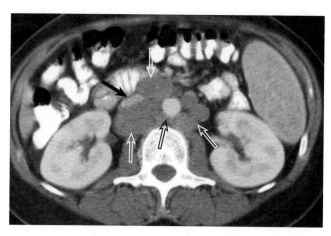

Figure 20-33. **Lymphoma.** *There is bulky, lobulated retroperitoneal adenopathy (open white arrows). The aorta (open black arrow) and inferior vena cava (closed black arrow) are displaced forward by additional nodes. Abdominal lymph nodes are considered pathologically enlarged if they exceed 1 cm in their short-axis dimension. Lymphadenopathy will classically displace the aorta or vena cava anteriorly.*

- **Recognizing an abdominal aortic aneurysm**
  - **Ultrasonography is the screening study of first choice** when an asymptomatic, pulsatile abdominal mass is palpated.
  - Unenhanced CT has the advantage over US of depicting the absolute size of the aneurysm but **in order to define**

the extent of mural thrombus and the presence of dissection, intravenous contrast should be used.

- **Mural thrombus** can be recognized as a **filling defect** in the contrast-filled aneurysm (Fig. 20-32A).
- Rupture can be inferred by **soft tissue encircling the aorta** (although other lesions can produce this finding) and is definite if **extravasation is identified** on a contrast-enhanced CT scan (Fig. 20-32B).

Adenopathy

- Lymphoma is classically divided into the **Hodgkin's and non-Hodgkin's (NHL) types.**
  - NHL features noncontiguous spread and extranodal involvement, especially in the gastrointestinal tract.
- **Recognizing the CT findings of lymphoma**
  - **Multiple enlarged lymph nodes**—pelvic lymph nodes are considered pathologically enlarged if they exceed 1 cm in their shortest dimension.
  - **Conglomerate masses of coalesced nodes** form bulky tumor masses that can encase and obstruct vessels.
  - Lymphadenopathy will classically **displace the aorta or vena cava anteriorly** (Fig. 20-33).
- Other malignancies can produce abdominal or pelvic adenopathy besides lymphoma and even benign disease such as sarcoid can produce abdominal adenopathy.

WebLink

More information about abdominal CT is available to registered users on StudentConsult.com.

⊞ TAKE-HOME POINTS: Recognizing the Basics on CT of the Abdomen

CT scans are used extensively in evaluation of the abdomen and pelvis and are the diagnostic modality of choice for most abdominal abnormalities, including trauma.

CT has had a profound impact in traumatized patients by distinguishing those patients who can be managed conservatively from those who need surgical or other interventions.

The most commonly affected solid organs in blunt abdominal trauma (in order of decreasing frequency) are the spleen, liver, kidney, and urinary bladder.

Evaluation of liver masses is frequently done utilizing a ***triple phase scan*** that includes a pre-contrast scan and two post-contrast scans, one in the hepatic arterial phase and then another in the portal venous phase.

Fatty infiltration of the liver is very common and can produce focal or diffuse areas of decreased attenuation that characteristically do not displace or obstruct the hepatic vessels; the liver appears less dense than the spleen.

In its later stages, ***cirrhosis*** produces a small liver (especially the right lobe) with a lobulated contour, inhomogeneous appearance of the parenchyma, prominent left and caudate lobes, splenomegaly, and ascites.

Metastases are the most common malignant hepatic masses originating mostly from the GI tract and appearing as multiple, low-density masses that may necrose as they become larger.

Hepatocellular carcinoma is the most common primary hepatic malignancy; these carcinomas are usually solitary and typically enhance with IV contrast.

Cavernous hemangiomas are usually solitary, are more common in females, and typically produce no symptoms; they have a characteristic centripetal pattern of enhancement and frequently retain contrast longer than the remainder of the liver.

The liver is commonly injured in both blunt and penetrating trauma and may demonstrate lacerations, hematomas, wedge-shaped defects, pseudoaneurysms, and acute hemorrhage; liver injury accounts for the majority of the deaths from abdominal trauma.

Ultrasound is the imaging study of first choice for the biliary system and the female pelvis.

Because the spleen is highly vascular, hemorrhage is the most serious sequela of splenic trauma; findings of splenic trauma include hematoma, laceration, contusion, and rupture.

(Continued)

TAKE-HOME POINTS: Recognizing the Basics on CT of the Abdomen—cont'd

Unenhanced CT scanning has replaced conventional radiography and intravenous urography in identifying renal and ureteral calculi, which may be calcified or produce secondary signs of obstruction or inflammation.

Pyelonephritis is secondary to an ascending lower urinary tract infection from gram-negative bacteria, which can produce enlarged kidney(s), wedge-shaped areas of low attenuation secondary to decreased perfusion, perinephric stranding, and hydronephrosis.

Renal cysts are a very common finding, are frequently multiple and bilateral, do not enhance, and typically have sharp margins where they meet the normal renal parenchyma.

Renal cell carcinoma is the most common primary renal malignancy and shows a propensity for extension into the renal vein and metastasizing to lung and bone; on CT, these carcinomas are usually solid masses that enhance with IV contrast but remain less dense than the normal kidney.

Patients who have had renal trauma almost all have hematuria and may show contusions, lacerations, fractures, subcapsular hematomas, or vascular pedicle injuries on CT. They may also demonstrate extraluminal contrast from an injury to the collecting system or ureter.

The two most common causes of **pancreatitis** are gallstones and alcoholism; pancreatitis is a clinical diagnosis with CT serving to document a cause or a complication of the disease; CT findings include enlargement of the pancreas, peripancreatic stranding, pancreatic necrosis, and pseudocyst formation.

Amorphous calcifications throughout the pancreas are pathognomonic of **chronic pancreatitis.**

Pancreatic adenocarcinoma has a very unfavorable prognosis, occurs most often in the pancreatic head, and usually manifests as a focal hypodense mass that may be associated with dilatation of the pancreatic or biliary ducts.

Key findings of bowel disease on CT are thickening of the wall, submucosal edema or hemorrhage, hazy infiltration of fat, and extraluminal air or contrast.

Shock bowel occurs with profound hypotension and shows diffuse small bowel wall thickening with enhancement of dilated and fluid-filled loops.

Uterine leiomyomas are commonly seen on pelvic CT scans, avidly enhance with contrast, and present as lobulated soft tissue masses frequently containing amorphous calcifications and areas of necrosis.

Pelvic inflammatory disease can produce haziness of pelvic fat, thickened fallopian tubes, enlarged and enhancing ovaries, an enlarged uterus with increased endometrial enhancement, pyosalpinx, tubo-ovarian abscess, and pelvic ascites.

Transitional cell carcinoma is the most common malignancy of the urinary bladder and appears as either a focal thickening of the bladder wall or a filling defect in the bladder.

Bladder ruptures may be either extraperitoneal (more common) or intraperitoneal, the former showing contrast around the bladder and the latter showing contrast that may flow freely in the peritoneal cavity.

Abdominal aortic aneurysms usually occur below the renal arteries and end in the iliac arteries; when they reach 4–5 cm they have a significant chance of rupture.

Abdominal or pelvic adenopathy may be caused by lymphoma, other malignancies, or, rarely, by benign diseases (e.g., sarcoid); multiple enlarged nodes or conglomerate masses of nodes may be seen on CT.

21 Recognizing Abnormalities of Bone Density

Normal Bone Anatomy

- On conventional radiographs, bones consist of a dense *cortex* of **compact bone** that completely envelopes a less dense *medullary cavity* containing **cancellous bone** arranged as *trabeculae,* separated primarily by blood vessels and fat.
  - The ratio of the amount of cortical versus trabecular bone varies in different skeletal sites and even at different locations in the same bone, i.e., the **cortex is naturally thicker is some places than in others.**
- When viewed in tangent on conventional radiographs, the **cortex** produces a **smoothly contoured, dense white shell** of varying thickness visualized best as a dense white band along the outer margins of the bone.
- The **medullary cavity** on conventional radiographs appears as a core of less dense, **grayish material inside the cortical shell, interlaced with a fine network of bony trabecular markings.**
  - There are relatively **fewer trabeculae in the midshaft** of long bones *(diaphysis)* than there are at the ends of the bones in the *metaphysis* and *epiphysis.*

- The *corticomedullary junction* is the edge between the inner margin of the cortex and the medullary cavity (Fig. 21-1).
- It is important to remember that **the cortex completely surrounds the entire bone** but is best seen where it is viewed in tangent (in profile).
- Almost all **examinations of bone still include conventional radiographs** obtained with at least **two views exposed at a 90° angle to each other** (called *orthogonal views*) so as to localize abnormalities better and to visualize as much of the circumference of the bone as possible (see Fig. 22-25).
- Still, **conventional radiographs cannot visualize the entire circumference of a tubular bone** and they are not particularly sensitive for demonstrating musculoskeletal soft tissue abnormalities.
  - Certain abnormalities, such as soft tissue swelling, can be seen on conventional studies.
- Generally speaking, **there must be a reduction of bone mass of almost 50% to produce a recognizable abnormality on conventional radiographs.**

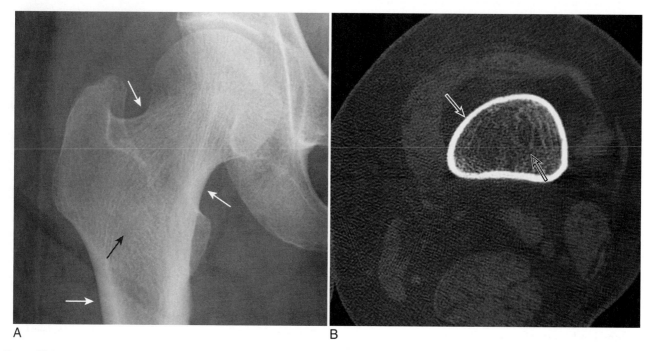

A   B

Figure 21-1. **Normal appearance of bone. A,** *In this anteroposterior view of the hip, the cortex is seen as a white line in tangent, varying in thickness in different parts of the bone (closed white arrows). In the medullary cavity, cancellous bone is seen to contain an interlacing network of trabeculae (closed black arrow).* **B,** *In this axial CT scan through the proximal femur, the entire 360° circumference of the cortex (open white arrow) is seen surrounding the less dense medullary cavity containing both bony trabeculae and fat (open black arrow). The image is optimized to display bone so that the muscles and subcutaneous fat are less well seen.*

• CT and MRI are able, by virtue of computer-aided reformatting and their superior ability to display more subtle differences in tissue densities, to demonstrate the entire circumference and internal matrix of bone including, especially with MRI, surrounding soft tissues not visible on conventional radiographs.

The Effect of Bone Physiology on Bone Anatomy

• Bones are continuously undergoing remodeling processes that include **resorption of old or diseased bone by osteoclasts** and **formation of new bone by osteoblasts.**

• Both osteoclastic and osteoblastic activity depend on the presence of a viable blood supply.
  - **Osteoblasts are responsible for bone matrix production.**
  - **Osteoclasts resorb both the matrix and mineral as well.**

• Bones reflect the general metabolic status of the individual.
  - Their composition requires a **protein-containing, collagenous matrix (osteoid)** upon which **bone mineral,** principally *calcium phosphate,* is transformed into cartilage and bone.

• **Bones** also **respond to mechanical forces**—for example, the contractions of muscles and tendons, the process of bearing weight, constant use or prolonged disuse—that help to form and maintain the shape as well as the content of each bone.

• There are **four major forces that affect bone density**
  - **Osteoblastic activity**
  - **Osteoclastic activity**
  - Production of normal **osteoid on which calcification can occur**
  - **Mechanical stress**

• In this chapter, we arbitrarily divide abnormalities of bone density into two major categories—those that produce a pattern of either **increased** or **decreased** bone density—and then subdivide those two patterns by **extent of disease** into those that produce **focal** versus **generalized** (or **diffuse**) changes (Table 21-1).

• Fractures and dislocations, arthritis, and spinal diseases are discussed in subsequent chapters.

Recognizing a *Generalized Increase* in Bone Density

• **Recognizing the findings of diffusely increased bone density**
  - An **overall whiteness (sclerosis)** to all or most of the bones
  - **Diffuse loss of visualization of the normal network of bony trabeculae in the medullary cavity** because of replacement of the normal intertrabecular fatty marrow by bone
  - **Loss of visualization of the normal corticomedullary junction** because of abnormally increased density of the normally gray-appearing medullary cavity relative to the cortex (Fig. 21-2)

• **The following are some examples of diseases that cause a diffuse increase in bone density.**

Table 21-1

CHANGES IN BONE DENSITY

Density	Extent	Examples
Increased density	Generalized	Diffuse osteoblastic metastases
		Osteopetrosis (rare)
	Focal	Localized osteoblastic metastases
		Avascular necrosis of bone
		Paget's disease
Decreased density	Generalized	Osteoporosis
		Hyperparathyroidism
		Rickets and osteomalacia
	Focal	Localized osteolytic metastases
		Multiple myeloma
		Osteomyelitis

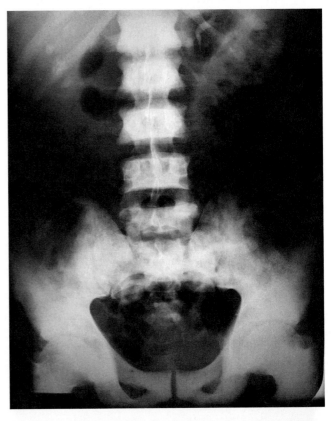

*Figure 21-2. **Diffuse metastatic disease from carcinoma of the prostate.** Notice that you can no longer see the normal trabeculae or the junction between the medullary cavity and the cortex as the medullary cavities have been filled in from osteoblastic metastatic disease that obscures these normal boundaries and increases the overall bone density. Contrast this picture with that of Paget's disease of the pelvis (see Fig. 21-11).*

CARCINOMA OF THE PROSTATE: DIFFUSE ↑ BONE DENSITY

- Diffuse, blood-borne, bony metastatic disease from *carcinoma of the prostate* is the **prototype for generalized increase in bone density.**
  - Osteoblastic activity occurs **beyond the control** of normal physiologic constraints.
  - Metastatic disease to bone **occurs in over 80% of autopsied patients with carcinoma of the prostate.**
  - **Multiple bone metastases** from carcinoma of the prostate occur much **more frequently** than do **solitary bone lesions.**
  - With diffuse bone metastases, a so-called *superscan* may be seen on radionuclide bone scan.
    - This superscan demonstrates high radiotracer uptake throughout the skeleton, with poor or absent renal excretion of the radiotracer (Fig. 21-3).

OSTEOPETROSIS: DIFFUSE ↑ BONE DENSITY

- *Osteopetrosis* (also called *marble bone disease* for obvious reasons) is a **rare** hereditary **defect in** osteoclastic activity that ultimately results in an **increase in bone density** affecting the entire skeleton (Fig. 21-4).
  - Although the bones are increased in density, they are **mechanically inferior** to normal bone and subject to **pathologic fractures.**
  - In the **infantile form** of this disease, the defective osseous material can **replace normal bone marrow** leading to **anemia, thrombocytopenia, and leukopenia** (*pancytopenia*).

Recognizing a *Focal Increase* in Bone Density

- **Recognizing the findings of localized increase in bone density**
  - **Focal sclerotic lesions** may affect the cortex or medullary cavity
    - Those that affect the cortex will usually produce **periosteal new-bone formation (periosteal reaction),** which leads to an appearance of **thickening of the cortex.**
    - Those that affect the medullary cavity will result in **punctate, amorphous sclerotic lesions** surrounded by the normally uniformly gray-appearing medullary cavity (Fig. 21-5).
- **The following are examples of diseases that cause a focal increase in bone density.**

CARCINOMA OF THE PROSTATE: FOCAL ↑ BONE DENSITY

- A substance secreted by tumor cells from **metastatic carcinoma of the prostate may stimulate osteoblastic**

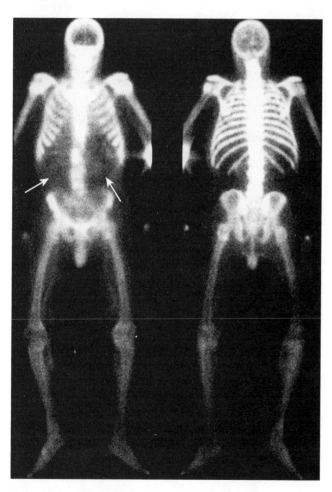

*Figure 21-3. **Radionuclide bone superscan.** AP and PA views of the axial and appendicular skeleton show the distribution of bone radiotracer uptake throughout the skeleton. This is the picture of the so-called **superscan** produced by osteoblastic metastatic disease involving every bone in the patient's body, leading to high uptake throughout the skeleton, with poor or absent renal excretion of the radiotracer (closed white arrows).*

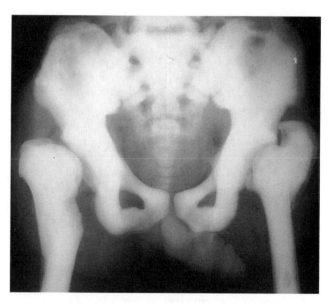

*Figure 21-4. **Osteopetrosis (marble bone disease).** A frontal view of the pelvis demonstrates diffuse sclerosis of the bones in this 22-year-old patient with osteopetrosis, a rare defect in osteoclastic activity that results in an increase in bone density. Although the bones are increased in density, they are mechanically inferior to normal bone and subject to pathologic fractures. In the infantile form of this disease, the defective osseous material can replace normal bone marrow leading to anemia, thrombocytopenia, and leukopenia (pancytopenia).*

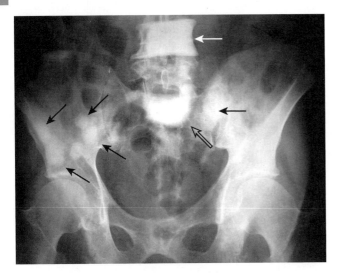

Figure 21-5. **Focal sclerotic metastases from carcinoma of the prostate.** *Sclerotic lesions are seen in the L4 (closed white arrow) and S1 (open black arrow) vertebral bodies. It is no longer possible to distinguish the junction between the cortex and the medullary cavity in either of those vertebral bodies. Also present, are multiple sclerotic lesions in the right ilium and the left ilium near the sacroiliac joint (closed black arrows). Sclerotic lesions in bone are a common finding in metastatic carcinoma of the prostate.*

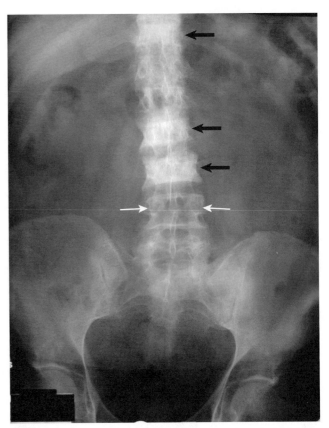

Figure 21-6. **Focal increase in bone density from carcinoma of the breast.** *A frontal view of the lumbar spine and pelvis demonstrates abnormally dense vertebral bodies, most marked at L2 and L3 but also involving T1 through L1 (closed black arrows). Notice how the pedicles of the involved vertebral bodies are obscured by the abnormally increased density of the vertebral body compared to the normal pedicles at L4 (closed white arrows). Dense, white vertebrae are called* **ivory vertebrae.** *Osteoblastic carcinoma of the breast and prostate are two causes of an ivory vertebra.*

Box 21-1

Finding Metastases to Bone—Bone Scan
Technetium-99m is the radionuclide used to tag methylene diphosphonate (MDP), the entity that directs the tracer to bone.
A minute amount of technetium-99m MDP is administered intravenously and affixes to the surface of bone.
Activity in bone depends, in part, on its blood supply and rate of bone turnover: processes with extremely high or extremely low bone turnover may produce false negative scans.
Metastases usually show increased uptake (activity), even if they are mostly osteolytic, because of the repair that occurs in most, but not all, osteolytic processes.
Bone scans are highly sensitive but not very specific—a positive scan almost always requires another imaging procedure (conventional radiographs, CT, or MRI) to rule out other causes of the positive bone scan (e.g., fractures, infection).
The bone scan is much less sensitive in detecting multiple myeloma or purely lytic metastases, so conventional radiographic surveys of the skeleton are the initial study of choice when searching for myeloma lesions.

activity and produce focal areas of localized increased density, i.e., **sclerotic bone lesions.**

- These lesions are **most often seen in the vertebrae, ribs, pelvis, humeri, and femurs.**
- The **radionuclide bone scan is currently the study of choice for detecting skeletal metastases,** regardless of the suspected primary cancer (Fig. 21-6, Box 21-1).

AVASCULAR NECROSIS OF BONE: FOCAL ↑ BONE DENSITY

- The continuous process of bone resorption and formation depends upon a balance between osteoclastic and osteoblastic activity.
- In *avascular necrosis of bone* (also called *ischemic necrosis, aseptic necrosis, osteonecrosis),* the blood supply to a particular part of the bone is interrupted (Table 21-2).
- On conventional radiographs, the **region of avascular necrosis appears more dense than the surrounding bone.**
  - Because of peculiarities of vascularization, a fracture through the midportion **(waist) of the scaphoid (navicular)** bone in the wrist **interrupts blood supply to the proximal pole** while the remainder of the bones of the wrist continue to undergo the process of bone turnover.
  - The result is an **apparent relative increase in the density of the devascularized part compared to the remainder of the bone** (Fig. 21-7).
- In other areas of the body as well, the **devascularized bone becomes denser** and thus appears more sclerotic than the remainder of the bone.
- This process especially occurs in two sites:
  - **Femoral head** (Fig. 21-8)
  - **Humeral head** (Fig. 21-9)

Table 21-2

SOME CAUSES OF AVASCULAR NECROSIS OF BONE

Location	Example of Disease
Intravascular	Sickle cell disease
	Polycythemia vera
Vascular	Vasculitis (lupus and radiation-induced)
Extravascular	Trauma (fractures)
Idiopathic	Exogenous steroids and Cushing's disease
	Legg-Calvé-Perthes disease

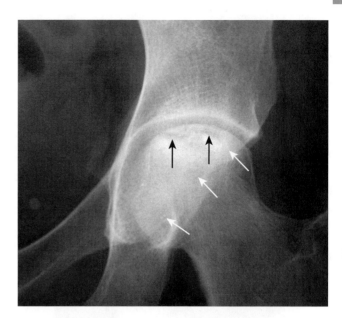

Figure 21-8. ***Avascular necrosis of the left femoral head in a patient on long-term steroids for lupus erythematosus.*** *A close-up view of the left femoral head shows a zone of increased sclerosis in the superior aspect of the femoral head (closed white arrows), a characteristic finding of avascular necrosis of the head. The linear, subcortical lucency (closed black arrows) represents subperiosteal hemorrhage seen in avascular necrosis, called the* **crescent sign.** *Notice that the disease is isolated to the femoral head and involves neither the joint space nor the acetabulum. This is not an arthritis.*

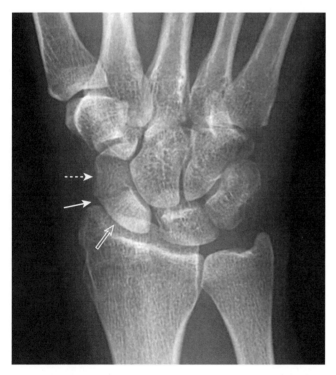

Figure 21-7. ***Avascular necrosis of the proximal pole of the scaphoid.*** *A close-up frontal view of the wrist demonstrates that the proximal pole of the scaphoid (open white arrow) is denser than the distal pole (dotted white arrow). There is a fracture through the waist of the scaphoid (closed white arrow). Because of the peculiar blood supply of the scaphoid (from distal to proximal), fractures through the waist may interrupt the proximal blood supply while the remainder of the bones of the wrist, having normal blood supply, become demineralized. This makes the proximal pole of the scaphoid appear denser relative to the other bones of the wrist.*

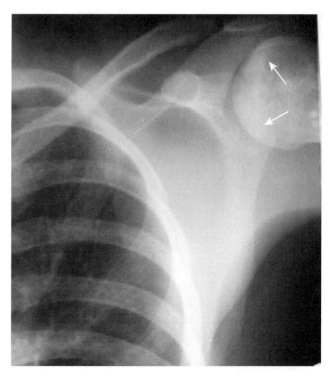

Figure 21-9. ***Avascular necrosis of humeral head.*** *Increased density is seen at the very top of the humeral head (closed white arrows) in this patient with sickle cell disease who developed avascular necrosis of the humeral head. Because the white cap on the bone looks like snow on a mountaintop, this sign of avascular necrosis has been called* **snow-capping.**

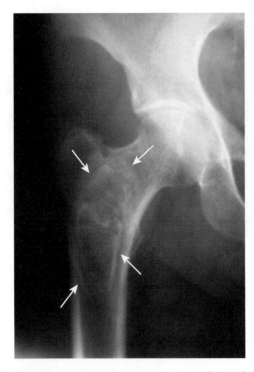

Figure 21-10. **Medullary bone infarct.** *An amorphous calcification is seen in the medullary cavity of the proximal femur (closed white arrows). In general, the differential diagnosis for such an intramedullary calcification includes bone infarct and enchondroma. The characteristic thin sclerotic membrane surrounding this lesion identifies it as a bone infarct.*

- *Medullary bone infarcts* are recognized as dense, serpiginous collections of bone within the medullary cavities of long bones frequently marginated by a thin, sclerotic membrane (Fig. 21-10).
- Today, **MRI is the study of choice in diagnosing avascular necrosis** because it is able to recognize changes in signal detected from the marrow much earlier than any findings become visible on conventional radiographs.

PAGET'S DISEASE: FOCAL ↑ BONE DENSITY

- Paget's disease is a **chronic disease of bone,** most often occurring in older men, now believed due to chronic paramyxoviral infection.
- It is **characterized by varying degrees of increased bone resorption and increased bone formation,** with the latter predominating in those cases seen in more progressive forms of the disease.
- The end result is almost always a **denser bone** which, despite its density, is **mechanically inferior** to normal bone and thus **prone to pathologic fractures** or bone-softening abnormalities such as *bowing.*
- The **pelvis is most frequently involved,** followed by the **lumbar spine, thoracic spine, proximal femur, and calvarium.**
- The **imaging hallmarks of Paget's disease**
  - **Thickening of the cortex**—compare the thickness of the cortex of the suspicious area with another part of the same bone or, if visible, the same bone on the opposite side of the body.

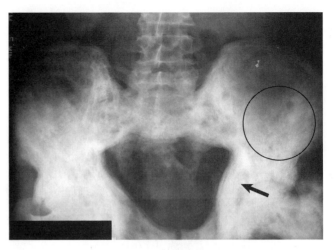

Figure 21-11. **Paget's disease of the pelvis.** *A frontal view of the pelvis shows a diffuse increase in bony density, accentuation and coarsening of the trabeculae (black circle), and thickening of the cortex (closed black arrow), the hallmark characteristics of Paget's disease of bone. Contrast this picture with that of diffuse metastatic disease from carcinoma of the prostate (see Fig. 21-2). Although they may look alike at first, the cortex is thickened in Paget's disease and trabeculae are accentuated, rather than obscured as they are in prostate carcinoma. The cortex is not thickened by metastatic disease as it is by Paget's disease.*

- **Accentuation of the trabecular pattern**—coarsening and thickening of the trabeculae occur (Fig. 21-11).
- **Increase in the size of the bone involved**—the "classical" history for Paget's disease, rendered less useful as fashions have changed, was a gradual increase in a man's hat size as the calvarium increased in size because of Paget's disease.

Recognizing a *Generalized Decrease* in Bone Density

- Several important diseases result in a generalized decrease in bony density.
- **Recognizing the findings of diffuse decrease in bone density**
  - The bones have an **overall increase in lucency.**
  - **Diffuse loss of the normal network of bony trabeculae in the medullary cavity** because of the loss and thinning of many of the smaller trabecular structures
  - **Accentuation of the normal corticomedullary junction** in which the **cortex,** although thinner than normal, **stands out more strikingly** because of the decreased density of the medullary cavity (Fig. 21-12)
  - **Compression of vertebral bodies** (see Fig. 24-7)
  - **Pathologic fractures** in the hip, pelvis, or vertebral bodies
- **The following are examples of diseases that cause a diffuse decrease in bone density.**

OSTEOPOROSIS: DIFFUSE ↓ BONE DENSITY

- *Osteoporosis* is defined as a systemic skeletal disorder **characterized by low bone mineral density** (BMD) and generally divided into postmenopausal and age-related bone loss.

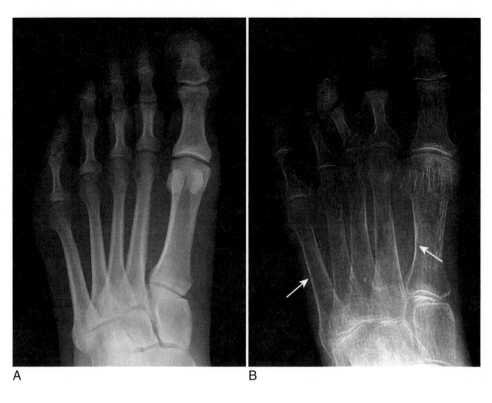

A   B

Figure 21-12. **Normal and osteoporotic foot.** *Contrast this normal frontal view of the foot (**A**) with an osteoporotic foot (**B**), which shows overall lucency in the bone and thinning of the cortices (closed white arrows). Conventional radiographs are insensitive in diagnosing osteoporosis, and they are subject to technical variations that can mimic the disease even in a healthy individual. More sensitive methods, such as a DEXA scan, should be used to confirm the diagnosis.*

- *Postmenopausal osteoporosis* is characterized by **increased bone resorption** due to osteoclastic activity.
- **Age-related bone loss** begins around age 45 to 55 and is characterized by a **loss of total bone mass.**
- Additional factors that increase the risk of osteoporosis include exogenous steroid administration, Cushing's disease, estrogen deficiency, inadequate physical activity, and alcoholism.
- Osteoporosis **predisposes to pathologic fractures** involving such bones as the femoral neck, compression fractures of the vertebral bodies, and fractures of the distal radius (Colles fractures).
- **Conventional radiographs** are relatively **insensitive for detecting osteoporosis.**
  - Almost **50% of the bone mass must be lost** before it is **recognizable** on conventional radiographs.
  - Findings on conventional radiographs include **overall lucency of bone, thinning of the cortex, and decrease in the visible number of trabeculae in the medullary cavity** (see Fig. 21-12).
- Bone mineral density measurements
  - Currently, **DEXA (*d*ual-*e*nergy *x*-ray *a*bsorptiometry) scans are the most accurate** and widely recommended method for BMD measurement.
  - DEXA scans are obtained by using a filtered x-ray source that produces two distinct energies that are differentially absorbed by bone and soft tissue, respectively, allowing for the more accurate calculation of bone density by subtracting out the error introduced by varying amounts of overlying soft tissue.

- X-ray dose is very low and density measurements of the spine or hip are used.

HYPERPARATHYROIDISM: DIFFUSE ↓ BONE DENSITY
- *Hyperparathyroidism* is a condition caused by excessive secretion of *parathormone (PTH)* by the parathyroid glands.
- Parathormone exerts its effects on bones, the kidneys, and the GI tract.
  - Its **effect on bones is to increase resorption** by stimulating osteoclastic activity.
  - Calcium is removed from the bone and deposited in the bloodstream.
- There are three forms of hyperparathyroidism (Table 21-3).

Table 21-3

FORMS OF HYPERPARATHYROIDISM

Type	Remarks
Primary	Usually caused by a single adenoma in most patients (80–90%) and almost always results in hypercalcemia
Secondary	Results from hyperplasia of the glands secondary to imbalances in calcium and phosphorus levels seen mostly with chronic renal disease
Tertiary	Occurs in patients with long-standing secondary hyperparathyroidism in whom autonomous hypersecretion of parathormone develops, leading to hypercalcemia

- The **diagnosis of hyperparathyroidism is based on clinical and laboratory findings,** but there are numerous findings of the disease on conventional radiographs and there are other imaging studies utilized to guide surgery on the glands, if indicated.
  - Imaging studies of the parathyroid glands may include ultrasound, nuclear medicine parathyroid scans, and MRI scans.
- Some of the many **findings of hyperparathyroidism on conventional radiographs**
  - **Overall decrease in bone density**
  - *Subperiosteal bone resorption,* especially on the radial side of the middle phalanges of the index and middle fingers (Fig. 21-13)
  - **Erosion of the distal clavicles** (Fig. 21-14)
  - **Well-circumscribed lytic lesions** in the long bones called *brown tumors* and a *salt-and-pepper appearance* of the skull (Fig. 21-15)

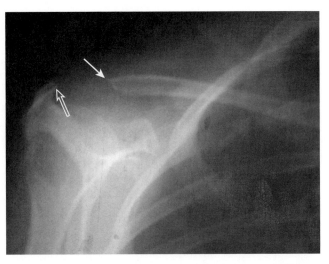

Figure 21-14. *Erosion of distal clavicle in hyperparathyroidism.* *Another relatively common site of bone resorption in hyperparathyroidism is the distal end of the clavicle. Here the distal clavicle (closed white arrow), which should articulate with the acromion (open white arrow), has been resorbed, increasing the distance between it and the acromion. Other sites of bone resorption might include the terminal phalanges (acro-osteolysis), the lamina dura of the teeth, and the medial aspect of the proximal tibia.*

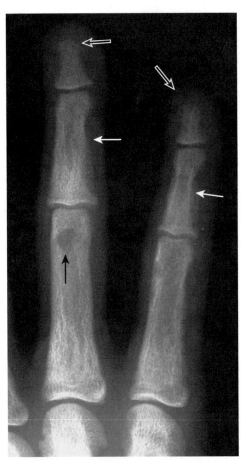

Figure 21-13. *Subperiosteal resorption in hyperparathyroidism.* *The radiologic hallmark of hyperparathyroidism is subperiosteal bone resorption, seen especially well on the radial aspect of the middle phalanges of the index and middle fingers (closed white arrows). Here the cortex appears shaggy and irregular, compared to the cortex on the opposite side of the same bone, which is well-defined. This patient also displays other findings of hyperparathyroidism: a small brown tumor (closed black arrow) and resorption of the terminal phalanges (open white arrows).*

RICKETS: DIFFUSE ↓ BONE DENSITY

- Rickets is caused by a wide variety of disorders mostly related to abnormalities in vitamin D ingestion, absorption, or activation, the end result of which is a **failure to calcify the osteoid matrix of bone, especially at the sites of maximal growth in children.**
- Rickets usually **results either from a deficiency, or abnormal metabolism, of vitamin D or from abnormal metabolism or excretion of inorganic phosphate.**
- By definition, **rickets occurs only in children** whose growth plates have not closed (which occurs at approximately 17 years of age in females and 19 years of age in males).
- **The imaging hallmarks of rickets**
  - **Fraying and cupping at the metaphyses of long bones,** including the anterior ends of the ribs (*rachitic rosary*) (Fig. 21-16)
    - This is especially pronounced at the ends of bones where the maximum growth occurs such as at the knees, wrists, and ankles.
  - **Widening and irregularity of the epiphyseal plates**
  - **Bones are soft and pliable** so there can be **bowing** of the femur and tibia.

OSTEOMALACIA: DIFFUSE ↓ BONE DENSITY

- *Osteomalacia* is characterized by the failure to calcify the osteoid matrix of bone in **adults,** most commonly as the result of chronic renal disease.
- **Findings of osteomalacia on conventional radiographs**
  - **Overall decrease in bone density**

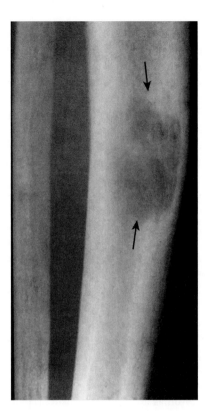

Figure 21-15. **Brown tumor.** *This geographic, lytic lesion is in the midshaft of the tibia (closed black arrows). Brown tumors (also called* **osteoclastomas**) *are benign lesions that represent the osteoclastic resorption of a localized area of (usually) cortical bone and replacement with fibrous tissue and blood. Their high hemosiderin content gives them a characteristic brown color; they were not named after a ''Dr. Brown.'' The lesions can look like osteolytic metastases or multiple myeloma, so that the clinical history of hyperparathyroidism is key. They can be seen with both primary and secondary hyperparathyroidism.*

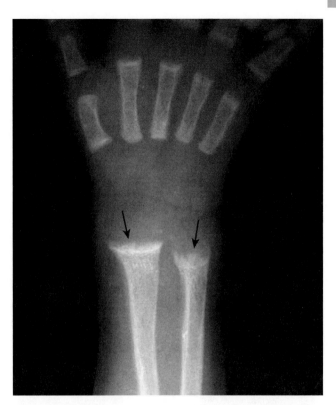

Figure 21-16. **Rickets.** *Frontal view of the wrist shows cupping and fraying (closed black arrows) of the metaphyses of the distal radius and ulna, characteristic findings of rickets. Rickets will first affect the bones growing fastest so that it is most common around the knee, distal tibia, and distal radius. It may also be seen at the growing end of the ribs.*

- **Thinning of the cortex**
- **Coarsening of the trabecular pattern** due to resorption of secondary trabeculae
- The **imaging hallmark of osteomalacia is the** *pseudofracture (Looser line),* which is a fracture that frequently occurs at multiple sites at the same time and is associated with nonunion due to inadequate calcification of the healing fracture.
  - **Common locations for pseudofractures** are the medial femoral neck and shaft, pubic and ischial rami, metatarsals, and calcaneus.
  - They are typically **short, lucent bands, at right angles to the cortex** with **sclerotic margins in later stages.**
  - They are **frequently bilateral and symmetrical** (Fig. 21-17).

Recognizing a *Focal Decrease* in Bone Density
- Several common lesions can produce a focal decrease in bone density.
- These lesions are most often produced by **focal infiltration of bone by cells other than osteocytes.**

- In lytic metastatic disease and multiple myeloma, malignant cells (plasma cells in the case of myeloma) replace normal bone cells.
- **The following are examples of diseases that cause a focal decrease in bone density.**

OSTEOLYTIC METASTATIC DISEASE: FOCAL ↓ BONE DENSITY
- **Osteolytic metastatic disease** can produce focal destruction of bone (Box 21-2).
- The **medullary cavity is almost always involved,** and from this cavity the disease may erode into and destroy the cortex as well.
  - When only the medullary cavity is involved, almost a 50% reduction in mass is required in order for the lesion to be recognizable on conventional radiographs when viewed *en face.*
- In **some cases, only the cortex is involved.**
  - Cortical metastases may be easier to visualize because relatively less cortical destruction is needed for it to become apparent, especially if the lesion is viewed in tangent.
- The **classical findings of osteolytic metastases** on conventional radiographs:
  - **Irregularly shaped, lucent bone lesions,** which can be single or multiple

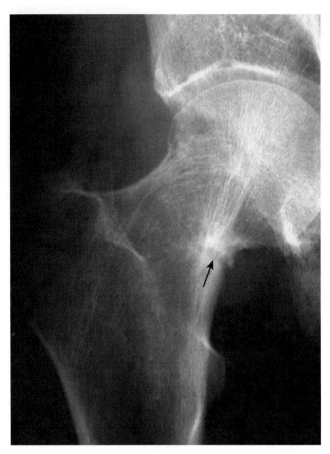

*Figure 21-17. **Looser line (pseudofracture).** A close-up view of the femoral neck shows the typical features of a Looser line: short, lucent bands, at right angles to the cortex with sclerotic margins (closed black arrow). Looser lines are the hallmark of osteomalacia in adults. They are frequently bilateral and symmetrical.*

Box 21-2

Metastatic Disease to Bone

Metastases to bone are far more common than primary bone tumors.

Metastases to bone fall into two major categories: those that stimulate the production of new bone are called *osteoblastic,* and those that destroy bone are called *osteolytic;* some metastases include lesions in which osteoblastic and osteolytic changes are both present.

Metastatic bone lesions from any source are very uncommon distal to the elbow or the knee; when present in these locations, they are usually widespread and due to lung or breast cancer.

The radionuclide bone scan is currently the study of choice for detecting skeletal metastases.

- These lytic lesions are frequently characterized as belonging to one (or sometimes more) of three patterns: *geographic, mottled,* or *permeative,* in order of decreasing size to the smallest and most discrete lesion visible (Fig. 21-18).

- They typically **incite little or no reactive bone formation** around them.
- They may be **expansile** and *soap-bubbly* (i.e., contain bony septations), especially in renal and thyroid carcinoma (Fig. 21-19).
- In the spine, they may preferentially **destroy the pedicles,** because of their blood supply (the *pedicle sign*), which can help to differentiate metastases from multiple myeloma (see below), which tends to spare the pedicle early in the disease (Fig. 21-20).
- The most common causes of osteoblastic and osteolytic bone metastases are listed in Table 21-4.

MULTIPLE MYELOMA: FOCAL ↓ BONE DENSITY

- **Multiple myeloma,** the most common primary malignancy of bone in adults, can occur in a **solitary form,** often seen as a soap-bubbly, expansile lesion in the spine or pelvis (called a *solitary plasmacytoma*) or a **disseminated form** with multiple, *punched-out* lytic lesions throughout the axial and proximal appendicular skeleton.
- **Findings of multiple myeloma on conventional radiographs**
  - The most common early manifestation is **diffuse and usually severe osteoporosis.**
  - **Plasmacytomas** appear as **expansile, septated lesions, frequently with associated soft tissue masses** (Fig. 21-21).
  - Later, in its disseminated form, **multiple, small, sharply circumscribed,** *punched-out* **lytic lesions of approximately the same size** are present, usually without any accompanying sclerotic reaction around them (Fig. 21-22).
- Classically, **conventional radiographs are more sensitive in detecting the lesions of multiple myeloma than radionuclide bone scans,** which tend to underestimate the number and extent of lesions due to the absence of reactive bone formation.

OSTEOMYELITIS: FOCAL ↓ BONE DENSITY

- *Osteomyelitis* refers to the **focal destruction of bone,** most often by a blood-borne **infectious agent,** the most common of which is *Staphylococcal aureus.*
- **In children,** the osteolytic lesion **tends to occur at the metaphysis** because of its exuberant blood supply.
- **Findings of acute osteomyelitis on conventional radiographs**
  - **Focal cortical bone destruction**
  - **Periosteal new bone formation** (Fig. 21-23)
  - Inflammatory changes accompanying the infection may produce **soft tissue swelling** and **focal osteoporosis** from hyperemia.
- In **adults,** the **infection tends to involve the joint space more** often than in children, producing not only osteomyelitis but also *septic arthritis* (see Chapter 24).
- **Conventional radiographs can take up to 10 days to display the first findings of osteomyelitis,** so other imaging modalities, such as MRI and nuclear medicine studies, are frequently used for earlier diagnosis.

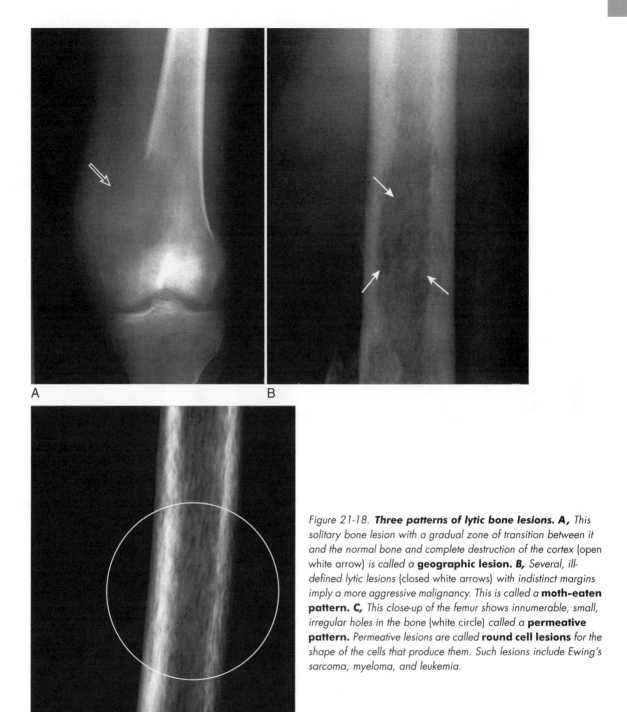

Figure 21-18. ***Three patterns of lytic bone lesions. A,*** *This solitary bone lesion with a gradual zone of transition between it and the normal bone and complete destruction of the cortex (open white arrow) is called a* **geographic lesion. B,** *Several, ill-defined lytic lesions (closed white arrows) with indistinct margins imply a more aggressive malignancy. This is called a* **moth-eaten pattern. C,** *This close-up of the femur shows innumerable, small, irregular holes in the bone (white circle) called a* **permeative pattern.** *Permeative lesions are called* **round cell lesions** *for the shape of the cells that produce them. Such lesions include Ewing's sarcoma, myeloma, and leukemia.*

- There are a variety of radionuclide bone scans that can demonstrate osteomyelitis, the most specific of which is currently a **tagged, white blood cell scan,** in which a sample of the patient's white blood cells is removed, tagged with a radioactive isotope (frequently indium), and injected back into the patient, who is then imaged with a camera specific for nuclear studies to detect a site of abnormally increased radioactive tracer uptake, which harbors infection.

Pathologic Fractures

- Pathologic fractures are those that **occur in bone with a preexisting abnormality.**

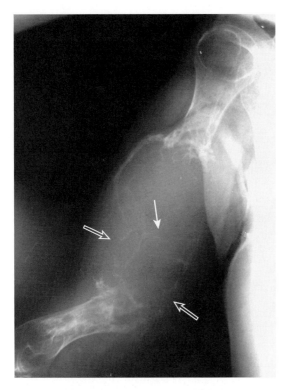

Figure 21-19. **Expansile renal cell carcinoma metastasis.** *This is a very aggressive and expansile osteolytic metastasis in the humerus from a primary renal cell carcinoma. Notice that the cortex has been destroyed in several areas (open white arrows) and the lesion has a* **soap-bubbly** *appearance produced by fine septa (closed white arrow). Thyroid carcinoma and a solitary plasmacytoma could also produce these findings.*

- Diseases that produce both an **increase** in bone density or a **decrease** in bone density tend to **weaken the normal architecture** of bone and predispose to pathologic fractures.
  - Diseases that predispose to pathologic fractures may be **local** (metastases, bone cysts) or **diffuse** (rickets).

Table 21-4

SITES OF ORIGIN OF OSTEOBLASTIC AND OSTEOLYTIC BONE METASTASES

Osteoblastic	Osteolytic
Prostate carcinoma (most common in older men)	Lung cancer (most common osteolytic lesion in males)
Breast carcinoma (especially if treated)	Breast cancer (most common osteolytic lesion in females)
Lymphoma	Renal cell carcinoma
Carcinoid tumors	Thyroid carcinoma

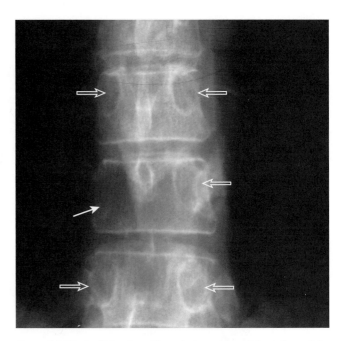

Figure 21-20. **Pedicle sign.** *There is destruction of the right pedicle of T10 (closed white arrow). Each vertebral body should have two oval pedicles, one on each side, visible on the frontal radiograph of the spine (open white arrows). In the spine, osteolytic metastases may preferentially destroy the pedicles, because of their blood supply, producing the* **pedicle sign,** *although most metastatic lesions to the spine will involve the body. In multiple myeloma, the pedicle tends to be spared early in the disease.*

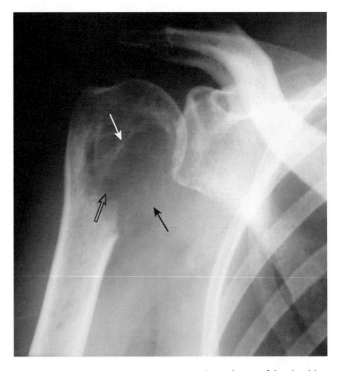

Figure 21-21. **Solitary plasmacytoma.** *Frontal view of the shoulder. A lytic lesion on the proximal humerus (open black arrow) destroys the cortex (closed black arrow) and contains multiple septations (closed white arrow). This is the so-called* **soap-bubbly** *appearance that can be seen with solitary plasmacytomas, a precursor to the more disseminated form of multiple myeloma.*

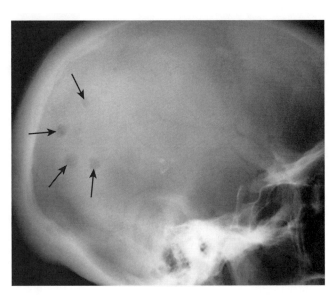

Figure 21-22. **Multiple myeloma.** *Several lytic lesions (closed black arrows) are seen in the skull. They are small, uniform in size, and have sharply marginated edges, the so-called* **punched-out** *lytic defect seen in multiple myeloma.*

- They occur more often in the **ribs, spine, and proximal appendicular skeleton** (humeri and femurs).
- **Recognizing pathologic fractures** (Fig. 21-24)
  - The underlying bone demonstrates abnormal density or architecture.
  - Pathologic fractures tend to be transverse in orientation.
- Their treatment depends in large part on treatment of the underlying condition that produced them.

WebLink

More information on recognizing changes in bone density is available to registered users on StudentConsult.com.

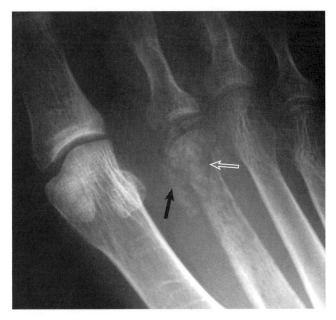

Figure 21-23. **Acute osteomyelitis of second metatarsal.** *Frontal view of the second toe shows the hallmarks of bone destruction (open white arrow) and periosteal new bone formation (closed black arrow) in osteomyelitis of the head of the second metatarsal in this 59-year-old female with diabetes.*

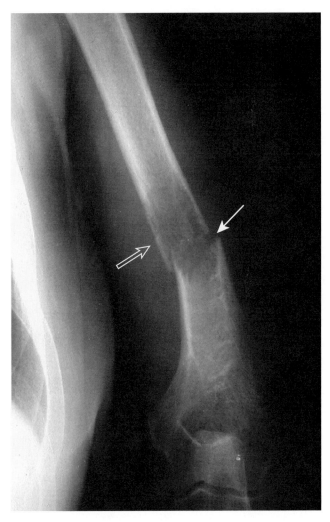

Figure 21-24. **Pathologic fracture.** *Pathologic fractures occur with minimal stress in bones with preexisting abnormalities. In this patient with metastatic renal cell carcinoma to the humerus, there is a geographic, lytic lesion seen in the distal humerus (open white arrow) through which a fracture (closed white arrow) has occurred that traverses the lytic lesion.*

- Attempts to predict "impending" fractures in diseased bone have, by and large, proved to be unreliable.
- Pathologic fractures tend to occur with **minimal or no trauma.**

TAKE-HOME POINTS: Recognizing Abnormalities of Bone Density

Bone is undergoing continuous change from a combination of forces including biochemical and mechanical.

Increased osteoclastic activity can produce focal or generalized decrease in bone density, and increased osteoblastic activity can produce focal or diffuse increased bone density.

Osteoblastic metastases, especially from carcinoma of the prostate and breast, can produce focal or generalized increase in bony density.

Other diseases that can increase bone density include osteopetrosis, avascular necrosis of bone, and Paget's disease.

Osteolytic metastases, especially from lung, renal, thyroid, and breast cancer, can produce focal areas of decreased bone density, as can multiple myeloma, the most common primary tumor of bone.

Examples of diseases that can cause a generalized decrease in bone density include osteoporosis, hyperparathyroidism, rickets (in children), and osteomalacia (in adults).

Pathologic fractures occur with minimal or no trauma in bones that had a preexisting abnormality.

22 Recognizing Fractures and Dislocations

Recognizing an Acute Fracture

- Fractures are a favorite among those learning radiology; it seems that everyone is fascinated by a broken bone or two.
- A fracture is described as a **disruption in the continuity of all or part of the cortex of a bone.**
  - If the **cortex** is **broken through and through,** the fracture is called **complete.**
  - If **only a part of the cortex** is fractured, it is called **incomplete.**
    - Incomplete fractures tend to occur in bones that are "softer" than normal, such as those in children, or in adults with bone-softening diseases such as **osteomalacia** or **Paget's disease** (see Chapter 21, Recognizing Abnormalities of Bone Density).
  - Examples of incomplete fractures in children are the **greenstick fracture,** which involves only one part of, but not the entire, cortex, and the **torus fracture (buckle fracture),** which represents buckling of the cortex (Fig. 22-1).

- **Radiologic features of acute fractures** (Box 22-1)
  - There may be an **abrupt discontinuity of the cortex,** sometimes associated with **acute angulation of the normally smooth contour of bone** (see Fig. 22-1B).
  - **Fracture lines,** when viewed in the correct orientation, **tend to be "blacker" (more lucent)** than other lines normally found in bones, such as **nutrient canals** (Fig. 22-2).
  - Fracture lines tend to be **straighter in their course yet more acute in their angulation** than any naturally occurring lines (such as **epiphyseal plates**) (Fig. 22-3).
  - The **edges of a fracture tend to be jagged and rough.**
- **Pitfalls: sesamoids, accessory ossicles, and unhealed fractures** (Table 22-1)
  - **Sesamoids** (bones which form in a tendon as it passes over a joint)
  - **Accessory ossicles** (accessory epiphyseal or apophyseal ossification centers that do not fuse with the parent bone)

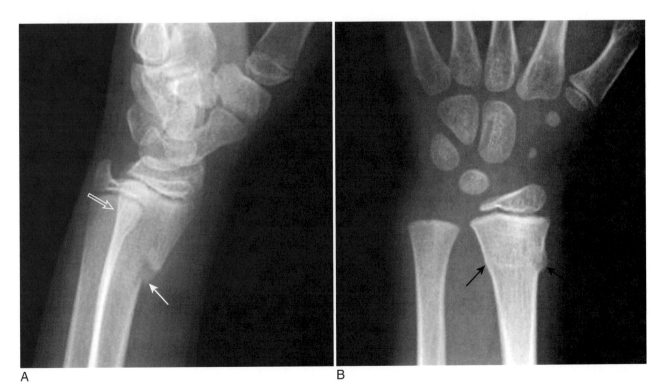

Figure 22-1. **Greenstick and torus fractures.** *Incomplete fractures involve only a portion of the cortex. They tend to occur in bones that are "softer" than normal, such as those in children, or in adults with bone-softening diseases such as osteomalacia or Paget's disease.* **A,** *This greenstick fracture* (closed white arrow) *involves only one part of, but not the entire, cortex* (open white arrow *shows the cortex to be intact*). **B,** *In this torus fracture* (buckle fracture) *there is buckling of the cortex* (closed black arrows).

Box 22-1

Characteristics of an Acute Fracture

| Abrupt disruption of all or part of the cortex |
| Acute changes in the smooth contour of a normal bone |
| Fracture lines are black and linear |
| Where fracture lines change their course, they tend to be sharply angulated |
| Fracture fragments are jagged and not corticated |

- **Old, unhealed fracture fragments** (sometimes mimic acute fractures) (Fig. 22-4A)
- Unlike fractures, these small bones are **corticated** (there is a white line that completely surrounds the bony fragment) and their edges are usually **smooth.**
- In the case of sesamoids and accessory ossicles, they are **usually bilaterally symmetrical** so that a view of the opposite extremity will usually demonstrate the same bone in the same location.
  - They **occur at anatomically predictable sites.**
    - There are almost always sesamoids present in the thumb, the posterolateral aspect of the knee (*fabella*), and the great toe (Fig. 22-4B).

- Accessory ossicles are most common in the foot (Fig. 22-4C).

Recognizing Dislocations and Subluxations

- In a **dislocation,** the bones that originally formed the two components of a joint are no longer in apposition to each other (Fig. 22-5A).
  - Dislocations occur only at joints.
- In a **subluxation,** the bones that originally formed the two components of a joint are in **partial contact** with each other.
  - Subluxations occur only at joints (Fig. 22-5B).
- Some characteristics of dislocations of the shoulder and hip are shown in Table 22-2.

Describing Fractures

- There is a common lexicon used in describing fractures to facilitate a reproducible description and to assure reliable and accurate communication.
- **Fractures are described** (Table 22-3)
  - By the **number of fragments**
  - By the **direction of the fracture line**
  - By the **relationship of the fragments** to each other
  - By **communication of the fracture with the outside**
- **Describing fractures by the number of fracture fragments**
  - **Two** fragments—**simple**
  - **More than two** fragments—**comminuted**

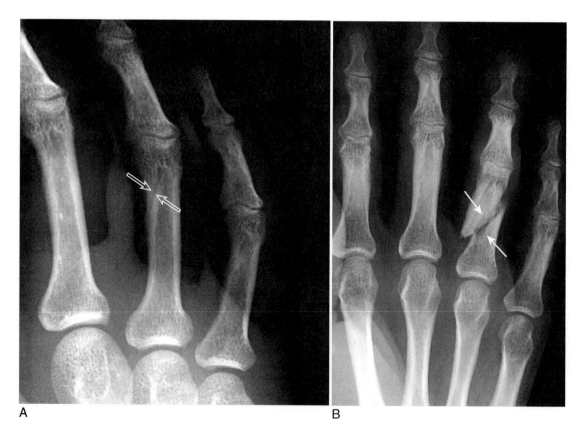

A   B

*Figure 22-2. **Nutrient canal versus fracture.** Fracture lines, when viewed in the correct orientation, tend to be "blacker" (more lucent) than other lines normally found in bones, such as nutrient canals. Compare a nutrient canal **(A)** (open white arrows) to a true fracture seen in another patient **(B)** (closed white arrows). Notice how the nutrient canal has a sclerotic (whiter) margin, which is not the case with fracture lines. The edges of a fracture tend to be jagged and rough.*

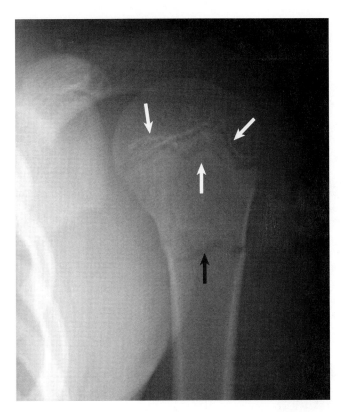

Figure 22-3. **Fracture versus epiphyseal plate.** *Fracture lines (closed black arrow)* tend to be straighter in their course and more acute in their angulation than any naturally occurring lines, such as the epiphyseal plate in the proximal humerus. Because the top of the metaphysis has irregular hills and valleys, the epiphyseal plate has an undulating course that will allow you to see it in tangent on both the anterior and posterior margins of the humeral head *(closed white arrows)*. This may give the mistaken impression that there is a fracture present.

Table 22-1

DIFFERENTIATING FRACTURES, OSSICLES, AND SESAMOIDS		
Finding	**Acute Fracture**	**Sesamoids and Accessory Ossicles**
Abrupt disruption of cortex	Yes	No
Bilaterally symmetrical	Almost never	Almost always*
"Fracture line"	Unsharp, jagged	Smooth
Bony fragment has a cortex completely around it	No	Yes

*Old, unhealed fractures will not be bilaterally symmetrical.

- **Segmental fracture**—a comminuted fracture in which a portion of the shaft exists as an isolated fragment (Fig. 22-6A).
- **Butterfly fragment**—a comminuted fracture in which the central fragment has a triangular shape (Fig. 22-6B).
- **Describing fractures by the direction of the fracture line** (Table 22-4)
  - **Transverse**—the fracture line is perpendicular to the long axis of the bone.
    - Transverse fractures are caused by a force directed perpendicular to shaft (Fig. 22-7A).
  - **Diagonal or oblique**—the fracture line is diagonal in orientation relative to the normal axis of the bone.
    - Diagonal or oblique fractures are caused by a force usually applied in the same direction as the long axis of the bone (Fig. 22-7B).
  - **Spiral**—a twisting fracture caused by a torque injury, such as might be caused by planting the foot in a hole while running.
    - Spiral fractures are often associated with soft tissue injuries such as tears in ligaments or tendons (Fig. 22-7C).
- **Describing fractures by the relationship of one fracture fragment to another**
  - By convention, abnormalities of the position of bone fragments secondary to fractures describe **the relationship of the distal fracture fragment relative to the proximal fragment.**
    - These descriptions are based on the position the distal fragment would have normally assumed had the bone not been fractured.
  - Four parameters are most commonly used to describe the relationship of the fracture fragments:
    - **Displacement**
    - **Angulation**
    - **Shortening**
    - **Rotation**
  - Many fractures display more than one of these abnormalities of position.
- **Displacement**
  - Describes **the amount by which the distal fragment is offset,** front-to-back and side-to-side, from the proximal fragment
  - Most often described in terms of either *percent* (*the distal fragment is displaced by 50% of the width of the shaft*) or *fractions* (*the distal fragment is displaced half the width of the shaft of the proximal fragment*) (Fig. 22-8A).
- **Angulation**
  - Describes **the angle between the distal and proximal fragments** as a function of the degree to which the distal fragment is deviated from its normal position
  - Described in degrees and by position (*the distal fragment is angulated 15° anteriorly relative to the proximal fragment*) (Fig. 22-8B)

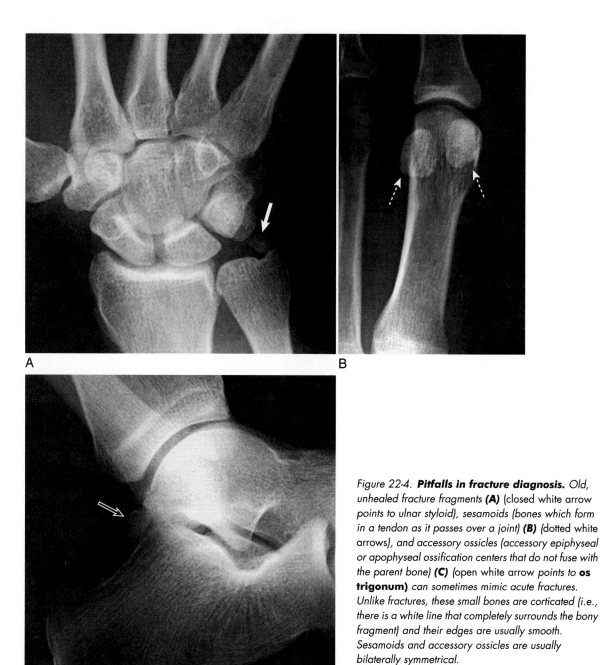

Figure 22-4. **Pitfalls in fracture diagnosis.** *Old, unhealed fracture fragments **(A)** (closed white arrow points to ulnar styloid), sesamoids (bones which form in a tendon as it passes over a joint) **(B)** (dotted white arrows), and accessory ossicles (accessory epiphyseal or apophyseal ossification centers that do not fuse with the parent bone) **(C)** (open white arrow points to **os trigonum**) can sometimes mimic acute fractures. Unlike fractures, these small bones are corticated (i.e., there is a white line that completely surrounds the bony fragment) and their edges are usually smooth. Sesamoids and accessory ossicles are usually bilaterally symmetrical.*

- **Shortening**
  - Describes **how much, if any, overlap there is of the ends of the fracture fragments,** which translates into how much shorter the fractured bone is than it would be had it not been fractured
    - The opposite term from shortening is *distraction* which refers to **the distance the bone fragments are separated from each other.**

- Shortening (overlap) and distraction (lengthening) are usually described in centimeters (*there are 2 cm of shortening of the fracture fragments*) (Fig. 22-8C and D).
- **Rotation**
  - An unusual abnormality in fracture positioning almost always involving the long bones, such as the femur or humerus, which describes the orientation of the joint at one end of the fractured bone relative

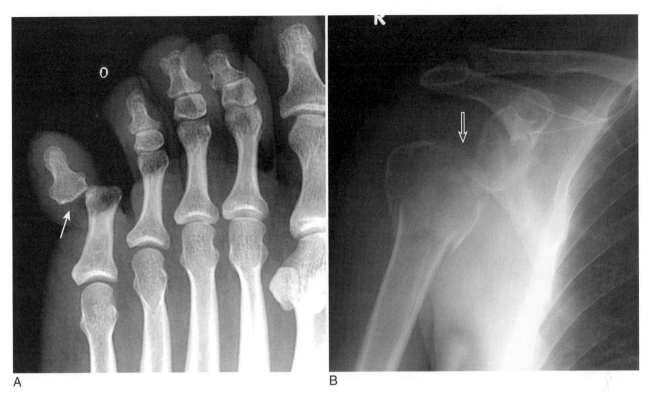

A   B

Figure 22-5. **Dislocation and subluxation.** *In a dislocation **(A)**, the bones that originally formed the two components of a joint are no longer in apposition to each other (closed white arrow). In a subluxation **(B)**, the bones that originally formed the two components of a joint are in partial contact with each other (open white arrow). In **A**, the terminal phalanx is dislocated lateral to the middle phalanx. In **B**, the humeral head is subluxed inferiorly in the glenoid because of large a hematoma in the joint from a fracture of the surgical neck of the humerus.*

to the orientation of the joint at the other end of the same bone
- Normally, for example, when the hip joint is oriented with the leg pointing forward, the knee joint is also oriented with the leg pointing forward.
  - If there is **rotation** about a fracture of the femoral shaft, the hip joint and the knee joint would no longer be oriented in the same plane (Fig. 22-9).

- To appreciate rotation, both the joint above and the joint below a fracture must be visualized, preferably on the same radiograph.
- **Describing fractures by the relationship of the fracture to the atmosphere.**
  - **Closed**—the more common type of fracture in which there is **no communication** between the fracture fragments and the outside atmosphere.

Table 22-2

DISLOCATIONS OF THE SHOULDER AND HIP

Features	Shoulder	Hip
Locations	Anterior, subcoracoid more common	Posterior and superior more common
Cause	Combination of abduction, external rotation, and extension	Frequently caused by knee striking dashboard, transmits force to hip
Associated fractures	Associated with fractures of humeral head (Hill-Sachs) and glenoid (Bankart's)	Associated with fractures of posterior rim of the acetabulum

Table 22-3

HOW FRACTURES ARE DESCRIBED

Parameter	Terms Used
Number of fracture fragments	Simple or comminuted
Direction of fracture line	Transverse, oblique, spiral
Relationship of one fragment to another	Displacement, angulation, shortening, and rotation
Open to the atmosphere (outside)	Closed or open (compound)

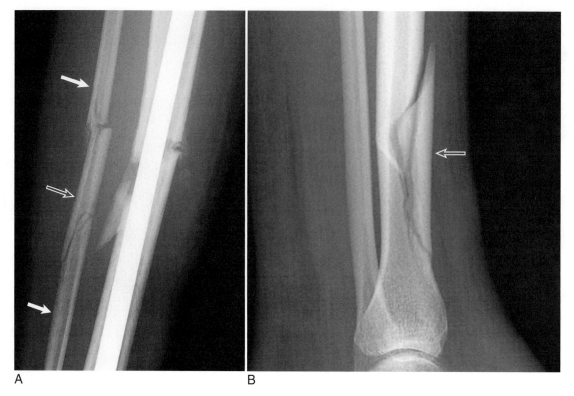

Figure 22-6. **Segmental fractures.** *Two comminuted fractures are shown.* **A,** *This segmental fracture is a comminuted fracture in which a portion of the shaft exists as an isolated fragment. Notice how the fibula has a center section now (open white arrow) and two additional fragments, one on either side (closed white arrows). A butterfly fragment* **(B)** *is a comminuted fracture in which the central fragment has a triangular shape (open white arrow) resembling a butterfly.*

- **Open or compound**—there is **communication between the fracture and the outside** atmosphere (Fig. 22-10).
  - This is best evaluated clinically.
  - Compound fractures have implications regarding the way in which they are treated in order to avoid the complication of osteomyelitis.

Table 22-4

DIRECTION OF FRACTURE LINE AND MECHANISM OF INJURY	
Direction of Fracture Line	**Mechanism**
Transverse	Force applied perpendicular to long axis of bone; fracture occurs at site of force
Diagonal (also known as oblique)	Force applied along the long axis of bone; fracture occurs somewhere along shaft
Spiral	Twisting or torque injury

Avulsion Fractures

- A **common mechanism of fracture production** in which the fracture fragment (*avulsed fragment*) is pulled from its parent bone by contraction of a tendon or ligament.
- Although avulsion fractures can and do occur at any age, they are **particularly common in younger individuals** engaging in athletic endeavors; in fact, they derive many of their names from the type of athletic activity that produces them, e.g., *dancer's fracture, skier's fracture, sprinter's fracture* (Fig. 22-11).
- They **occur in anatomically predictable locations** (tendons insert on bones in a known location) and they are **typically small fragments** (Table 22-5).
- They sometimes **heal with such exuberant callus formation** that they can be mistaken for a bone tumor (Fig. 22-12).

Salter-Harris Fractures: Epiphyseal Plate Fractures in Children

- In growing bone, the hypertrophic zone in the *growth plate* (*epiphyseal plate* or *physis*) is most vulnerable to shearing injuries.
- Epiphyseal plate fractures are common and **account for as many as 30% of childhood fractures.**
  - By definition, because these are all fractures through an open epiphyseal plate, they **can occur only in children.**

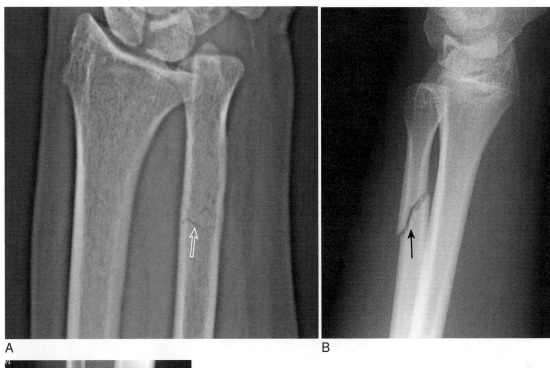

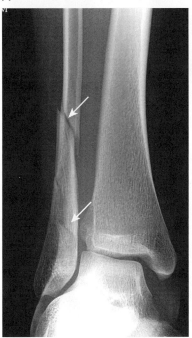

Figure 22-7. **Transverse, diagonal, and spiral fracture lines. A,** *In a transverse fracture (open white arrow), the fracture line is perpendicular to the long axis of the bone.* **B,** *Diagonal or oblique fractures (closed black arrow) are diagonal in orientation relative to the normal axis of the bone.* **C,** *Spiral fractures (closed white arrows) are usually caused by twisting or torque injuries.*

- The **Salter-Harris classification of epiphyseal plate injuries** is a commonly used method of describing such injuries that helps identify the type of treatment required and recognizes the likelihood of complications based on the type of fracture (Fig. 22-13 and Table 22-6).
  - Types I and II heal well.
  - Type III can develop arthritic changes or asymmetrical growth plate fusion.
  - Types IV and V are more likely to develop early fusion of the growth plate with angular deformities and shortening of that bone.

- Type I—fractures of the epiphyseal plate alone
  - Often **difficult to detect without the opposite side for comparison,** these fractures have a **favorable prognosis.**
  - *Slipped capital femoral epiphysis (SCFE)* is a manifestation of a Salter-Harris type I injury.
    - Slipped capital femoral epiphysis **occurs most often in taller and heavier teenage boys** and involves the inferior, medial, and posterior slippage of the proximal femoral epiphysis relative to the neck of the femur (Fig. 22-14).
  - It is **bilateral in about 25% of cases.**

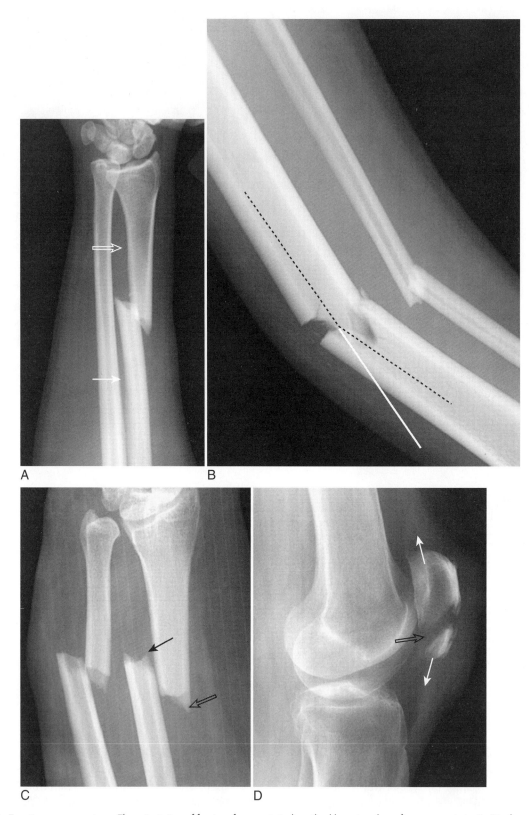

Figure 22-8. **Fracture parameters.** *The orientation of fracture fragments is described by using these four parameters.* **A,** *Displacement describes the amount by which the distal fragment (open white arrow) is offset, front-to-back and side-to-side, from the proximal fragment (closed white arrow).* **B,** *Angulation describes the angle between the distal and proximal fragments (dotted black line) as a function of the degree to which the distal fragment is deviated from its normal position (white line).* **C,** *Shortening describes how much, if any, overlap there is of the ends of the fracture fragments (open and closed black arrows). The opposite term from shortening is distraction* **(D),** *which refers to the distance the bone fragments are separated from each other (two white arrows show pull of tendons on fracture fragments of patella; open black arrow points to distraction of fracture).*

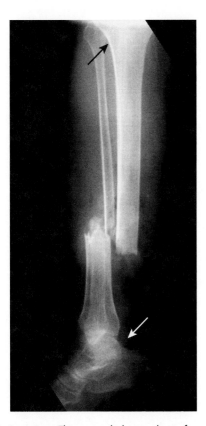

Figure 22-9. **Rotation.** *This unusual abnormality in fracture positioning almost always involves the long bones; rotation describes the orientation of the joint at one end of the fractured bone relative to the orientation of the joint at the other end of the fractured bone. To appreciate rotation, both the joint above and the joint below a fracture must be visualized, preferably on the same radiograph. In this patient, the proximal tibia (closed black arrow) is oriented in the frontal plane while the distal tibia and ankle (closed white arrow) are oriented laterally. The foot is rotated 90° to the plane of the knee.*

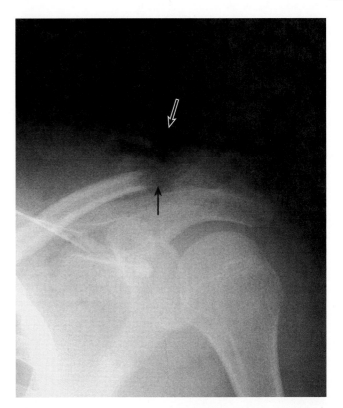

Figure 22-10. **Open (compound) fracture.** *Most fractures are closed, in which there is no communication between the fracture fragments and the outside atmosphere. Open or compound fractures have communication between the fracture (closed black arrow) and the outside atmosphere (open white arrow points to air entering through a wound above the fractured clavicle). Whether a fracture is open or not is best evaluated clinically. Compound fractures have implications for treatment in order to avoid the complication of osteomyelitis*

- It can result in **avascular necrosis** of the slipped femoral head because of interruption of the blood supply **in up to 15% of cases.**
- **Type II—fracture of the epiphyseal plate and fracture of the metaphysis**
  - **Most common type of Salter-Harris fracture (75%),** often involving the distal radius.
  - The small metaphyseal fracture fragment produces the so-called *corner sign* (Fig. 22-15).
- **Type III—fracture of the epiphyseal plate and the epiphysis**
  - There is a **longitudinal fracture through the epiphysis itself,** which means the fracture invariably enters the joint space and fractures the articular cartilage.
  - This can have long-term implications for the development of **secondary osteoarthritis** (see Chapter 24) and can result in **asymmetrical and premature fusion of the growth plate** with subsequent deformity of the bone (Fig. 22-16).
- **Type IV—fracture of the epiphyseal plate, metaphysis and epiphysis**

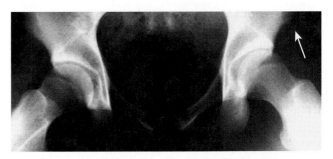

Figure 22-11. **Avulsion fracture, ASIS.** *Avulsion fractures are common fractures in which the fracture fragment (avulsed fragment) is pulled from its parent bone by contraction of a tendon or ligament. Although avulsion fractures can occur at any age, they are particularly common in younger individuals who engage in athletic endeavors. In this 9-year-old, there is an avulsion of the anterior superior iliac spine (ASIS) (closed white arrow), which is the site of the insertion of the sartorius muscle, forcefully contracted when this patient tried to jump over a hurdle in a race.*

Table 22-5

AVULSION FRACTURES AROUND THE PELVIS

Avulsed Fragment	Muscle that Inserts on Avulsed Fragment
Anterior, superior iliac spine	Sartorius muscle
Anterior, inferior iliac spine	Rectus femoris muscle
Ischial tuberosity	Hamstring muscles
Lesser trochanter of femur	Iliopsoas muscle

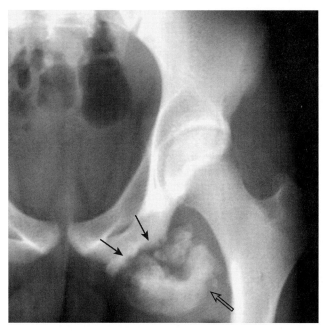

*Figure 22-12. **Healing avulsion fracture of ischial tuberosity.** Avulsion fractures of the pelvis occur in anatomically predictable locations (tendons insert on bones in known locations) and they are typically small fragments. Sometimes they heal with such exuberant callus formation that they can be mistaken for a bone tumor. In this healing fracture (closed black arrows) of the ischial tuberosity caused by contraction of the hamstring muscles there is a great deal of external callus present (open black arrow).*

- This type has a **poorer prognosis** than other Salter-Harris fractures; premature and possibly asymmetrical closure of the epiphyseal plate, especially in bones of the lower extremity, may lead to differences in leg length, angular deformities, and secondary osteoarthritis (Fig. 22-17).
- **Type V—crush fracture of epiphyseal plate**
  - **Rare,** crush-type injury of the epiphyseal plate **produces associated vascular injury** and almost always **results in**

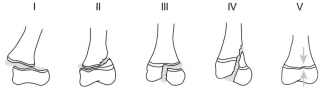

*Figure 22-13. **Salter-Harris classification of epiphyseal plate fractures.** The Salter-Harris classification helps to recognize the likelihood of complications based on the type of fracture. All these fractures involve the epiphyseal plate (growth plate). Type I fractures are of the epiphyseal plate alone. Type II fractures, the most common of the epiphyseal plate fractures, involve the epiphyseal plate and metaphysis. These first two types have a favorable prognosis. Type III fractures involve the epiphyseal plate and the epiphysis and have a less favorable prognosis. Type IV fracture involves the epiphyseal plate, epiphysis, and metaphysis. It has an even less favorable prognosis. Type V is a crush injury of the epiphyseal plate. It has the worst prognosis. (From The Johns Hopkins Hospital:* The Harriet Lane Handbook, *17th ed. Philadelphia, Mosby, 2005.)*

Table 22-6

SALTER-HARRIS CLASSIFICATION OF EPIPHYSEAL PLATE FRACTURES

Type	Fracture Site	Remarks
I	Epiphyseal plate	Seen in phalanges, distal radius, SCFE; good prognosis
II	Epiphyseal plate and metaphysis	Most common of all Salter-Harris fractures; frequently distal radius; corner sign; good prognosis
III	Epiphyseal plate and epiphysis	Intra-articular fracture; especially distal tibia; less favorable prognosis
IV	Epiphyseal plate, epiphysis and metaphysis	Seen in distal humerus and distal tibia; poor prognosis
V	Crush injury of epiphyseal plate	Worst prognosis; difficult to diagnose until healing begins

growth impairment through early focal fusion of the growth plate.
- **Most common in distal femur,** proximal tibia and distal tibia, it is **difficult to diagnose on conventional radiographs,** even with the opposite side for comparison, until later in its course when complications ensue (Fig. 22-18).
- CT with multiplanar reconstruction and MRI may be helpful in treatment planning, but conventional radiography remains the method of choice for initial diagnosis in most cases of epiphyseal fractures.

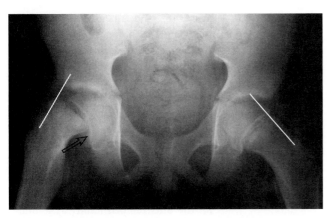

Figure 22-14. **Slipped capital femoral epiphysis.** *Slipped capital femoral epiphysis (SCFE) is a manifestation of a Salter-Harris type I injury. It occurs more often in taller or heavier teenage boys and produces inferior, medial, and posterior slippage of the proximal femoral epiphysis relative to the neck of the femur (open black arrow). A line drawn parallel to the neck of the femur (white lines) should intersect a portion of the head. It does on the normal left side, but does not on the right side because the epiphysis has slipped.*

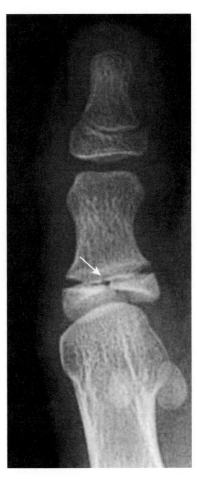

Figure 22-16. **Salter-Harris III fracture.** *With type III fractures, there is a fracture of the epiphyseal plate as well as a longitudinal fracture through the epiphysis itself (closed white arrow), which means the fracture invariably enters the joint space and fractures the articular cartilage. This can have long-term implications for the development of secondary osteoarthritis and can result in asymmetrical and premature fusion of the growth plate with subsequent deformity of the bone. This type of fracture most commonly occurs in the distal tibia.*

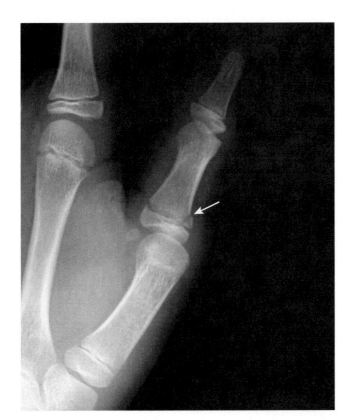

Figure 22-15. **Salter-Harris II fracture.** *In type II fractures, there is a fracture of the epiphyseal plate and a fracture of the metaphysis. This is the most common type of Salter-Harris fracture. The small metaphyseal fracture fragment (closed white arrow) produces the so-called* **corner sign.**

Stress Fractures

- Stress fractures **occur as a result of numerous microfractures** in which bone is subjected to repeated stretching and compressive forces.
- Although **conventional radiographs should be the study of first choice,** they may **initially appear normal in as many as 85% of cases,** so it is common for a patient to complain of pain yet have a normal-appearing radiograph.
- The **fracture may not be diagnosable** until after periosteal new bone formation occurs or, in the case of a healing stress fracture of cancellous bone, **the appearance of a thin, dense zone of sclerosis across the medullary cavity** (Fig. 22-19).
- Radionuclide **bone scan will usually be positive much earlier** than conventional radiographs: **within 6 to 72 hours after the injury.**

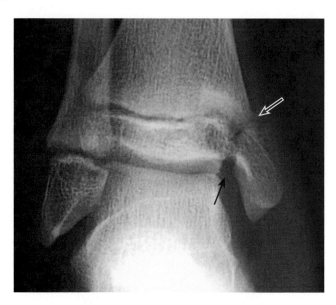

Figure 22-17. **Salter-Harris IV fracture.** *In type IV fractures, there is a fracture of the epiphyseal plate, metaphysis (open white arrow), and the epiphysis (closed black arrow). These fractures have a poorer prognosis than other Salter-Harris fractures because of increased likelihood of premature and possibly asymmetrical closure of the epiphyseal plate. Salter-Harris IV fractures are most often seen in the distal humerus and distal tibia.*

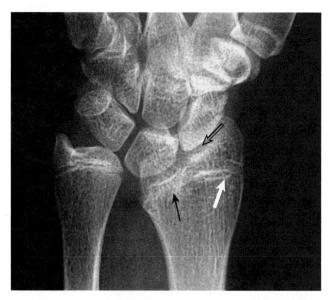

Figure 22-18. **Salter-Harris V fracture.** *Type V fractures are crush fractures of the epiphyseal plate. They are frequently not diagnosed until after they produce their growth impairment through early focal fusion of the growth plate leading to angular deformity. In this child, the medial portion of the distal radial epiphyseal plate has fused (closed black arrow) while the lateral portion remains open (closed white arrow). This premature fusion of the medial growth plate has resulted in an angular deformity of the distal radius (open black arrow).*

- Some **common locations for stress fractures** are the **shafts of long bones** such as the proximal femur or proximal tibia, as well as the calcaneus and the second and third metatarsals (***march fractures***).

Common Fracture Eponyms

- There are almost as many fracture eponyms as there are types of fractures.
- We will concentrate on five of the most commonly used eponyms.
- **Colles fracture**
  - A Colles fracture is a **fracture of the distal radius** with dorsal angulation of the distal radial fracture fragment caused by a **fall on the outstretched hand** (sometimes abbreviated as ***FOOSH***).
    - There is frequently an associated fracture of the ulnar styloid (Fig. 22-20).
- **Smith fracture** is a fracture of the distal radius with palmar angulation of the distal radial fracture fragment (a reverse Colles fracture).
  - It is caused by a fall on the back of the flexed hand (Fig. 22-21).
- **Jones fracture** is a transverse, avulsion fracture of the base fifth metatarsal at the insertion of the peroneus brevis tendon.
  - It is caused by plantar flexion of the foot and inversion of the ankle, a combination frequently caused by missing a step at a curb (Fig. 22-22).
- **Boxer's fracture** is a fracture of the head of the fifth metacarpal (little finger) with palmar angulation of the distal fracture fragment.
  - It is most often the result of punching a person or wall (Fig. 22-23).
- **March fracture** is a type of ***stress fracture*** caused by repeated microfractures to the foot from trauma (such as marching), affecting the **shafts of the second and third metatarsals** especially.
  - The **fracture line is frequently *invisible*** when the patient first begins to complain of foot pain, with the sensitivity of conventional radiographs as low as 15%.
  - Radionuclide **bone scan will usually be positive within 6 to 72 hours after the injury.**
  - Fracture may only become evident when **periosteal new bone** (secondary union) begins to appear in about 10 to 14 days (see Fig. 22-19).

Some Easily Missed Fractures or Dislocations

- Look at these areas carefully when evaluating for a possible fracture; then look a second and third time.
- **Scaphoid fractures (common)**
  - Clinically suspected if there is tenderness in the ***anatomic snuff box*** after fall on outstretched hand
  - Look for **hairline-thin radiolucencies** on special angled views of the scaphoid (Fig. 22-24).
  - Fractures across the waist of the navicular can lead to avascular necrosis of proximal pole of that bone.
- **Buckle fractures of radius or ulna in children (common)**
  - Common fractures in children

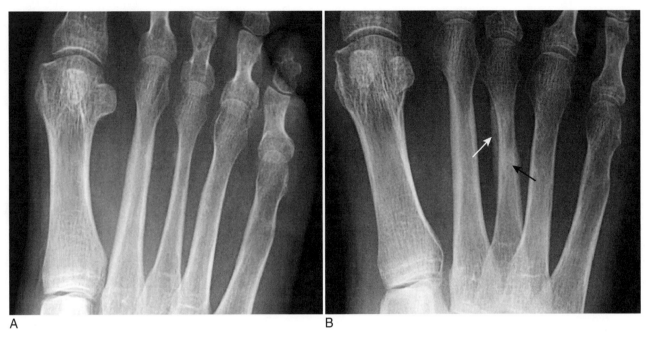

A   B

Figure 22-19. **Stress fracture.** *These two frontal views were taken 5 weeks apart. Although conventional radiographs should be the study of first choice, they may initially appear normal* **(A)** *in as many as 85% of cases, so it is common for a patient to complain of pain yet have a normal-appearing radiograph. Radionuclide bone scan will usually be positive much earlier than conventional radiographs: within 6 to 72 hours after the injury.* **B,** *The fracture may not be diagnosable until after periosteal new bone formation occurs (closed white arrow) or, in the case of a healing stress fracture of cancellous bone, the appearance of a thin, dense zone of sclerosis across the medullary cavity (closed black arrow).*

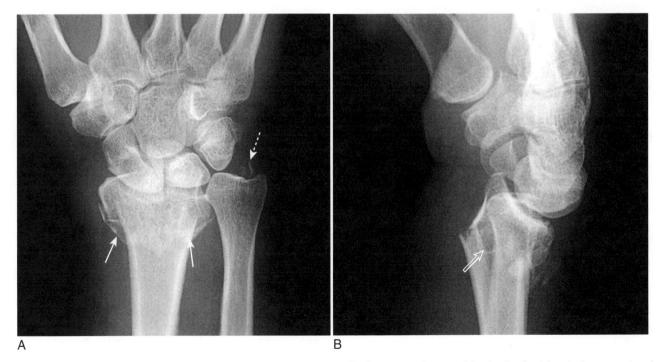

A   B

Figure 22-20. **Colles fracture, frontal (A) and lateral (B) views.** *A Colles fracture is a fracture of the distal radius (closed white arrows) with dorsal angulation of the distal radial fracture fragment (open white arrow) caused by a fall on the outstretched hand (sometimes abbreviated as FOOSH). There is frequently an associated fracture of the ulnar styloid (dotted white arrow).*

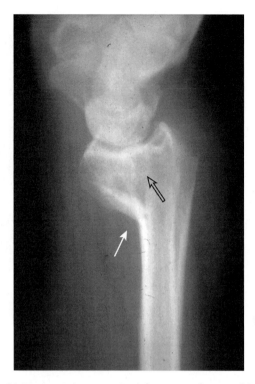

Figure 22-21. **Smith fracture.** Smith fracture is a fracture of the distal radius (closed white arrow) with palmar angulation of the distal radial fracture fragment (open black arrow), the reverse of a Colles fracture. It is caused by a fall on the back of the flexed hand.

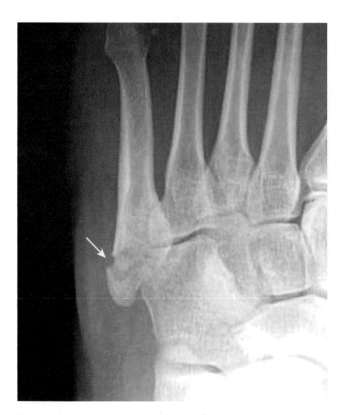

Figure 22-22. **Jones fracture.** A Jones fracture is a transverse, avulsion fracture of the base fifth metatarsal at the insertion of the peroneus brevis tendon (closed white arrow). It is caused by plantar flexion of the foot and inversion of the ankle.

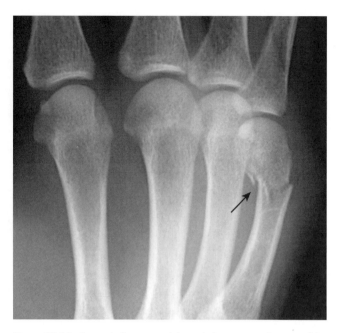

Figure 22-23. **Boxer's fracture.** A boxer's fracture is a fracture of the head of the fifth metacarpal (little finger) with palmar angulation of the distal fracture fragment (closed black arrow). It is most often the result of punching a person (or a wall).

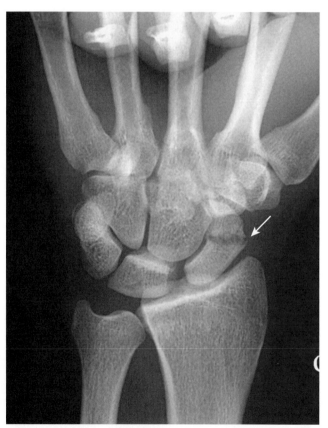

Figure 22-24. **Scaphoid fracture.** Scaphoid fractures are common. They are suspected clinically if there is tenderness in the anatomic snuff box after a fall on an outstretched hand. Look for hairline-thin radiolucencies on special angled views of the scaphoid (closed white arrow). Fractures across the waist of the scaphoid can lead to avascular necrosis of proximal pole of that bone (see Fig. 21-7).

- Look for **acute and sudden angulation of the cortex**, especially near the wrist (see Fig. 22-1B).
- Impacted fractures heal quickly.
- **Radial head fracture (common)**
  - **Most common fracture of the elbow in an adult**
  - Look for fat appearing as a crescentic lucency along the dorsal aspect of the distal humerus caused by intracapsular, extrasynovial fat that is lifted away from the bone by swelling of the joint capsule due to a traumatic hemarthrosis—the *positive posterior fat-pad sign* (Fig. 22-25).
- **Supracondylar fracture of the distal humerus in children (common)**
  - **Most common fracture of the elbow in a child**
  - Most of these fractures produce **posterior displacement** of the distal humerus.
  - On a true lateral film, the **anterior humeral line** (a line drawn tangential to the anterior humeral cortex) **should bisect the middle third of the ossification center of capitellum** (Fig. 22-26).
  - **With a supracondylar fracture this line passes anterior to its normal location**
- **Posterior dislocation of the shoulder (uncommon)**
  - Humeral head looks like "lightbulb" in all views of the shoulder.
  - Look at a view like the axillary or Y view to see if head still lies within glenoid fossa (Fig. 22-27).
    - On the Y view, the head will lie lateral to the glenoid when posteriorly dislocated.

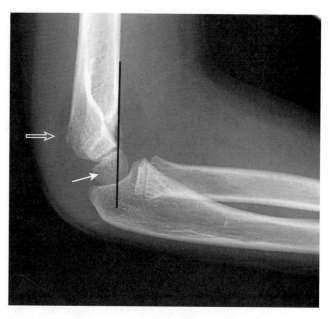

Figure 22-26. *Supracondylar fracture.* *A supracondylar fracture of the distal humerus is a common fracture in children and its findings may be subtle. Most of these fractures produce posterior displacement of the distal humerus. On a true lateral film, the **anterior humeral line** (a line drawn tangential to the anterior humeral cortex and shown here in black) should bisect the **middle** portion of the capitellum (closed white arrow). With a supracondylar fracture, this line will pass more **anteriorly,** as it does here. There is a positive posterior fat-pad sign present (open white arrow).*

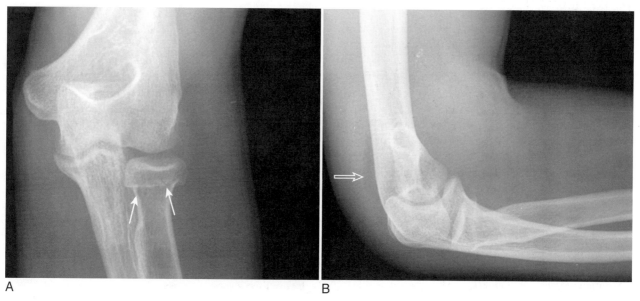

A   B

Figure 22-25. *Fracture of radial head with joint effusion, frontal (A) and lateral (B) views.* *Radial head fractures (closed white arrows) are the most common fractures of the elbow in an adult. Look for fat appearing as a crescentic lucency along the dorsal aspect of the distal humerus (open white arrow) caused by intracapsular, extrasynovial fat that is lifted away from the bone by swelling of the joint capsule due to a traumatic hemarthrosis—the **positive posterior fat-pad sign.** Virtually all studies of bones will include at least two views at 90° angles to each other, called **orthogonal views.** Many protocols call for two additional oblique views, which enable you to visualize more of the cortex in profile.*

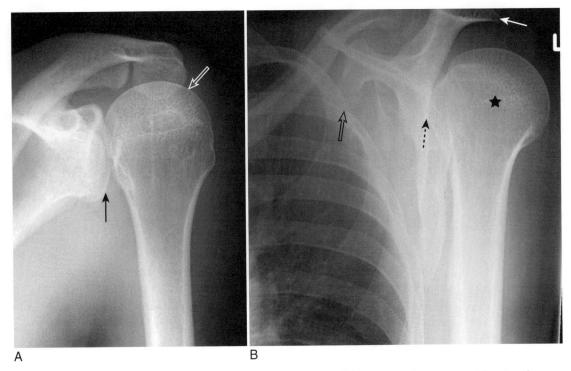

A   B

Figure 22-27. **Posterior dislocation.** *Posterior dislocations of the shoulder are much less common than anterior dislocations but more difficult to diagnose. On the frontal view (A), look for the humeral head to be persistently fixed in internal rotation and resemble a "lightbulb" (open white arrow) no matter how the patient turns the forearm. There is also an increased distance between the head and the glenoid (closed black arrow). On the Y view (B), the head (black star) will lie under the acromion (closed white arrow), a posterior structure of the scapula. Normally, the head is centered between the coracoid (open black arrow) and the acromion in the glenoid fossa (dotted black arrow).*

- **Hip fractures in the elderly (common)**
  - Common and frequently related to osteoporosis
  - Look for **angulation of the cortex,** zones of **increased density indicating impaction** (Fig. 22-28).
  - Conventional radiographs of the femoral neck should be obtained with the patient's leg in internal rotation so as to display the neck in profile.
  - May be very subtle and require bone scan or MRI for diagnosis
- **Rib fractures**
  - Rib fractures are **important only for the complications they might produce** or the clues they might provide to unsuspected pathology (Fig. 22-29).
  - Fractures of the **first three ribs** are relatively uncommon and, if they occur following blunt trauma, **indicate a considerable amount of force** that could have produced other internal injuries.
  - Fractures of **ribs 4 through 9 are common** and important if they are displaced (pneumothorax) or if there are anterior and posterior fractures of three or more contiguous ribs *(flail chest).*
  - Fractures of **ribs 10 through 12** may indicate the presence of **underlying trauma** to the **liver** (on the right) or the **spleen** (on the left).
  - It is **not unusual for rib fractures to be undetectable on the initial examination** but to become visible in time after callus begins to form.
- **Look for indirect signs indicating the possibility of an underlying fracture** (Table 22-7 and Fig. 22-30).

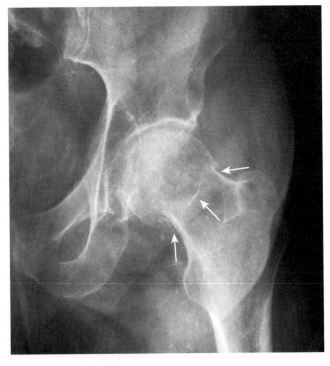

Figure 22-28. **Impacted subcapital hip fracture.** *Hip fractures are relatively common fractures in the elderly and are frequently related to osteoporosis. Look for angulation of the cortex and zones of increased density (closed white arrows) indicating impaction. Conventional radiographs of the femoral neck should be obtained with the patient's leg in internal rotation (as shown here) so as to display the neck in profile. Hip fractures can be very subtle and sometimes require additional imaging such as bone scan or MRI for their diagnosis.*

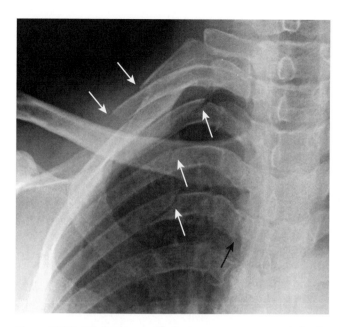

Figure 22-29. **Rib fractures.** *Rib fractures are important only for the complications they might produce or the unsuspected pathology they might herald. Fractures of the first three ribs (closed white arrows) are relatively uncommon and, following blunt trauma, their presence is a clue that the force to the chest was considerable and might have produced other internal injuries. Don't mistake the normal costovertebral junction (closed black arrow) for a fracture.*

Table 22-7

INDIRECT SIGNS OF FRACTURE

Sign	Remarks
Soft tissue swelling	Frequently accompanies a fracture but does not necessarily mean that a fracture is present
Disappearance of normal fat stripes	One of the most consistent is the **pronator quadratus fat stripe** on the volar aspect of the wrist; it may become displaced with a fracture of the distal radius (see Fig. 22-30)
Joint effusion	The most "famous" is the **positive posterior fat pad sign** seen on the dorsal aspect of the distal humerus from a traumatic joint effusion (see Fig. 22-25B)
Periosteal reaction	Sometimes the healing of a fracture will be the first manifestation that a fracture was present, especially with march fractures of the foot (see Fig. 22-19B)

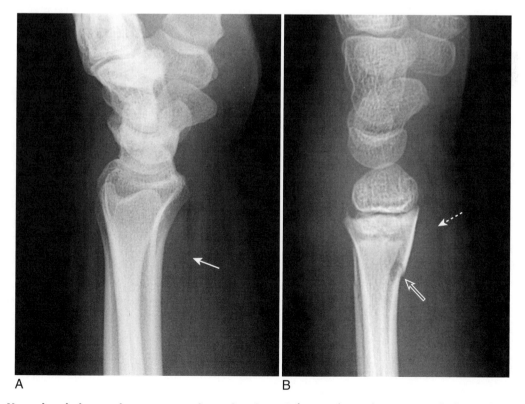

A   B

Figure 22-30. **Normal and abnormal pronator quadratus fat plane.** *Soft tissue abnormalities can provide clues to the presence of subtle fractures or help confirm the significance of a questionable finding. Compare this normal fascial plane (**A**) produced by the pronator quadratus (closed white arrow) on the volar aspect of the wrist to a bulging fascial plane (**B**) (dotted white arrow) that has occurred because of soft tissue swelling accompanying a fracture of the distal radius (open white arrow).*

Fracture Healing

- Fracture healing is determined by many factors including the age of the patient, the fracture site, the position of the fracture fragments, the degree of immobilization, and the blood supply to the fracture site (Table 22-8).
- Immediately following a fracture, there is hemorrhage into the fracture site.
- Over the next several weeks, osteoclasts act to remove the diseased bone.
  - The **fracture line may actually minimally widen** at this time.
- Over the next several weeks, **new bone (*callus*) begins to** bridge the fracture gap (Fig. 22-31).
  - **Internal endosteal healing** is manifest by **indistinctness of the fracture line** leading to obliteration of the fracture line.
  - **External, periosteal healing** is manifest by external callus formation eventually leading to **bridging of the fracture site.**
- **Remodeling** of bone **begins at about 8 to 12 weeks** after fracture as mechanical forces, in part, begin to adjust the bone to its original shape.
  - In **children, this occurs much more rapidly** and usually produces a bone that appears normal.
  - In **adults, this process may take years** and the healed fracture may never assume a completely normal shape.
- **Complications of the healing process**
  - **Delayed union—fracture does not heal in the expected period** for a fracture at that particular site (e.g., 6–8 weeks for a fracture of the shaft of the radius).
    - **Most cases of delayed union will eventually progress to complete healing** with further immobilization.
  - **Malunion**—healing of the fracture fragments occurs in a **mechanically or cosmetically unacceptable position.**
  - **Nonunion**—**fracture healing will never occur.**

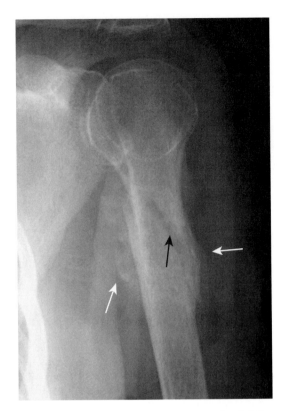

*Figure 22-31. **Healing humeral fracture.** Immediately following a fracture, there is hemorrhage into the fracture site. Over the next several weeks, new bone (callus) begins to bridge the fracture gap. Internal endosteal healing is manifest by indistinctness of the fracture line (closed black arrow) eventually leading to obliteration of the fracture line. External, periosteal healing is manifest by external callus formation (closed white arrows), leading to bridging of the fracture site.*

Table 22-8

FACTORS AFFECTING FRACTURE HEALING	
Factors that Accelerate Fracture Healing	**Factors that Delay Fracture Healing**
Youth	Old age
Early immobilization	Delayed immobilization
Adequate duration of immobilization	Too short a duration of immobilization
Good blood supply	Poor blood supply
Physical activity after adequate immobilization	Steroids
Adequate mineralization	Osteoporosis, osteomalacia

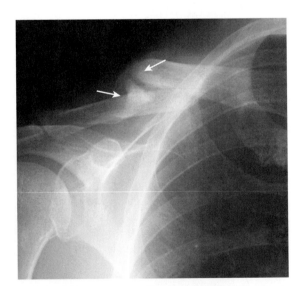

*Figure 22-32. **Nonunion of clavicular fracture.** Nonunion is a radiologic diagnosis that implies fracture healing is not likely to occur as the processes leading to the repair of bone have ceased. It is characterized by smooth and sclerotic fracture margins with distraction of the fracture fragments (closed white arrows). A **pseudarthrosis,** complete with a synovial lining, may form at the fracture site.*

- Characterized by **smooth and sclerotic fracture margins** with **distraction of the fracture fragments** (Fig. 22-32)
- **Motion at the fracture site** may be demonstrated under fluoroscopic manipulation or on stress views.
- A *pseudarthrosis,* complete with a synovial lining, may form at the fracture site.

WebLink
More information on recognizing fractures and dislocations is available to registered users on StudentConsult.com.

 TAKE-HOME POINTS: Recognizing Fractures and Dislocations

A **fracture** is described as a disruption in the continuity of all or part of the cortex of a bone.

Complete fractures involve the entire cortex, are more common, and typically occur in adults; **incomplete fractures** involve only a part of the cortex and typically occur in bones that are softer, such as those of children; **torus** and **greenstick fractures** are incomplete fractures.

Fracture lines tend to be blacker, more sharply angled, and more jagged than other lucencies in bones (e.g., nutrient canals or epiphyseal plates).

Sesamoids, accessory ossicles, and unhealed fractures may mimic acute fractures but all will have smooth and corticated margins, hallmarks of a "nonfracture".

Dislocation is present when two bones that originally formed a joint are no longer in contact with each other; **subluxation** is present when two bones that originally formed a joint are in partial contact with each other.

Fractures are described in many ways including the number of fracture fragments, direction of the fracture line, relationship of the fragments to each other, and whether or not they communicate with the outside atmosphere.

Simple fractures have two fragments; **comminuted fractures** have more than two fragments; segmental and butterfly fractures describe two types of comminuted fracture.

The direction of fracture lines is described as **transverse, diagonal, or spiral**.

The relationships of the fragments of a fracture are described by four parameters: **displacement, angulation, shortening, and rotation**.

Closed fractures are those in which there is no communication between the fracture and the outside atmosphere; they are much more common than **open or compound fractures** in which there is a communication with the outside atmosphere.

Avulsion fractures are produced by the forceful contraction of a tendon or ligament; they can occur at any age but are particularly common in younger, athletic individuals.

The Salter-Harris classification categorizes fractures through the epiphyseal plate that are graded by severity and prognosis, the more severe having an increased risk of resulting in angular deformities or shortening of the affected bone.

Stress fractures, such as march fractures in the metatarsals, occur as a result of numerous microfractures and frequently are not visible on conventional radiographs taken when the pain first begins; after some time, bony callus formation or a dense zone of sclerosis becomes visible.

Some common named fractures are **Colles fracture** (of the radius), **Smith fracture** (of the radius), **Jones fracture** (of the base of the fifth metatarsal), **boxer's fracture** (of the head of the fifth metacarpal), and **march fracture** (of the metatarsals).

Some fractures are more difficult to detect than others; the easily missed fractures (and how common they are) include scaphoid fractures (common), buckle fractures of the radius and ulna (common), radial head fractures (common), supracondylar fractures (common), posterior dislocations of the shoulder (uncommon), hip fractures (common), and rib fractures (common).

Soft tissue swelling, the disappearance of normal fat stripes and fascial planes, joint effusions, and periosteal reaction are indirect signs that should alert you to the possibility of an underlying fracture.

Fractures heal with a combination of endosteal callus, recognized by a progressive indistinctness of the fracture line, and external callus that bridges the fracture site; many factors affect fracture healing, including the age of the patient, the degree of mobility of the fracture, and its blood supply.

Delayed union refers to a fracture that is taking longer to heal than is usually required for that site; **malunion** means the fracture is healing but in a mechanically or cosmetically unacceptable way; **nonunion** is a radiologic diagnosis that implies there is little, if any, likelihood the fracture will heal.

23 Recognizing Joint Disease: An Approach to Arthritis

- Imaging studies play a key role in the diagnosis and management of arthritis.
  - Many arthritides are first diagnosed through imaging studies.
  - Still others are initially diagnosed on clinical and laboratory grounds, and imaging is used to document the severity, extent, and course of the disease (Table 23-1).
- Conventional radiographs demonstrate abnormalities of the bone but provide only indirect and usually delayed evidence of abnormalities involving the soft tissues such as the synovial lining of the joint, the articular cartilage, muscles, ligaments, and tendons surrounding the joint.
  - MRI is now used to demonstrate those soft tissue abnormalities.
- First, let's define **what an arthritis is** and then we'll develop a classification of arthritides.
  - An **arthritis is a disease that affects a joint and usually the bones on either side the joint.**
  - Arthritis is almost always accompanied by **joint space narrowing** (Fig. 23-1).

Classification of Arthritis

- We will divide arthritides into **three main categories** (Table 23-2).
  - **Hypertrophic arthritis** is characterized, in general, by **bone formation** at the site of the involved joint(s).
    - The bone may form within the confines of the parent bone *(subchondral sclerosis)* or protrude from the parent bone *(osteophyte).*
  - **Infectious arthritis** is characterized by joint swelling, osteopenia, and **destruction of long, contiguous segments of the articular cortex.**
  - **Erosive arthritis** indicates underlying inflammation and is characterized by tiny, marginal, irregularly shaped lytic lesions in or around the joint surfaces called *erosions.*
- Many different arthritides have been described, but we will look at only a few of the more common types that have characteristic imaging findings.

Anatomy of a Joint

- Figure 23-2 is a representation of a synovial joint.
- The *articular cortex* is the thin, white line within the joint capsule that is usually capped by *hyaline cartilage,* which is called the *articular cartilage.*
- The bone immediately beneath the articular cortex is called *subchondral bone.*
- Within the *joint capsule* is the *synovial membrane* and *synovial fluid.*
  - The synovial membrane is frequently the earliest structure involved by an arthritis.

- On conventional radiographs, the synovial membrane, synovial fluid, and the articular cartilage are usually not directly visible.
- Conventional radiographs will demonstrate abnormalities of the articular cortex and the subchondral bone and will provide late, indirect evidence of the integrity of the articular cartilage.
- Although MRI is more sensitive in directly visualizing the soft tissues in and around a joint, **conventional radiographs remain the study of first choice** in evaluating for the presence of an arthritis.

Hypertrophic Arthritis

- **Hypertrophic arthritis is characterized by bone formation,** either **within** the confines of preexisting bone *(subchondral sclerosis)* or by bony protrusions **extending from** the normal bone *(osteophytes).*
- **Hypertrophic** arthritides
  - **Osteoarthritis (degenerative arthritis)**
    - **Primary**
    - **Secondary**

Table 23-1

ARTHRITIS—WHO MAKES THE DIAGNOSIS?
Usually Diagnosed Clinically
Septic (pyogenic) arthritis
Psoriatic arthritis
Gout
Hemophilia
Frequently Diagnosed Radiologically
Osteoarthritis
Early rheumatoid arthritis
Calcium pyrophosphate deposition disease
Ankylosing spondylitis
Septic (tuberculosis)
Charcot (neuropathic) joint (late)

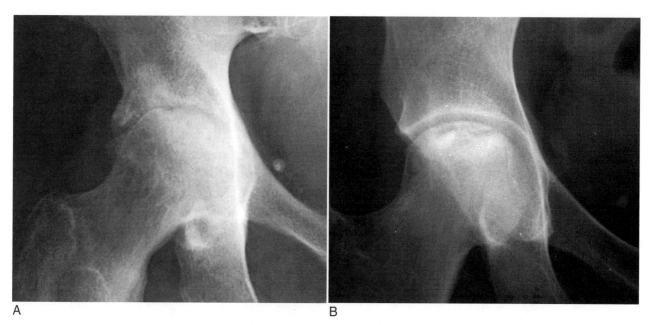

A   B

Figure 23-1. **Arthritis or not?** *An arthritis is a disease that affects a joint and usually the bones on either side of the joint, almost always accompanied by joint space narrowing. The disease depicted in* **A** *meets those specifications.* **A,** *There is narrowing of the hip joint and both the bones of the femoral head and the acetabulum are abnormal. This is osteoarthritis of the hip.* **B,** *Abnormality of the femoral head (sclerosis) is evident, but the joint space is normal, as is the acetabulum. This is avascular necrosis of the femoral head, without arthritis.*

Table 23-2

CLASSIFICATION OF ARTHRITIS

Category	Hallmarks	Types	Remarks
Hypertrophic arthritis	Bone formation, osteophytes	Primary osteoarthritis	Most common; mechanical stress; hands, hips and knees most common
		Secondary osteoarthritis	Degeneration secondary to prior trauma, or avascular necrosis
		Charcot arthropathy	Fragmentation; joint destruction; sclerosis; most often secondary to diabetes
		Calcium pyrophosphate deposition disease	Chondrocalcinosis; degenerative joint disease in unusual sites
Infectious arthritis	Osteopenia and soft tissue swelling; early and marked destruction of most or all of the articular cortex	Pyogenic	Early destruction of articular cortex; osteoporosis
		Nonpyogenic (tuberculosis)	Gradual and late destruction of articular cortex; marked osteoporosis
Erosive arthritis	Erosions	Rheumatoid arthritis	Carpals, MCPs, PIPs of hands; osteoporosis; soft-tissue swelling
		Gout	Juxta-articular erosions with overhanging edges; long latency; MTP joint of big toe; no osteoporosis
		Psoriatic arthritis	Juxta-articular erosions of DIP joints of hands; pencil-in-cup deformity; enthesophytes
		Hemophilia	Remodeling from hemarthroses and hyperemia; same changes in female—think of juvenile rheumatoid arthritis
		Ankylosing spondylitis	HLA-B27+, bilateral SI joints, syndesmophytes
		Seronegative spondyloarthropathies	HLA-B27+, SI joints; syndesmophytes, Reiter's syndrome, psoriasis; rheumatoid factor−

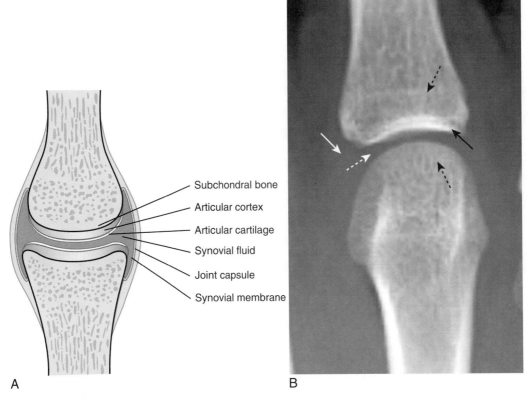

Figure 23-2. **Diagram (A) and radiograph (B) of a true joint.** *A representation of a synovial joint shows the* **articular cortex,** *which corresponds to the thin, white line* (closed black arrow) *within the* **joint capsule** (closed white arrow) *that is usually capped by* **articular cartilage** (dotted white arrow). *The bone immediately beneath the articular cortex is called* **subchondral bone** (dotted black arrows). *Within the joint capsule is the* **synovial membrane** *and* **synovial fluid.**

- **Erosive osteoarthritis**
- **Charcot arthropathy (neuropathic joint)**
- **Calcium pyrophosphate deposition disease (CPPD)**

PRIMARY OSTEOARTHRITIS

- Primary osteoarthritis is also known as **primary degenerative arthritis** and as **degenerative joint disease (DJD).**
- This is the **most common form of arthritis,** estimated to affect over 20 million Americans.
- It results from **intrinsic degeneration of the articular cartilage,** mostly from the mechanical stress of **excessive wear and tear** in weight-bearing joints.
- A disease that increases in prevalence with increasing age, it mostly involves the **hips, knees, and hands.**
- The **imaging findings in osteoarthritis**
  - **Marginal osteophyte formation**—a **hallmark of hypertrophic arthritis,** osseous transformation of cartilaginous excrescences and metaplasia of synovial lining cells lead to the production of bony protrusions at or near the joint called *osteophytes* (Fig. 23-3).
  - **Subchondral sclerosis**—this is a reaction of the bone to the mechanical stress to which it is subjected when its protective cartilage has been destroyed.

- **Subchondral cysts**—as a result of chronic impaction, necrosis of bone, or imposition of synovial fluid into the subchondral bone, cysts of varying sizes form in the subchondral bone.
- **Narrowing of the joint space** (as in all forms of arthritis):
  - In osteoarthritis, destruction of the cartilaginous buffer between the apposing bones of a joint leads to narrowing of the joint space most often on the weight-bearing side of the joint: hip (superior and lateral) and knee (medial) (Fig. 23-4).
  - In most patients with osteoarthritis of the interphalangeal joints of the hands, the first carpometacarpal joint (base of thumb) is also affected (Fig. 23-5).

SECONDARY OSTEOARTHRITIS (SECONDARY DEGENERATIVE ARTHRITIS)

- This form of degenerative arthritis of synovial joints occurs because of an underlying, predisposing condition, **most frequently trauma,** that damages or leads to damage of the articular cartilage.
- The radiographic findings of secondary osteoarthritis are the same as those for the primary form, along with several special clues to help suggest secondary osteoarthritis.

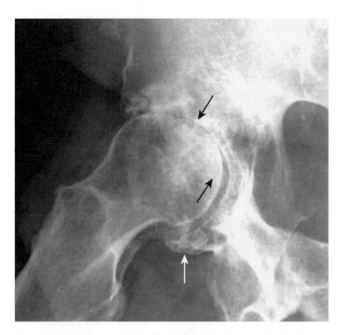

Figure 23-3. **Osteoarthritis.** *The hallmarks of osteoarthritis are demonstrated in this patient's right hip. There is marginal osteophyte formation (closed white arrow), a process by which there is osseous transformation of cartilaginous excrescences and metaplasia of synovial lining cells leading to the production of bony protrusions at or near the joint. There is also subchondral sclerosis (closed black arrows), representing reaction of the bone to the mechanical stress to which it is subjected when its protective cartilage has been destroyed.*

- It **occurs at an atypical age** for primary osteoarthritis (for example, a 20-year-old with osteoarthritis). (Box 23-1).
- It has an **atypical appearance for primary osteoarthritis** (for example, primary osteoarthritis is usually bilateral and often symmetrical; severe osteoarthritic changes of one hip at the same time the opposite appears perfectly normal should alert you to the possibility of secondary osteoarthritis) (Fig. 23-6).
- It may **appear in an unusual location** for primary arthritis (for example, the elbow joint).
- **Eventually, any arthritis that affects the articular cartilage, no matter what the cause, can lead to changes of secondary osteoarthritis.**

EROSIVE OSTEOARTHRITIS

- This type of **primary osteoarthritis** is characterized by more **severe inflammation** and by the development of **erosive changes.**
  - Erosive osteoarthritis occurs most often in **perimenopausal females.**
  - Erosive osteoarthritis may feature bilaterally symmetrical changes (e.g., the osteophytes of DJD) but with **marked inflammation (swelling and tenderness) and centrally located erosions at the affected joints.**
    - The **erosions are typically centrally located within the joint** and, combined with the small osteophytes associated with the disease, may produce the so-called *gull-wing deformity* (Fig. 23-7).

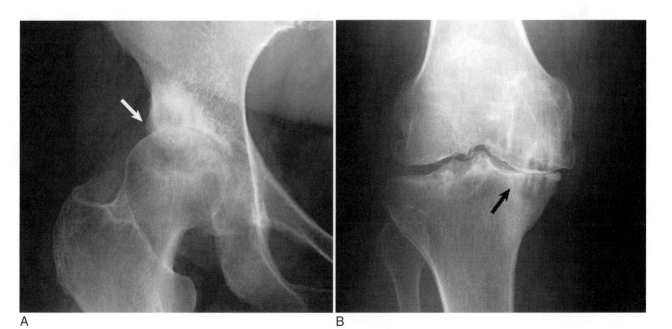

A   B

Figure 23-4. **Osteoarthritis of hip and knee.** *In osteoarthritis, destruction of the cartilaginous buffer between the apposing bones of a joint leads to narrowing of the joint space most often on the weight-bearing side of the joint. In the hip (A), the superior and lateral surfaces are most affected (closed white arrow), but in the knee (B), the medial compartment is more affected (closed black arrow).*

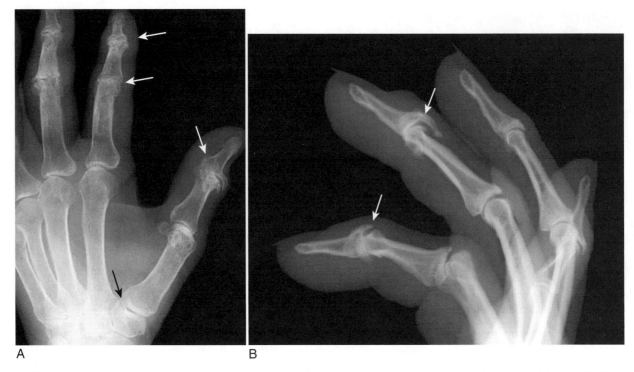

A   B

Figure 23-5. **Osteoarthritis of the hands.** *In the hands, osteoarthritis affects the distal and proximal interphalangeal joints primarily. There are small osteophytes in small joints (closed white arrows) and the joint space is narrowed. Also, subchondral sclerosis is present at the carpal-metacarpal joint of the thumb (closed black arrow). Osteoarthritis of the hands occurs most often in older women.*

- It most commonly occurs at the **proximal and distal interphalangeal joints of the fingers, first carpal-metacarpal and the IP joint of the thumb.**
- **Bony ankylosis may occur,** an uncommon finding in primary osteoarthritis.

CHARCOT ARTHROPATHY (NEUROPATHIC JOINT)
- Charcot arthropathy develops from a **disturbance in sensation,** which leads to **multiple microfractures,** as well as an autonomic imbalance, which leads to **hyperemia, bone resorption, and fragmentation of bone.**

Box 23-1

Some Causes of Secondary Osteoarthritis
Trauma
Infection
Avascular necrosis
Calcium pyrophosphate deposition disease
Rheumatoid arthritis

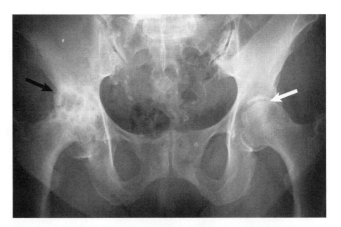

Figure 23-6. **Secondary osteoarthritis, right hip.** *There is a marked discrepancy between the two hips with severe and advanced osteoarthritis of the right hip (closed black arrow) and a normal left hip (closed white arrow). The radiographic findings of secondary osteoarthritis are the same as those for the primary form except it occurs at an atypical age for primary osteoarthritis, it has an atypical appearance for primary osteoarthritis (for example, primary osteoarthritis is usually bilateral and often symmetrical), and it may appear in an unusual location for primary arthritis, (for example, the elbow joint). This patient had a slipped capital femoral epiphysis on the right, and it was never attended to medically.*

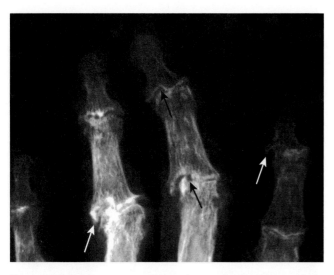

Figure 23-7. **Erosive osteoarthritis.** *A type of primary osteoarthritis characterized by more severe inflammation and by the development of erosive changes, it may feature bilaterally symmetrical changes like the osteophytes of DJD but with marked inflammation (swelling and tenderness). The erosions are typically centrally located within the joint* (closed black arrows) *and, combined with the small osteophytes associated with the disease* (closed white arrows), *may produce the so-called* **gull-wing deformity.**

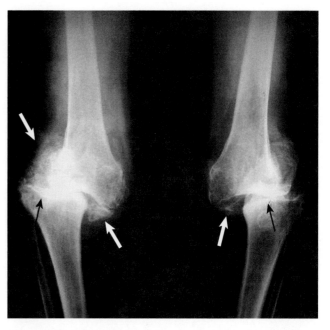

Figure 23-8. **Charcot arthropathy of knees.** *As a hypertrophic arthritis, a Charcot joint will demonstrate extensive subchondral sclerosis The hallmark findings of a Charcot joint, however, are fragmentation* (closed white arrows) *of the bones surrounding the joint that produce numerous small, bony densities within the joint capsule and joint space destruction* (closed black arrows). *The most common cause of Charcot joint of the knee formerly had been syphilis but is now diabetes.*

- Even though the joint lacks sensory feedback, almost three fourths of patients with a Charcot joint **complain of some degree of pain,** although it is usually far less than would be expected for the degree of joint destruction present.
- **Soft tissue swelling is a prominent feature.**
- The **most common cause of a Charcot joint today is diabetes,** and most Charcot joints are found in the **lower extremities, particularly in the feet and ankles.**
- **Causes of Charcot joints** by location
  - **Shoulders**—syrinx, spinal tumor, and syphilis
  - **Hips**—tertiary syphilis, diabetes
  - **Ankles and feet**—diabetes (common) and syphilis (uncommon)
- **Radiographic findings in Charcot arthropathy**
- As a hypertrophic arthritis, a Charcot joint will demonstrate **extensive subchondral sclerosis.**
- The **hallmark findings of a Charcot joint**
  - **Fragmentation** of the bones surrounding the joint produces numerous small, bony densities within the joint capsule.
    - Sometimes, **many—if not all—of the fragments may be resorbed** and no longer be visible (Fig. 23-8).
  - Eventual **destruction of the joint**—Charcot neuropathy is responsible for some of the **most dramatic examples of total joint destruction of any arthritis** (Fig. 23-9).
- A Charcot joint shares some of the same findings as osteomyelitis in that it produces **bone destruction** and **periosteal reaction (from fracture healing).**

- A radioactive indium-tagged white blood cell bone scan can help to differentiate infection from Charcot joint.

CALCIUM PYROPHOSPHATE DEPOSITION DISEASE

- This arthropathy results from the deposition of **calcium pyrophosphate dihydrate (CPPD)** crystals in and around joints, **mostly in hyaline cartilage and fibrocartilage** (especially the triangular fibrocartilage of the wrist and the menisci of the knee).
- The terminology associated with describing this disease can be confusing:
  - *Chondrocalcinosis* refers only to calcification of the articular cartilage or fibrocartilage and is seen in about 50% of adults over the age of 85, most of whom are **asymptomatic** (Fig. 23-10).
    - Chondrocalcinosis can occur with other diseases besides CPPD, such as hyperparathyroidism and hemochromatosis.
  - *Pseudogout* is a **clinical syndrome** consisting of **acute, monarticular arthropathy** characterized by **redness, pain, and swelling** of the affected joint (most commonly the knee) from which **calcium pyrophosphate dihydrate** crystals can be aspirated.
  - *Pyrophosphate arthropathy* is a radiologic diagnosis and the most common form of CPPD.
- Pyrophosphate arthropathy in its most common manifestation acts like a type of secondary osteoarthritis.

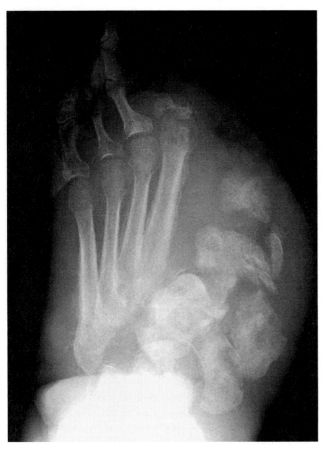

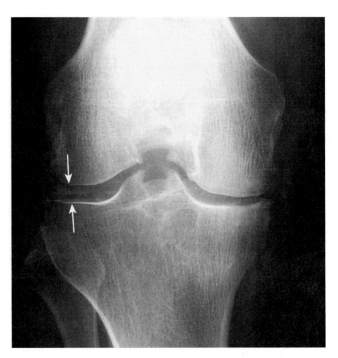

Figure 23-10. **Chondrocalcinosis.** *Chondrocalcinosis refers only to calcification of the articular cartilage (closed white arrows) or fibrocartilage and is seen in about 50% of adults over the age of 85, most of whom are asymptomatic. If this patient had acute pain, redness, swelling, and limitation of motion, the syndrome would be called pseudogout.*

Figure 23-9. **Charcot arthropathy of foot.** *This patient had previously undergone amputations of the phalanges of the first and second toes for diabetic gangrene but the destruction seen here is a manifestation of Charcot neuropathy. Charcot neuropathy can produce some of the most dramatic examples of total joint destruction of any arthritis. Note the severe fragmentation of the first metatarsal and tarsal bones.*

Infectious Arthritis

- It **produces changes similar to osteoarthritis** but differs from it in several important respects:
  - CPPD affects such joints as the **patellofemoral joint space of the knee,** the **radiocarpal joint,** the **MCP joints of the hands** and the **wrist, all joints not usually affected by primary osteoarthritis.**
  - **Chondrocalcinosis is usually present** in pyrophosphate arthropathy, but does not have to be.
  - **Subchondral cysts are common;** they are larger, more numerous, and more widespread than in primary osteoarthritis.
  - **Hook-shaped bony excrescences** along the second and third metacarpal heads are a common finding in this form of CPPD (Fig. 23-11A).
  - **In the wrist,** characteristic findings include calcification of the triangular fibrocartilage, narrowing of the radiocarpal joint, separation of the scaphoid and the lunate, and collapse of the distal carpal row toward the radius (Fig. 23-11B).

- **Infectious arthritis** usually **occurs as a result of hematogenous seeding of the synovial membrane from an infected source elsewhere in the body,** such as a wound infection, or **from direct, contiguous extension from osteomyelitis** adjacent to the joint.
- It is usually divided into **pyogenic (septic) arthritis,** due mostly to staphylococcal and gonococcal organisms and **nonpyogenic arthritis,** due mostly to infection with *Mycobacterium tuberculosis.*
- **Risk factors** include intravenous drug use, steroid injections or ingestion, joint prostheses, and recent joint trauma including surgery.
- **In children and adults, the knee is frequently affected; in children, the hip is** another **common** site of infection.
  - Hands may be infected from human bites, feet are prone to infection in diabetics.
- Although **conventional radiographs are** obtained as the initial study, they are **relatively insensitive** to the early findings of the disease except for soft tissue swelling and osteopenia.
  - If septic arthritis is strongly suspected, aspiration of the joint will usually confirm the diagnosis.
- The **hallmark of infectious arthritis,** especially the pyogenic form, **is destruction of the articular cartilage and long contiguous segments of the adjacent articular**

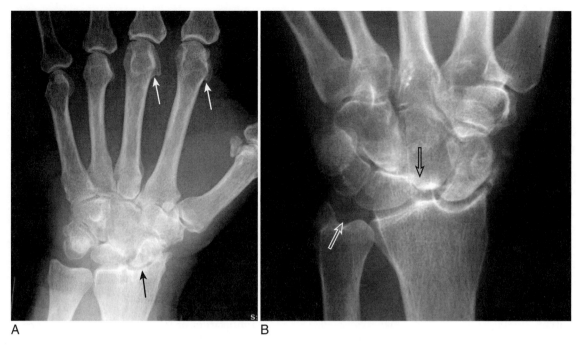

A   B

Figure 23-11. *Calcium pyrophosphate deposition disease.* *Calcium pyrophosphate deposition disease produces changes similar to osteoarthritis but differs from it in that it affects such joints as the patellofemoral joint space of the knee, the radiocarpal joint (closed black arrow), and the MCP joints of the hands and the wrist, joints not usually affected by primary osteoarthritis. Chondrocalcinosis is usually present (open white arrow), along with subchondral cysts. Hook-shaped bony excrescences along the second and third metacarpal heads are a common finding (closed white arrows). In the wrist, characteristic findings include calcification of the triangular fibrocartilage (open white arrow), narrowing of the radiocarpal joint (closed black arrow), separation of the scaphoid and the lunate, and collapse of the distal carpal row toward the radius (open black arrow).*

cortex from proteolytic enzymes released by the inflamed synovium.

- The **destruction,** unlike in other arthritides, **is usually quite rapid.**
- Infectious arthritis tends to **be monarticular** and is associated with **soft tissue swelling** and **osteopenia** from the hyperemia of inflammation (Fig. 23-12).
- **Nonpyogenic infectious arthritis** is most often caused by *Mycobacterium tuberculosis,* which **spreads via the bloodstream from the lung.**
- Unlike pyogenic arthritis, **tuberculous arthritis has an indolent and protracted course** resulting in **gradual loss of the joint space** and **late destruction of the articular cortex.**
  - **Usually monarticular, severe osteoporosis is a common finding.**
  - **In children, the spine is most often affected; in adults, it is the knee.**
- Healing with fibrous and bony ankylosis occurs in both pyogenic and nonpyogenic infectious arthritis.

Erosive Arthritis

- **Erosive arthritis** comprises a large number of different arthritides, all of which are associated with some degree of *inflammation* and *synovial proliferation (pannus formation),* which participates in the production of **lytic lesions in or near the joint** called *erosions,* especially in the small joints of the hands and feet.

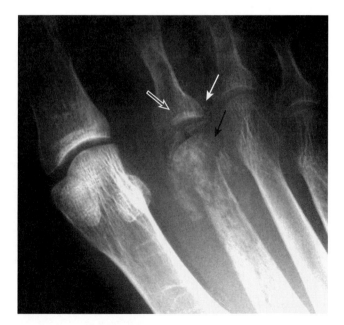

Figure 23-12. *Septic arthritis, second toe.* *The hallmark of infectious arthritis, especially the pyogenic form, is destruction of the articular cartilage and long contiguous segments of the adjacent articular cortex (closed black arrow) from proteolytic enzymes released by the inflamed synovium. The destruction, unlike other arthritides, is usually quite rapid. There is associated osteopenia from the hyperemia of inflammation (open white arrow). Small bubbles of gas (closed white arrow) are present in the soft tissues from gas-forming bacterial cellulitis.*

- **Pannus** acts like a mass of growing and enlarging synovial tissue and leads to **marginal erosions** of the **articular cartilage and underlying bone.**
- Box 23-2 lists some of the many causes of erosive arthritis. We shall talk about only four of the more common.

RHEUMATOID ARTHRITIS

- Rheumatoid arthritis (RA) is **more common in females,** frequently **involving the proximal joints of the hands and wrists.**
- It is **usually bilateral and symmetrical.**
- **Conventional radiographs remain the study of first choice in imaging RA.**
- The **earliest radiographic changes are soft tissue swelling** of the affected joints and **osteoporosis,** which tends to be most severe on both sides of the joint space (*periarticular osteoporosis* or *demineralization*).
- **In the hand,** the erosions tend to involve the proximal **joints:** the carpal-metacarpal, metacarpal-phalangeal, and proximal interphalangeal joints (Fig. 23-13).
- **In the wrist,** erosions of the **carpals, ulnar styloid,** and **narrowing with erosion of the radiocarpal joint** space are frequently seen.
  - **Late findings in the hands** include deformities such as **ulnar deviation of the fingers at the MCP joints,**

Box 23-2

Some Causes of Erosive Arthritis
Rheumatoid arthritis
Gout
Psoriatic arthritis
Ankylosing spondylitis (spine)
Rheumatoid variants
Reiter's syndrome
Sarcoid
Hemophilia

subluxation of the MCP joints, and ligamentous laxity leading to deformities of the fingers (*swan-neck and boutonnière deformities*).
- Elsewhere in the body, the **larger joints usually show no erosions,** but there may be **marked uniform narrowing of**

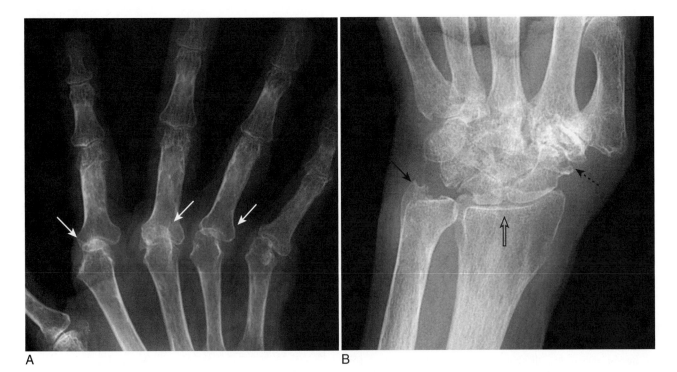

A   B

Figure 23-13. **Rheumatoid arthritis, hand (A) and wrist (B).** In the hand **(A),** the erosions tend to involve the proximal joints: the carpal-metacarpal, metacarpal-phalangeal (closed white arrows), and proximal interphalangeal joints. In the wrist **(B),** erosions of the carpals (dotted black arrow), ulnar styloid (closed black arrow), and narrowing of the radiocarpal joint space (open black arrow) are frequently seen. Late findings in the hands include deformities such as ulnar deviation of the fingers at the MCP joints, subluxation of the MCP joints, and ligamentous laxity leading to deformities of the fingers (all present in this case).

the joint space with little or no subchondral sclerosis (Fig. 23-14).

- **In the spine,** RA tends to involve the cervical spine by producing **ligamentous laxity,** which can lead to forward subluxation of C1 on C2 (*atlantoaxial subluxation*).
  - Atlantoaxial subluxation can produce cord compression if severe (Fig. 23-15).
  - **RA may also cause narrowing, sclerosis, and eventual fusion of the facet joints.**

GOUT

- Gout represents the **inflammatory changes incited by the deposition of calcium urate crystals in the joint.**
- There is **characteristically an extremely long latent period (5–7 years)** between onset of symptoms and the visualization of bone changes, so **gout is usually a clinical and not a radiologic diagnosis** (see Table 23-1).
- Gout tends to be **monarticular** at its onset and **asymmetrical later** in its course.
- It is **more common in males** and **most commonly affects the metatarsal-phalangeal joint of the great toe** at the time of symptom onset.
- **Imaging findings of gout**
  - As an erosive arthritis, the **hallmark of gout is the sharply marginated, juxta-articular erosion which tends to have a sclerotic border.**
    - The overhanging edges of gouty erosions have been called *rat-bite lesions.*

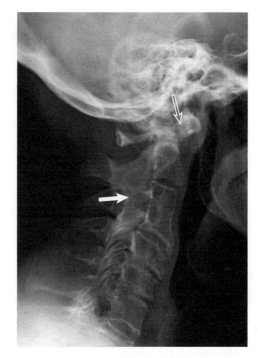

Figure 23-15. **Rheumatoid arthritis of the cervical spine.** RA tends to involve the cervical spine by producing ligamentous laxity that can lead to forward subluxation of C1 on C2 (atlantoaxial subluxation) (open white arrow shows widening of the space between the dens and the anterior tubercle of C1). RA may also cause fusion of the facet joints (closed white arrow).

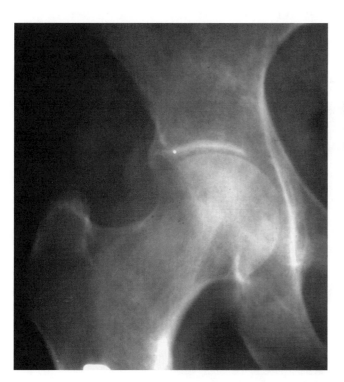

Figure 23-14. **Rheumatoid arthritis of the hip.** The larger joints (hip and knees) usually show no erosions but there may be marked uniform narrowing of the joint space with little or no subchondral sclerosis as in this patient.

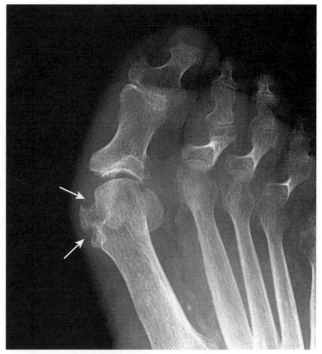

Figure 23-16. **Gout.** Gout most commonly affects the metatarsal-phalangeal joint of the great toe, as in this patient. As an erosive arthritis, the hallmark of gout is the sharply marginated, juxta-articular erosion, which tends to have a sclerotic border (closed white arrows). The overhanging edges of gouty erosions have been called **rat-bite** lesions. The metatarsal-phalangeal joint space is minimally narrowed and there is no periarticular osteoporosis.

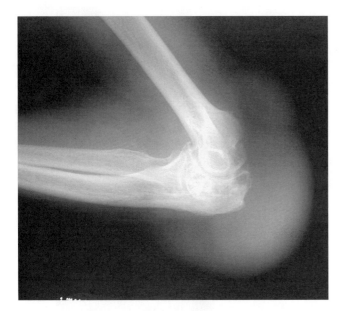

Figure 23-17. **Olecranon bursitis.** *Olecranon bursitis is a common manifestation of gout (large soft tissue mass around elbow) and its presence should alert you to the underlying possibility of gout.*

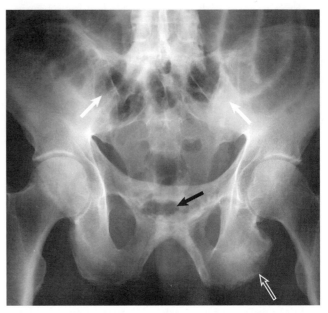

Figure 23-19. **Ankylosing spondylitis.** *Ankylosing spondylitis is an enthesopathy, a process that produces inflammation, with subsequent calcification and ossification at and around the* entheses, *which are the insertion sites of tendons, ligaments, and joint capsules (open white arrow). Bilaterally symmetrical* sacroiliitis *is the hallmark of ankylosing spondylitis. This eventually leads to bony fusion or ankylosis of the SI joints until they fuse together (closed white arrows). The symphysis pubis is also ankylosed (closed black arrow).*

- **Joint space narrowing may be a late finding** in the disease and there is **characteristically little or no periarticular osteoporosis** (Fig. 23-16).
- **Tophi rarely calcify.**
- **Olecranon bursitis is common** (Fig. 23-17).

PSORIATIC ARTHRITIS

- **Most patients** with psoriatic arthritis **also have skin and nail changes of psoriasis,** although for some, the joint

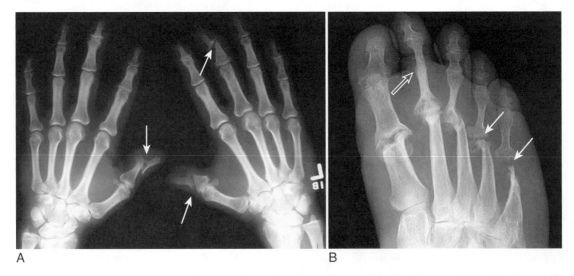

Figure 23-18. **Psoriatic arthritis. A,** *Psoriatic arthritis typically involves the small joints of the hands, especially the distal interphalangeal (DIP) joints (closed white arrows) and resorption of the terminal phalanges or the DIP joints with telescoping of one phalanx into another (pencil-in-cup deformity) (closed white arrows).* **B,** *There is ankylosis of the second toe (open white arrow) and more pencil-in-cup deformities (closed white arrows).*

manifestations may be the initial presentation of the disease.

- Psoriatic arthritis **typically involves the small joints of the hands, especially the distal interphalangeal (DIP) joints.**
- The **hallmarks of psoriatic arthritis**
  - **Juxtarticular erosions of the DIP joints** of the hands especially
  - **Bony proliferation at the sites of tendon insertions (enthesophytes)**
  - **Periosteal reaction along the shafts of the bone** (not common)
  - **Resorption of the terminal phalanges** or the DIP joints with telescoping of one phalanx into another *(pencil-in-cup deformity)* (Fig. 23-18)
  - **No osteoporosis**
- In the **sacroiliac joints,** psoriasis can produce **bilateral, but asymmetrical, sacroiliitis.**
  - The **SI joints do not usually completely fuse as in ankylosing spondylitis.**

ANKYLOSING SPONDYLITIS

- This chronic and progressive arthritis is characterized by **inflammation and eventual fusion of the sacroiliac (SI) joints** along with the spinal facet joints and involvement of the paravertebral soft tissues.

- Almost all patients with ankylosing spondylitis have the *human leukocyte antigen B27 (HLA-B27)* as opposed to only about 5% of the general population.
- More **common in young males,** the disease **characteristically ascends the spine starting in the SI joints** and moving to the lumbar, thoracic, and finally cervical spine.
- **Conventional radiographs** of the affected areas are the **usual study performed for diagnosis and follow-up** of patients with ankylosing spondylitis.
- Ankylosing spondylitis is an *enthesopathy,* a process that **produces inflammation, with subsequent calcification** and ossification at and around the *entheses,* which are the insertion **sites of tendons, ligaments, and joint capsules.**
- *Sacroiliitis* is the hallmark of ankylosing spondylitis.
  - It is usually **bilaterally symmetrical** and **eventually leads to bony fusion** or *ankylosis* of these joints until they either appear as a thin white line or disappear altogether (Fig. 23-19).

In the spine, there is **ossification of the outer fibers of the annulus fibrosis** producing **thin, bony bridges** from the corners of one vertebra to another called *syndesmophytes.*

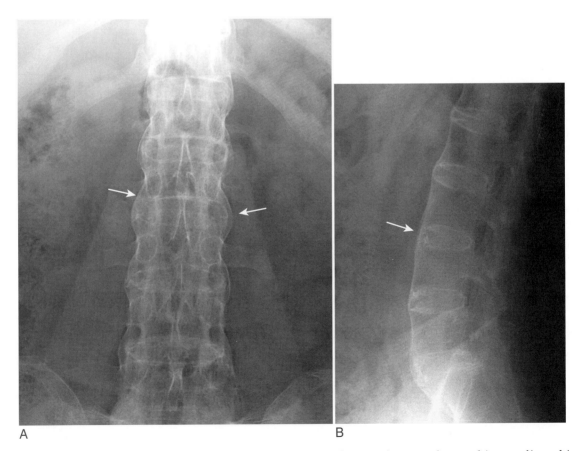

A   B

Figure 23-20. **Ankylosing spondylitis, frontal (A) and lateral (B) spine.** *In the spine, there is ossification of the outer fibers of the annulus fibrosis producing thin, bony bridges from the corners of one vertebra to another called syndesmophytes (closed white arrows). Progressive ossification of tissue connecting adjacent vertebral bodies produces the bamboo-spine appearance seen here.*

- Progressive ossification of tissue connecting adjacent vertebral bodies produces the ***bamboo-spine*** appearance (Fig. 23-20).

WebLink
More information about recognizing arthritis is available to registered users on StudentConsult.com.

 TAKE-HOME POINTS: Recognizing Joint Disease: An Approach to Arthritis

An arthritis is a disease of a joint that invariably leads to joint space narrowing and changes to the bones on both sides of the joint.

Arthritides can be roughly divided into hypertrophic, infectious, and erosive (inflammatory) categories.

Hypertrophic arthritis features subchondral sclerosis, marginal osteophyte production, and subchondral cyst formation.

Primary osteoarthritis, the most common form of arthritis, is a type of hypertrophic arthritis.

Other hypertrophic arthritidies include Charcot joints and osteoarthritis secondary to either prior trauma, avascular necrosis, or superimposed on another underlying arthritis.

Infectious arthritis features soft tissue swelling and osteopenia and, in the case of pyogenic arthritis, relatively early and marked destruction of most or all of the articular cortex.

Erosive (or inflammatory) arthritis is associated with inflammation and synovial proliferation (pannus formation), which produces lytic lesions in or near the joint called erosions.

Rheumatoid arthritis, gout, and psoriasis are three examples of erosive arthritis; the site of involvement is helpful in differentiating among the causes of erosive arthritides.

24 Recognizing Some Common Causes of Neck and Back Pain

Conventional Radiography, CT, and MRI

- **Conventional radiographs** remain an important method of evaluating selected spinal lesions for two primary reasons:
  - They are **inexpensive** and **rapidly available,** even on a portable basis, if needed.
  - They **demonstrate bony anatomy with great detail** and are utilized as a **screening method** for most spinal trauma.
- **CT,** with its ability to reformat images in different planes, now supplements, and in some cases **has replaced, conventional radiography in the evaluation of spinal trauma,** although the yield of discovering an unexpected traumatic lesion in an alert, asymptomatic patient remains a matter of question.
  - CT is utilized to determine **the extent of the injury** in any patient in whom a traumatic spinal injury has already been demonstrated by conventional radiographs.
- CT is also utilized to **detect bony lesions not visible on conventional radiographs** and, in some cases, to **evaluate soft tissue abnormalities** in patients who are unable to undergo an MRI examination.
- **MRI,** with its superior soft tissue differentiation, **is the study of choice for most diseases of the spine** for the following reasons:
  - Its **ability to visualize, and detect abnormalities in, soft tissues** such as bone marrow, the spinal cord and the intervertebral disks
  - Its **ability to display images in any plane**
  - The **lack of exposure to radiation** (Box 24-1)
- Still, **MRI has its limitations:**
  - The study **remains expensive** and its **availability is not as widespread** as CT or conventional radiographs.
  - **Patients with pacemakers** and certain internal ferromagnetic materials (aneurysm clips) **are not able to be scanned.**
  - Protocols designed to best demonstrate a particular abnormality or disease usually **require multiple scan sequences,** which means the procedure **takes more time** to complete.
  - Some patients cannot tolerate the **claustrophobia** they experience in some of the high-field strength MRI scanners.

The Normal Spine

- There are normally 7 cervical vertebra, 12 thoracic vertebra (all of which normally bear ribs), 5 lumbar vertebra, and 5 fused sacral vertebrae.
- The spinal cord normally terminates at the L1-L2 level as the *conus medullaris* and the *cauda equina* extends

inferiorly from that point as a collection of nerve roots with each root exiting below its respectively numbered vertebral body.

- Each neural foramen contains a **spinal nerve, blood vessels,** and **fat.**
- **Spinal nerves** are named and numbered **according to the site they exit** from the spinal canal.
  - **C1 to C7** nerves exit **above** their respective vertebrae.
  - **C8** exits **between the seventh cervical and first thoracic** vertebrae.
  - The **remaining nerves exit below** their respectively numbered vertebrae.
- The articular facets of the *superior and inferior articular processes* are lined with cartilage, and these facet joints are **true synovial joints.**

Box 24-1

Magnetic Resonance Imaging (MRI)

MRI produces images by using radiofrequency pulses deployed in defined sequences through a very strong, static magnetic field in a way that causes protons within the patient's body, most abundant in the hydrogen atoms of water, to first be "excited" and then "relaxed."

The change from the excited to relaxed state releases energy in the form of radiofrequency signals that are recorded by the scanner's receiving coil and then computer-processed to form an image.

Each tissue releases its energy at two different relaxation rates; this forms the basis for scans that are acquired with "weighting" toward either a T_1 or a T_2 relaxation time.

In addition, different tissues release their energies at different rates, which forms the basis for the differences in contrast that allow MRI to display a wide range of soft tissues.

MRI examinations utilize protocols designed to demonstrate certain abnormalities better than others, depending on the clinical situation; as such, the protocols are usually composed of multiple scan or pulse sequences, each lasting 2 to 15 minutes.

T_1-weighted images display anatomic details and make distinction between solid and cystic structures easier; T_2-weighted images tend to display pathologic changes better; together, they enable the detection and characterization of most tissues.

Occasionally, additional contrast enhancement is acquired through the use of gadolinium, which is a paramagnetic contrast agent that can be injected intravenously; gadolinium-enhanced tissues and fluids appear bright on T_1-weighted images and provide high sensitivity for detection of vascular tissues (e.g., tumors).

- From the level of **C3 through the level of L5,** generally speaking, the vertebral **bodies are rectangular** and of about equal height posteriorly as anteriorly.
- The **relative height of the disk space varies in each section of the spine.**
  - In the **cervical spine,** the **disk spaces** are about **equal** to each other in height.
  - In the **thoracic spine,** they are usually **decreased** in size from the **cervical spine,** but remain **equal** in height **to each other.**
  - In the **lumbar spine,** they **progressively increase in height** with each successive interspace, except for L5-S1, which can be equal to or slightly less than the height of L4-L5.
- The **end-plates of contiguous vertebral bodies are roughly parallel to each other.**
- In the frontal projection, **each vertebral body displays two ovoid pedicles** visible on each side of the vertebral body (Fig. 24-1).
  - **The pedicles of L5** are frequently **difficult to visualize, even in normal individuals,** owing to the lordosis of the lumbar spine.
- On conventional radiographs of the lumbar spine performed in the oblique projection, the anatomic structures combine to produce a shadow that resembles the front end of a Scottish terrier, the famous *Scottie dog* sign (Fig. 24-2).

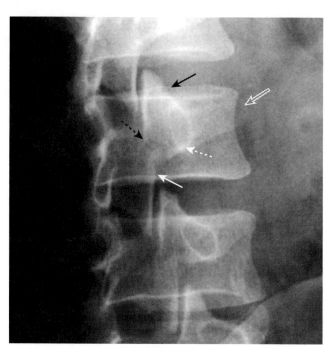

Figure 24-2. **Scottie dog sign.** This is a left posterior oblique view of the lumbar spine (the patient is turned about halfway toward her own left). The "Scottie dog" is made up of the following: the "ear" (closed black arrow) is the superior articular facet, the "leg" (closed white arrow) is the inferior articular facet, the "nose" (open white arrow) is the transverse process, the "eye" (dotted white arrow) is the pedicle, and the "neck" (dotted black arrow) is the pars interarticularis. All these structures are paired; an identical set should be visible on the patient's right side.

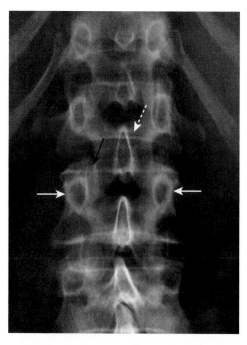

Figure 24-1. **Normal pedicles.** In the frontal projection, each vertebral body displays two ovoid pedicles visible on either side of the vertebral body (closed white arrows). The spinous process (dotted white arrow) may usually be visualized slightly below the body to which it is attached. The facet joint is seen here en face (closed black arrow).

- There are several ligaments that traverse the spine (Table 24-1).

Back Pain
- It has been estimated that **almost 80% of all Americans will have some episode of back pain** during their lifetime.
- The causes of back pain are numerous and the anatomic and physiologic interrelationships that produce it in many cases are still not known.

Table 24-1

LIGAMENTS OF THE SPINE

Ligament	Connects
Anterior longitudinal ligament	Anterior surfaces of vertebral bodies
Posterior longitudinal ligament	Posterior surfaces of vertebral bodies
Ligamentum flavum	Laminae
Interspinous ligament	Between spinous processes
Supraspinous ligament	Tips of spinous processes

- Some of the **more common causes of back pain**
  - **Muscle and ligament strain**
  - **Herniation of an intervertebral disk**
  - **Degeneration of an intervertebral disk**
  - **Arthritis involving the synovial joints of the spine**
  - **Compression fractures, usually from osteoporosis**
  - **Trauma to the spine**
  - **Malignancy involving the spine**
- We will discuss all except muscle and ligament strains.

Herniated Disks

- Only about 2% of patients with acute low back pain have a herniated disk.

- The **majority of disk herniations occur at the lower three lumbar disk levels,** L3-L4, L4-L5 (most common), and L5-S1.
- **More than 60% of disk herniations occur posterolaterally,** the location of the herniation determining the clinical presentation depending on the nerve roots compressed.
- In the **cervical spine, disk herniations occur most frequently at C4-C5, C5-C6, and C6-C7.**
- In the **lumbar region,** disk herniation may lead to **back pain** and **sciatica,** and herniation of a **cervical disk** may produce **radiculopathy** and **myelopathy.**
- The intervertebral disks have a central gelatinous *nucleus pulposus* surrounded by an outer *annulus fibrosus,* which is, in turn, made up of inner fibrocartilaginous fibers and outer cartilaginous fibers *(Sharpey's fibers).*
- **Degeneration** of the annular fibers or **trauma** can lead to an interruption in those fibers and allow the disk material to bulge, which may or may not be associated with back pain.
- When the annular fibers rupture, the **nucleus pulposus may herniate** (usually posterolaterally) **through a weakened area of the posterior longitudinal ligament.**
  - The herniated material may protrude but remain in contact with the disk from which it originated, or it may be completely *extruded* into the spinal canal.
- Symptoms are caused by acute compression of the nerve root.
- **MRI is the study of choice for evaluating herniated disks** (Fig. 24-3).
  - Conventional radiographs of the spine cannot identify the presence of a herniated disk.

Degenerative Disk Disease

- With increasing age, the normally gelatinous nucleus pulposus becomes dehydrated and degenerates.
  - This gradually leads to **progressive loss of the height of the intervertebral disk space.**
  - The end-plates of contiguous vertebral bodies become *eburnated* or sclerotic.
  - **Small osteophytes are produced** at the margins of the vertebral bodies at each disk space.
- At the same time, there is typically **degeneration of the outer annulus fibrosis.**

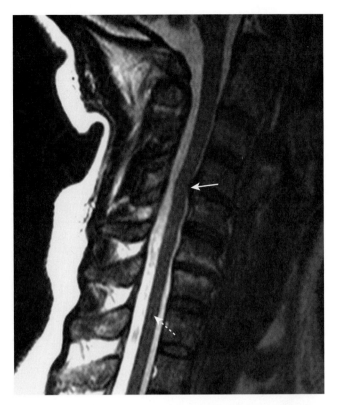

Figure 24-3. **Herniated disk, C4-C5 on MRI.** *The spinal cord is dark* (dotted white arrow) *relative to the high intensity (whiter) signal surrounding it which is the cerebrospinal fluid in the spinal canal. The closed white arrow points to a herniated disk extending posteriorly from the C4-C5 disk space compressing the cord.*

- This leads to the production of **larger marginal osteophytes** at the end-plates than those seen with degeneration of the nuclear material.
- At times, desiccation of the disk leads to **release of nitrogen** from tissues surrounding the disk space, resulting in the appearance of **air density in the disk space,** which is called a *vacuum-disk phenomenon.*
  - A vacuum-disk represents a **late sign of a degenerated disk** (Fig. 24-4).
- It should be noted that osteophytes are an extremely common finding, increasing in prevalence with increasing age and that most patients with osteophytes of the spine are **asymptomatic.**

Osteoarthritis of the Facet Joints

- The *facet joints* (also known as the *apophyseal joints)* are **true joints** in that they have cartilage, a synovial lining, and synovial fluid.
  - As such, they are **subject to osteoarthritis,** similar to the appendicular skeleton.
- Some consider the small joint-like structures at the lateral edges of C3 to T1, called the *uncovertebral joints* or the *joints of Luschka,* to be true joints, but others do not.
  - They are also frequent sites of osteophyte formation.
  - The **costovertebral joints,** representing the articulation between the posterior ribs and the thoracic vertebrae, also are **true joints.**

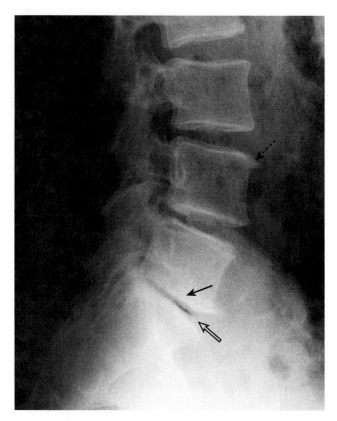

Figure 24-4. **Degenerative disk disease.** *With increasing age, there is progressive loss of the height of the intervertebral disk space. The end-plates of contiguous vertebral bodies become sclerotic (closed black arrow),* small osteophytes are produced at the margins of the vertebral bodies (dotted black arrow), and there is desiccation of the disk which can produce a vacuum-disk phenomenon (gas in the disk space) recognized by the air density in place of the disk seen here at L5-S1 (open black arrow).

- There is usually a **complex interrelationship between degenerative disk disease and facet arthritis** such that the two frequently occur together.
  - The **osteophytes** formed by osteoarthritis of the facet joints **may encroach on the neural foramina and produce radicular pain.**
- In the **cervical spine, osteophytes may also develop at the uncovertebral joints** and produce **protrusions of bone into the** normally oval-shaped **neural foramina,** which are visualized on conventional radiographs taken in the oblique projection (Fig. 24-5A).
  - **Osteophytes at the uncovertebral joints** are **frequently associated with both degenerative disk disease and osteophytes of the facet joints.**
- In the **lumbar spine,** facet osteoarthritis may cause **narrowing** and **sclerosis of the facet joints,** best seen on oblique views of the spine (see Fig. 24-5B).
  - Facet arthritis is easier to visualize on CT scans of the spine than conventional radiographs, but actual nerve compression is easier to visualize on MRI of the spine.

Diffuse Idiopathic Skeletal Hyperostosis (DISH)

- This common disorder is characterized by bone or calcium formation at the sites of ligamentous insertions *(enthesopathy).*
- DISH usually affects **men** over the age of **50,** and can occur **anywhere in the spine** but **most often** does so in the **lower thoracic and lower cervical spine.**
- Frequently patients with DISH complain of back stiffness but may have **no pain** or only **mild back pain.**
- **Conventional radiographs of the spine are sufficient** to make the diagnosis of DISH.
- DISH is manifest by **thick, bridging or flowing calcification/ossification** of the **anterior** or, sometimes, posterior **longitudinal ligaments.**
- This ossification is visualized along the anterior or anterolateral aspects **of at least four contiguous vertebral bodies.**
  - Unlike degenerative disk disease, **the disk spaces** and usually the **facet joints are preserved.**
  - The ossification is **separate from the vertebral body** (Fig. 24-6A).
  - Unlike ankylosing spondylitis, which may radiographically resemble DISH, the **sacroiliac joints are normal.**
- Patients with DISH are more prone to develop heterotopic bone at surgical sites.
- **Ossification of the posterior longitudinal ligament (OPLL)** is often present with DISH, is better visualized on CT and MRI than on conventional radiographs, and may cause compression of the spinal cord, especially in the cervical spine (Fig. 24-6B).

Compression Fractures of the Spine

- Vertebral compression fractures are **common,** affecting **women more than men,** and are typically secondary to **osteoporosis.**
- Osteoporotic compression fractures usually **involve the anterior and superior aspects** of the vertebral body **sparing the posterior aspect.**
- This produces a **wedge-shaped deformity** that leads to accentuation of the kyphosis in the thoracic spine and the lordosis in the lumbar spine (Fig. 24-7).
- Progressive **loss of overall body height is a common consequence** of multiple compression fractures in the elderly.
  - There is **usually no neurologic deficit** associated with osteoporotic compression fracture because the fracture involves the anterior part of the vertebral body.
- **Conventional spine radiographs are usually the study of first choice for identifying compression fractures.**
  - MRI can be utilized for differentiating osteoporotic compression fractures from malignancy.
  - Both MRI and nuclear bone scans can help in establishing the age of the compression abnormality.
- **Recognizing compression fractures on conventional radiographs**

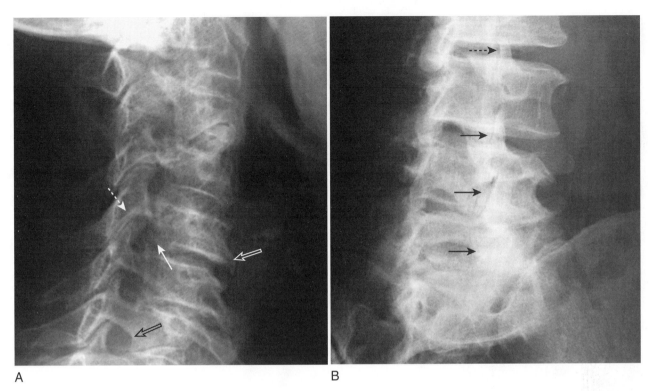

A   B

Figure 24-5. **Uncovertebral osteophytes and facet arthritis. A,** In the cervical spine, osteophytes may develop at the uncovertebral joints (closed white arrow), producing bony protrusions into the normally oval neural foramina (open black arrow points to a normal foramen), in this conventional radiograph taken in the oblique projection. Osteophytes at the uncovertebral joints are frequently associated with both degenerative disk disease (open white arrow points to thick marginal osteophyte) and osteophytes of the facet joints (dotted white arrow). **B,** Sclerosis and osteophyte formation involve the lower facet joints of the lumbar spine (closed black arrows). The dotted black arrow points to a normal facet joint.

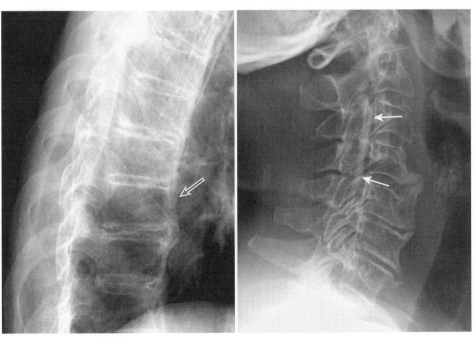

A   B

Figure 24-6. **Diffuse idiopathic skeletal hyperostosis (DISH) and ossification of the posterior longitudinal ligament (OPLL). A,** DISH is manifested by thick bridging or flowing calcification/ ossification of the anterior longitudinal ligaments (open white arrow). This ossification is visualized along the anterior or anterolateral aspects of at least four contiguous vertebral bodies. The ossification is separate from the vertebral body. **B,** OPPL (closed white arrows) can be associated with DISH and may contribute to the production of spinal stenosis.

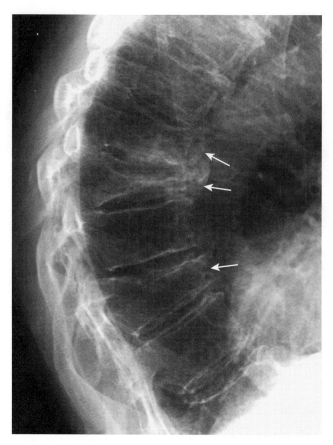

Figure 24-7. Compression fracture secondary to osteoporosis. *Vertebral compression fractures are common, affecting women more than men, and typically are secondary to osteoporosis. Osteoporotic compression fractures usually involve the anterior and superior aspects of the vertebral body sparing the posterior aspect (closed white arrows). This produces a wedge-shaped deformity that leads to accentuation of the kyphosis in the thoracic spine. Progressive loss of overall stature is a common sign of compression fractures in the elderly*

- Difference in the height between the anterior and posterior aspects of the same vertebral body in excess of **3 mm**
- Alternatively, the compressed body is typically >20% shorter than the body above or below it.

Spondylolisthesis and Spondylolysis

- *Spondylolisthesis* is defined as **slippage** (typically forward) **of one vertebral body** (and the spine above it) **on another.**
  - **Forward slipping** spondylolisthesis is also called *anterolisthesis.*
  - **Posterior slipping** of one vertebral body on another is called *retrolesthesis.*
  - Spondylolisthesis is graded according to the degree one body has slipped on the adjacent body (Fig. 24-8).
- In general, spondylolisthesis can occur if
  - There are **bilateral breaks in the pars interarticularis (spondylolysis)**
  - There is **osteoarthritis of the facet joints**

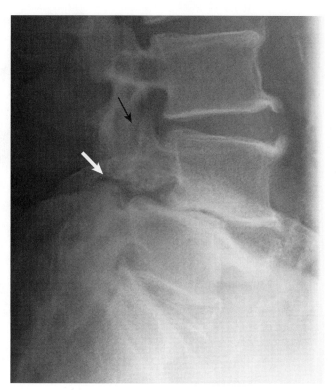

Figure 24-8. Spondylolisthesis and spondylolysis. *Spondylolisthesis is defined as slippage (typically forward) of one vertebral body (and the spine above it) on another. In this case, there is forward slippage of L4 on L5 equal to about half the anteroposterior diameter of L5, so this is graded as a grade II spondylolisthesis. There is both spondylolysis (closed white arrow) and degenerative arthritis of the facet joints (closed black arrow) in this patient.*

- **Spondylolysis** is believed to be due to a combination of a **congenitally dysplastic pars interarticularis** that is then subjected to the strains of an upright posture which eventually leads to a **stress fracture of the pars** (Fig. 24-9).
  - A **familial history** of spondylolisthesis or spondylolysis is relatively **common.**
- **Facet osteoarthritis** may be associated with spondylolisthesis *(degenerative spondylolisthesis)* through a complex interaction between the **ligaments, disks,** and **facet joints** wherein disease in any one (or more) of these components increases the stress on the others and leads to spondylolisthesis.
  - In **degenerative spondylolisthesis,** there is **no break in the pars interarticularis.**
  - The degree of spondylolisthesis is usually less in this group than in those with spondylolisthesis from bilateral spondylolysis.
  - The **L4-L5 disk space is most commonly affected** (Fig. 24-10).
  - **Posterior slippage** of one vertebral body on the body below may occur from **facet osteoarthritis**.
- Other causes of spondylolisthesis include trauma, malignancy, and a congenital vertebral anomaly.

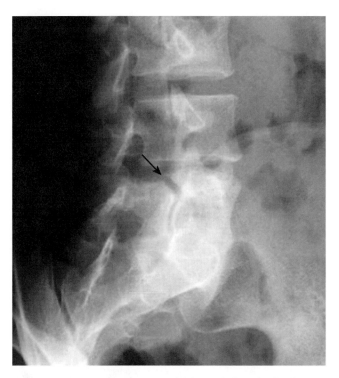

Figure 24-9. **Spondylolysis.** *Spondylolysis is believed to be due to a combination of a congenitally dysplastic pars that is then subjected to certain strains that eventually lead to a stress fracture of the pars (closed black arrow). You might recognize the break as a "collar" on the "neck" of the Scottie dog (see Fig. 24-2). When the spondylolysis is bilateral, this allows the affected vertebral body to slip forward on the one below it (spondylolisthesis).*

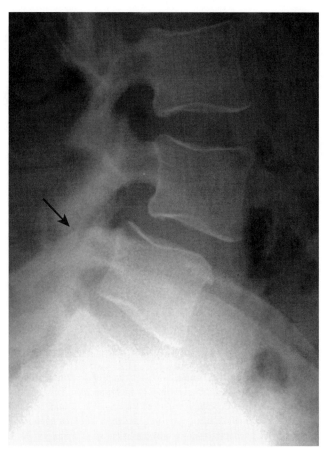

Figure 24-10. **Degenerative spondylolisthesis.** *Facet osteoarthritis (closed black arrow) may be associated with spondylolisthesis through a complex interaction between the ligaments, disks, and facet joints. In degenerative spondylolisthesis, there is no break in the pars interarticularis and the degree of spondylolisthesis is usually less in this group than in those with spondylolisthesis from bilateral spondylolysis. The L4-L5 disk space is most commonly affected, as in this patient.*

- **Conventional radiographs of the lumbar spine are usually the initial imaging study.**
  - CT may be more helpful in detecting **spondylolysis,** whereas MRI may demonstrate soft tissue abnormalities but be less effective in detecting spondylolysis.
- **Recognizing spondylolisthesis/spondylolysis on conventional radiographs**
  - The **lateral view is best** at demonstrating **spondylolisthesis,** which will be visible as (usually) anterior slippage of one vertebral body on the body below.
    - If the slippage approximates 25% of the AP diameter of the vertebral body below, it is called a grade I spondylolisthesis.
    - If the slippage approximates 50% of the AP diameter of the vertebral body below, it is called a grade II spondylolisthesis, and so on for grades III and IV.
  - **Spondylolysis** is easiest to visualize on an **oblique view of the lumbar spine** in which a **lucency** represented by the break in the neck of the Scottie dog (the "collar" on the Scottie dog) may be seen **in the pars interarticularis** (see Fig. 24-9).

Spinal Stenosis

- Spinal stenosis refers to **narrowing of the spinal canal** or the neural foramina secondary to **soft tissue or bony abnormalities,** either on an **acquired or congenital** basis.
  - Degenerative, **acquired etiologies are more common** than congenital causes.
- **Soft tissue abnormalities** can lead to spinal stenosis:
  - Hypertrophy of the ligamentum flavum
  - Bulging disk(s)
  - Ossification of the posterior longitudinal ligament (OPPL)
- **Bony abnormalities** can lead to spinal stenosis:
  - Congenitally narrow spinal canal
  - Osteophytes
  - Facet osteoarthritis
  - Spondylolisthesis
- Spinal stenosis is **most common in the cervical and lumbar areas** and can produce radicular pain, myelopathy, or in the lumbar region, neurogenic claudication, which is relieved by flexing the spine.
- **Conventional radiographic** findings may include an **AP diameter of the spinal canal of less than 10 mm, facet joint arthritis,** and **spondylolisthesis associated with spondylolysis** (Fig. 24-11).

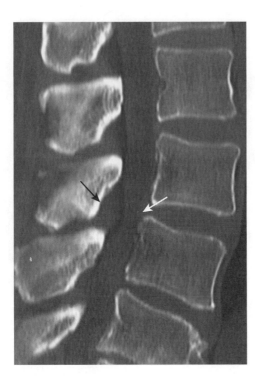

Figure 24-11. ***Spinal stenosis.*** *A combination of a protruding disk (closed white arrow) and hypertrophy of the ligamentum flavum (closed black arrow) combine to reduce the size of the spinal canal at L3-L4 to about 6 mm in this sagittally reformatted CT of the lumbar spine. Spinal stenosis refers to narrowing of the spinal canal or the neural foramina secondary to soft tissue or bony abnormalities, either on an acquired or congenital basis, usually to a diameter less than 10 mm.*

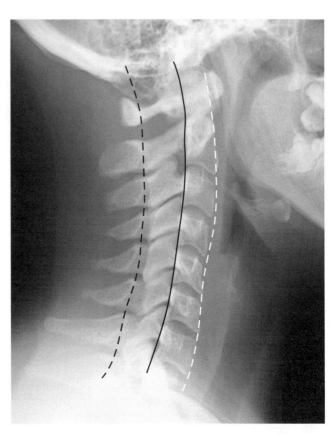

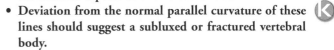

Figure 24-12. ***The cervical lines.*** *The lateral view of the cervical spine enables a quick assessment for spinal fracture/subluxation before further studies are performed which might involve motion of the patient's neck. Three parallel arcuate lines should smoothly join the spinolaminar white lines, which are the junctions between the laminae and the spinous processes (dotted black line), a second line should join the posterior aspects of the vertebral bodies (solid black line), and a third should join the anterior aspects of the vertebral bodies (dotted white line). Deviation from the normal parallel curvature of these lines should suggest a subluxed or fractured vertebral body.*

- **CT** provides an excellent method of demonstrating bony abnormalities.
- **Conventional radiographs are usually obtained first** in evaluating for spinal stenosis, but **MRI is the study of choice.**

Spinal Trauma

- Fractures of the spine are infrequent compared to fractures of other parts of the skeleton.
- When they occur, they have particular importance because of the implications for associated spinal cord injury.
- **The three cervical lines** (Fig. 24-12)
  - Many trauma protocols include a ***cross-table* lateral view of the cervical spine** (the patient's neck is immobilized, the patient remains on the stretcher or examining table, and the x-ray beam is directed **horizontally** so that the patient's **head is not moved).**
  - This view enables a **quick assessment for spinal fracture/subluxation** before further studies are performed that might involve motion of the patient's neck.
  - **Three, parallel arcuate lines** should first smoothly join the ***spinolaminar white lines*** (the junctions between the laminae and the spinous processes), a second line should join the **posterior aspects**

of the vertebral bodies, and a third should join the **anterior aspects of the vertebral bodies.**
- **Deviation from the normal parallel curvature of these lines should suggest a subluxed or fractured vertebral body.**
- **Some of the more common spinal fractures**
  - **Compression fractures,** which are the most common fractures of the spine, were previously discussed.
  - **Jefferson fracture**
  - **Hangman's fracture**
  - **Burst fracture**

Jefferson Fracture

- A Jefferson fracture is a **fracture of C1** usually involving both the anterior and posterior arches.
  - In its classical presentation, there are **bilateral fractures of both the anterior and posterior arches of C1** (four fractures in all).
- It is **caused by an axial loading injury** (such as diving into a swimming pool and hitting one's head on the bottom).

- On conventional radiographs, the hallmark of a Jefferson fracture is **bilateral,** *lateral* **offset of the lateral masses of C1 relative to C2 as seen on the** *open-mouth view* **of the cervical spine** (Fig. 24-13).
- The fracture is **confirmed utilizing CT.**
- A Jefferson fracture is a "self-decompressing" fracture in that the cervical canal at the level of the fracture is wide enough to accommodate any swelling of the cord.
  - There is usually **no neurologic deficit** associated with the fracture.

HANGMAN'S FRACTURE

- A hangman's fracture is a **fracture of the posterior elements of C2.**
- Hangman's fractures **result from a hyperextension-compression injury** typically occurring in an unrestrained occupant in a motor vehicle accident who strikes the forehead on the windshield.
- For conventional radiography, hangman's fractures are **best evaluated on the lateral view** of the cervical spine.
- The fracture effectively **separates the posterior aspect of the C2 vertebral body** from the **anterior aspect of C2,** allowing the **anterior aspect of C2 to sublux forward on the body of C3** (Fig. 24-14).
  - Some hangman's fractures are less displaced, so that CT may be needed for their detection.
- Because hangman's fractures lead to **widening of the bony canal,** they are usually **not associated with neurological deficits.**
  - This is in contrast to the injury after which this fracture is named, the fracture incurred during a *judicial hanging* in which there was hyperextension leading to a fracture of C2 **and marked distraction** of C2 from C3.

BURST FRACTURES

- Burst fractures are most common in the **cervical spine, thoracic spine, and upper lumbar spine.**
- They are **axial loading injuries** in which the disk above is driven into the vertebral body below and the vertebral body bursts.

- This drives bony fragments **posteriorly into the spinal canal** *(retropulsed fragments)* while the anterior aspect of the vertebral body is displaced forward.
- The **majority of burst fractures are associated with a neurologic deficit.**
- Findings include a **comminuted, compression fracture of the vertebral body** in which the **posterior aspect of the body is bowed backward toward the spinal canal** (Fig. 24-15).
  - **CT** is the **best method** for identifying **bony fragments** in the spinal canal.

LOCKED FACETS

- Bilateral locking of the facets in the cervical spine can occur as a result of a **hyperflexion injury** in which the **inferior facets of one vertebral body slide over and in front of the superior facets of the body below.**
- This results in **forward slippage** of the affected vertebral body on the body below it **by at least 50% of its AP diameter.**
- On a **lateral, conventional radiograph** of the cervical spine, the **inferior articular facets will lie in front of the superior facets** of the body below (Fig. 24-16).
  - Because the superior articular facets are no longer "covered" by the inferior facets above them, this was described on CT as the *naked facet sign.*
- This injury virtually **always results in neurologic impairment.**

Malignancy Involving the Spine

- Metastases to bone are 25 times more common than primary bone tumors.
- Metastases usually occur where red marrow is found, with 80% of metastatic bone lesions occurring in the axial skeleton (spine, pelvis, skull, and ribs).
- Because of the **rich blood supply** in the posterior vertebral body, hematogenous **metastatic deposits in that part of the body are common,** especially from **lung** and **breast** carcinoma.
  - Secondary spread to, and involvement of, the pedicle, is called the *pedicle sign* (see Fig. 21-20).

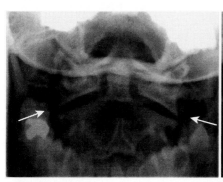
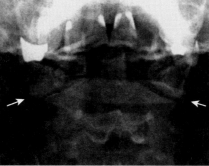
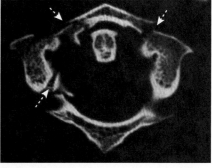

A   B   C

Figure 24-13. **Normal open-mouth view; Jefferson fracture, open-mouth view and CT.** *A Jefferson fracture is a fracture of C1 usually involving both the anterior and posterior arches. **A,** A normal "open-mouth" view of C1 and C2 is shown to demonstrate that the lateral margins of C1 (closed white arrows) line up with the lateral margins of C2. **B,** The hallmark of a Jefferson fracture is bilateral, lateral offset of the lateral masses of C1 (closed white arrows) relative to C2. The fracture is confirmed utilizing CT **(C),** which shows fractures of both the right and left anterior arch of C1 and the right posterior arch (dotted white arrows).*

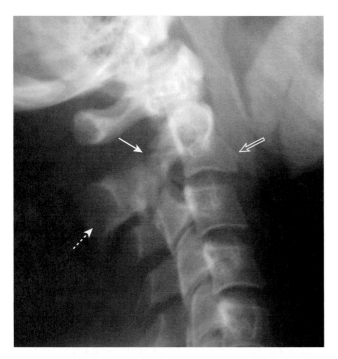

Figure 24-14. **Hangman's fracture.** A hangman's fracture results from a hyperextension-compression injury. It involves fractures through the posterior elements of C2 (closed white arrow shows fracture line) best evaluated on the lateral view. The fracture effectively separates the posterior aspect of the C2 vertebral body (dotted white arrow) from the anterior aspect of C2 (open white arrow) allowing the anterior aspect of C2 to sublux forward on the body of C3. Notice that the cervical lines, had they been drawn, cannot smoothly connect the spinolaminar white line of C2 or the anterior aspects of the vertebral bodies.

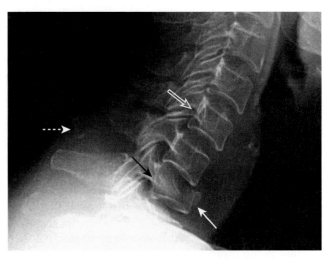

Figure 24-15. **Burst fracture, C7.** The vertebral body bursts and drives bony fragments posteriorly into the spinal canal (retropulsed fragments) while the anterior aspect of the vertebral body is displaced forward (closed white arrow). Findings include a comminuted, compression fracture of the vertebral body in which the posterior aspect of the body is bowed outward (closed black arrow) toward the spinal canal. Notice how the posterior aspects of the normal vertebral bodies are concave inward (open white arrow). The dotted white arrow points to calcification of the ligamentum nuchae.

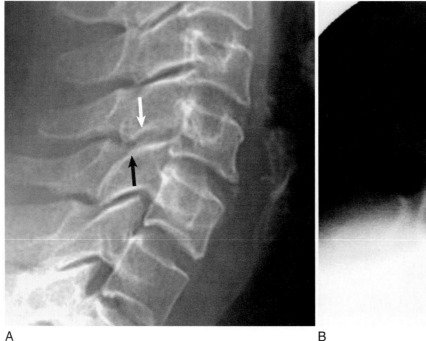
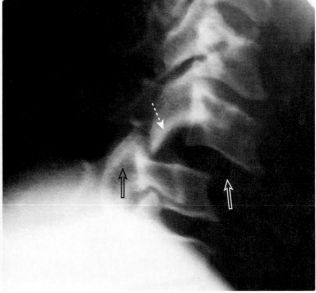

A   B

Figure 24-16. **Normal (A) and bilateral locked (B) facets.** Bilateral locking of the facets in the cervical spine can occur as a result of a hyperflexion injury in which the inferior facets of one vertebral body slide over and in front of the superior facets of the body below **(B).** This results in forward slippage of the affected vertebral body on the body below it by at least 50% of its AP diameter (open white arrow). The inferior articular facets (dotted white arrow) will lie in front of the superior facets (open black arrow) of the body below. Compare this with the normal relationship **(A)** between the inferior (closed black arrow) and superior articular facets (closed white arrow).

- In the spine, **metastases may produce compression fractures.**
  - **Metastases** tend to **destroy the vertebral body,** including and especially the posterior aspect and the pedicles, which is different from **osteoporotic compression fractures** in which **the posterior vertebral body and pedicles remain intact.**
- **Metastatic disease** can be either mostly bone-producing, i.e., *osteoblastic,* or mostly bone-destroying, i.e., *osteolytic.*
  - Metastases that contain both osteolytic and osteoblastic processes occurring simultaneously are called *mixed metastatic lesions.*
- **Recognizing an osteoblastic lesion of bone**
  - Osteoblastic metastases will appear **more dense**—that is, whiter—than the surrounding normal bone on conventional radiographs.
  - If **focal,** they may appear as **round regions of increased density.**
  - When **widespread,** they may **fill in the normal red marrow–containing medullary cavity** by stimulating bone-producing osteoblastic cells.
  - This will lead to **obliteration of the normal junction between the dense white cortex and the grayer medullary cavity** so that the cortex of the bone may seem to "disappear" because it now blends in with the medullary cavity (see Fig. 21-6).
- **Prostate cancer** is the prototypical example of a primary malignancy that produces **osteoblastic metastases;** the prototype of such a primary malignancy **in a female is breast cancer.**
- **Recognizing an osteolytic lesion of bone**
  - Osteolytic metastases will appear **less dense** (blacker), or more lucent, than the surrounding normal bone on conventional radiographs.
  - Osteolytic lesions will **destroy all or part of a bone;** e.g., the cortex of a bone may be absent, a rib may be destroyed, a pedicle may be missing.
  - Osteolytic lesions **may also be (but are usually not) *expansile;*** that is, they may cause enlargement of the portion of the bone they involve (see Fig. 21-19).
- The **most common** causes of primary malignancies that produce **osteolytic metastatic lesions** are **lung** and **breast cancer.**
  - **Thyroid and renal carcinomas** may **produce osteolytic lesions** that are also **expansile** (see Fig. 21-19).
- The spine is also a frequent site of **multiple myeloma,** the most common primary malignancy of bone.
  - Multiple myeloma is known for its tendency to produce almost totally lytic lesions.
  - One of the hallmarks of multiple myeloma is severe osteoporosis, so that myeloma may be associated with diffuse spinal osteoporosis and multiple compression fractures.

WebLink
More information about lesions that cause back pain is available to registered users on StudentConsult.com.

TAKE-HOME POINTS: Recognizing Some Common Causes of Neck and Back Pain

Conventional radiographs, CT, and MRI are all used to evaluate the spine, but MRI is the study of choice for most diseases of the spine.

Some of the more common causes of back pain are muscle and ligament strain, herniation of an intervertebral disk, degeneration of an intervertebral disk, arthritis involving the synovial joints of the spine, compression fractures from osteoporosis, trauma to the spine, and malignancy involving the spine.

Most herniated disks occur posterolaterally in the lower cervical or lower lumbar spine and are best evaluated through the use of MRI.

With increasing age, the nucleus pulposus becomes dehydrated and degenerates, leading to changes of degenerative disk disease such as progressive loss of the height of the disk space, marginal osteophyte production, sclerosis of the end-plates of the vertebral bodies, and occasionally, the appearance of air in the disk space.

The facet joints are true joints and so are subject to changes of osteoarthritis; facet osteoarthritis is frequently associated with degenerative disk disease and can lead to radicular pain.

Diffuse idiopathic skeletal hyperostosis is manifest by thick, bridging or flowing calcification/ossification of the anterior longitudinal ligaments usually occurring in men over the age of 50; the ossification is visualized along the anterior or anterolateral aspects of at least four contiguous vertebral bodies, separate from the vertebral body, but the disk spaces and usually the facet joints are, for the most part, preserved.

Spondylolisthesis is defined as slippage (typically forward) of one vertebral body (and the spine above it) on another; in general it is caused by either bilateral breaks in the pars interarticularis (spondylolysis) or osteoarthritis of the facet joints (degenerative spondylolisthesis).

Spondylolysis is believed secondary to a congenitally dysplastic pars interarticularis that eventually develops a stress fracture; when this occurs bilaterally, the vertebral body is able to slip forward on the body below it.

Degenerative spondylolisthesis, which is most common at L4-L5, may occur through a complex interaction between the ligaments, disks, and facet joints; there is no break in the pars interarticularis and the degree of slip is usually less than that seen with bilateral spondylolysis.

Spinal stenosis is a narrowing of the spinal canal or the neural foramina secondary to soft tissue or bony abnormalities, either on an acquired (more common) or congenital basis; in general, the canal is less than 10 mm in diameter.

(Continued)

TAKE-HOME POINTS: Recognizing Some Common Causes of Neck and Back Pain—cont'd

Three parallel arcuate lines should smoothly connect important landmarks on the lateral cervical spine view to quickly assess for the presence of fracture/subluxation before the patient is moved for further studies.

Jefferson fracture, hangman's fracture, burst fracture, and locked facets are common spinal traumatic injuries; the first two are self-decompressing fractures that are usually not associated with neurologic deficit, but the latter two are frequently associated with neurologic impairment.

Metastatic lesions to the spine are very common, especially to the blood-rich posterior aspect of the vertebral body including the pedicles; lung (mixed), breast (mixed), and prostate (osteoblastic) metastases are the most common causes.

Multiple myeloma also frequently involves the spine either with severe osteoporosis, which can produce compression fractures, or lytic destruction of the vertebral body.

25 Recognizing Abnormal Head CT Findings

Normal Anatomy and General Considerations

- CT and MRI are utilized for studying the brain and spinal cord, with MRI being the study of first choice for most clinical scenarios (Table 25-1).
- The anatomy and pathology are somewhat easier to understand on CT (Fig. 25-1), and many of the same general principles carry over to MRI scans.
- On an unenhanced CT scan of the brain, anything that appears "white" will either be bone (calcium) density or blood.
- **Nonpathologic calcifications**
  - **Pineal gland**
  - **Choroid plexus** (Fig. 25-2A)
  - **Falx and tentorium**
  - **Basal ganglia**
- After administration of iodinated intravenous contrast, several **normal structures can enhance:**
  - **Venous sinuses**
  - **Choroid plexus**
  - **Pituitary gland and stalk**
- Metallic densities in the head can cause artifacts on CT scans.
  - Dental fillings, aneurysm clips, and bullets can all cause *streak artifacts,*
- **White matter** appears **blacker than the gray matter** and **gray matter appears gray.**
  - Cerebrospinal fluid (CSF) appears **black,** and bone appears **white** (Fig. 25-2B).

- In general, **MRI is the study of choice** for detecting and staging intracranial and spinal cord abnormalities.

Head Trauma

- **Unenhanced CT is the study of choice in acute head trauma.**
- The primary goal is to identify is a life-threatening but treatable lesion.

FRACTURES

- In order to visualize skull fractures, you must view the CT scan using the "bone windows" (Fig. 25-3).
- **Linear skull fractures** have little importance other than for the intracranial abnormalities that may have occurred at the time of the fracture, such as epidural hematomas.
  - Fractures of the cranial vault are most apt to occur in the **temporal** and **parietal bones.**
- **Depressed skull fractures** can be associated with underlying brain injury.
  - They result from a high-energy blow to a small area of the skull and usually must be depressed more than the thickness of the skull itself to require elevation.
- **CT is the imaging study of choice** for evaluating **facial fractures.**
  - Multislice scanners allow for reconstruction in the coronal plane so that the patient does not have to be repositioned in the scanner.
  - Care must be taken in diagnosing fractures based on viewing one image because CT scans by their nature

Table 25-1

INDICATIONS FOR CT AND MRI STUDIES

Problem	CT	MRI
Hemorrhage	Better at detecting acute subarachnoid hemorrhage	More sensitive than CT in detecting most of the various temporal phases of hemorrhage, especially later
Head trauma	Nonenhanced CT is readily available and the study of first choice in head trauma; more sensitive than MRI in detecting fractures and acute intracranial bleeding	Better at finding diffuse axonal injury but requires more time; difficult to monitor the patient and not always available
Acute stroke	Initial study—differentiate hemorrhagic from ischemic infarct	Diffusion-weighted imaging for acute or small strokes
Masses	Useful, but less sensitive than MRI	More sensitive than CT
Aneurysms	Either can be used but most will use CT initially to evaluate for subarachnoid hemorrhage	

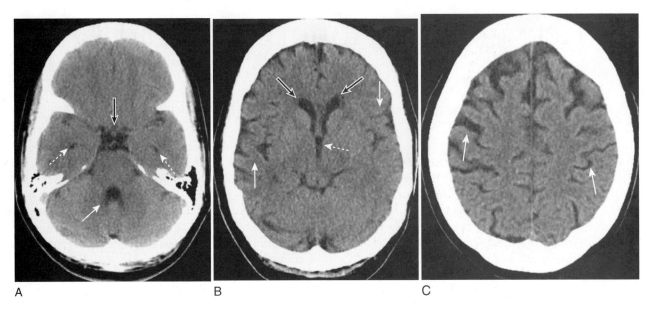

A   B   C

Figure 25-1. **Normal CT scans of the head.** *Normal unenhanced CT scans of the head demonstrate the fourth ventricle* (closed white arrow) *and basilar cisterns* (open white arrow) **(A).** *Notice the size of the temporal horns* (dotted white arrows). **B,** *The frontal horns of the lateral ventricle* (open white arrows) *are seen along with the third ventricle* (dotted white arrow) *and the sulci* (closed white arrows). *In the most superior scan* **(C),** *the sulci* (closed white arrows) *are again seen, slightly prominent but still within normal limits.*

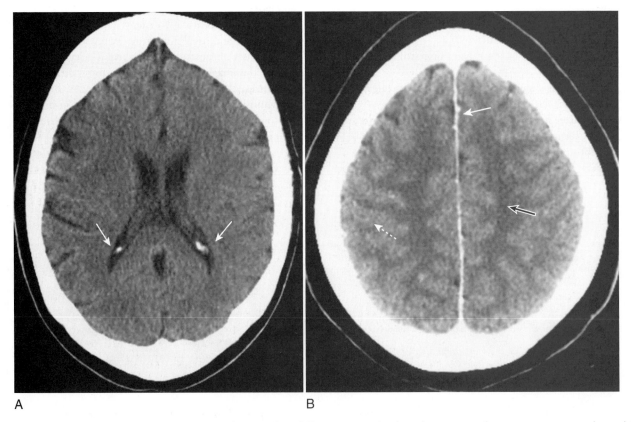

A   B

Figure 25-2. **Choroid plexus calcification, normal gray-white differentiation.** *Anything that appears white on a non-contrast-enhanced CT of the brain is either calcium or blood.* **A,** *Note the normal calcifications* (closed white arrows) *of the choroid plexus of the posterior horns of the lateral ventricles. The contrast-enhanced scan* **(B)** *shows normal opacification of the falx* (closed white arrow) *and the normal differentiation between the more superficial (and whiter appearing) gray matter* (dotted white arrow) *and the deeper (gray appearing) white matter* (open white arrow).

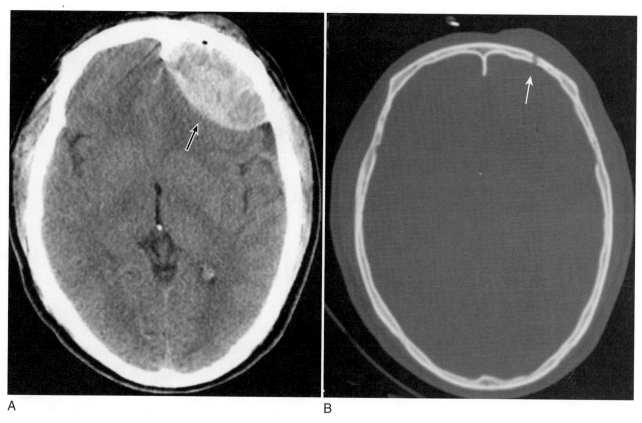

A   B

Figure 25-3. **CT, brain and bone windows.** *In order to visualize skull fractures, you must view the CT scan using the "bone" windows. **A,** The "brain window" shows a lenticular band of increased attenuation in the left frontal region (open white arrow) having the typical appearance of an epidural hematoma. **B,** The same scan viewed at the "bone window" shows a fracture (closed white arrow) of the frontal bone at the site of the epidural hematoma.*

produce thin, axial, or coronal sections that may not demonstrate the entire extent of the bone in question.

- The most common orbital fracture is the **"blow-out" fracture,** which is produced by **direct impact on the orbit** (baseball in the eye), which produces a sudden increase in intraorbital pressure causing a fracture of the inferior orbital floor (into the maxillary sinus) or the medial wall of the orbit (into the ethmoid sinus).

- **Recognizing a blow-out fracture of the orbit**
  - **Orbital emphysema**—air in the orbit from communication with one of the adjacent air-containing sinuses, either the ethmoid or maxillary sinus
  - **Fracture** through either the medial wall or floor of the orbit
  - **Entrapment of fat or extraocular muscle** that project downward as a soft tissue mass into the maxillary sinus
  - **Fluid (blood)** in the maxillary sinus.

- A *tripod fracture* is a common facial fracture that involves **separation of the frontozygomatic suture, fracture of the floor of the orbit,** and fracture of the **lateral wall of the ipsilateral maxillary sinus** (Fig. 25-4).

HEMORRHAGE

- There are **three types of extra-axial, intracranial hemorrhages:**
  - **Epidural hematoma**
  - **Subdural hematoma**

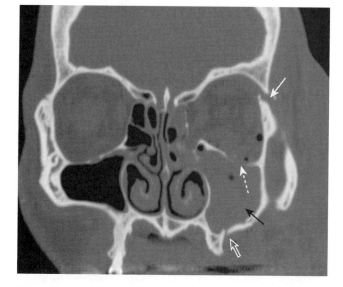

Figure 25-4. **Multiple facial fractures, CT.** *This is a coronal reconstruction of images acquired in the axial plane. Numerous facial fractures are present, including separation of the frontozygomatic suture (closed white arrow), fracture through the floor of the left orbit (dotted white arrow), and a fracture through the lateral wall of the left maxillary sinus (open white arrow). The little black dots in the orbit are bubbles of air in the orbit, and the left maxillary sinus is opacified by blood (closed black arrow). The medial wall of the orbit is also fractured.*

- **Subarachnoid hemorrhage** (discussed with aneurysms)

EPIDURAL HEMATOMA

- Epidural hematomas represent **hemorrhage** into the potential space **between the dura mater and the inner table of the skull** (Table 25-2).
  - The dura is **fused to the calvarium** at the **margins of the sutures,** making it impossible for an epidural hematoma to cross suture lines.
- Most cases are due to **injury to the middle meningeal artery or vein** from blunt head trauma, classically a motor vehicle accident.
- **Almost all epidural hematomas (95%) have an associated skull fracture.**
  - Epidural hematomas may also be caused by disruption of the dural venous sinuses adjacent to a skull fracture.
- **Recognizing an epidural hematoma**
  - **High-density, extra-axial, biconvex lens-shaped mass lesion** most often found in the temporoparietal region of the brain (Fig. 25-5).
  - Does not cross sutures (subdurals do)
  - Can cross tentorium (subdurals don't)

SUBDURAL HEMATOMA

- **More common** than epidural hematomas
- Most commonly a **result of deceleration injuries in motor vehicle or motorcycle accidents** (younger patients) **or falls** (older patients).
- They represent hemorrhage into the potential space **between the dura mater and the arachnoid.**
- **Acute subdural hematomas (SDHs)** herald more severe parenchymal brain injury and increased intracranial pressure and are **associated with a high mortality rate.**
- Subdural hematomas are usually produced by **damage to the bridging veins** that cross from cerebral cortex to the venous sinuses of the brain.
- **Recognizing an acute subdural hematoma**
  - **Crescent-shaped, extracerebral band of high attenuation** that **may** cross suture lines and enter the interhemispheric fissure.

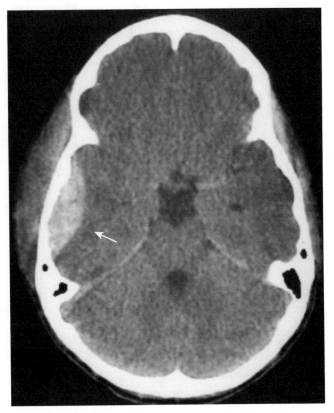

Figure 25-5. Epidural hematoma. *Acute epidural hematomas usually occur as a result of trauma-induced skull fractures. Findings include a high-density, extra-axial, biconvex, lens-shaped mass lesion often found in the temporoparietal region of the brain (closed white arrow). They do not cross sutures (subdurals do) but can cross the tentorium (subdurals don't). This patient also has associated extracranial soft-tissue swelling.*

- They **do not cross the midline.**
- Typically SDH is **concave** inward to the brain (epidural hematomas are **convex** inward) (Fig. 25-6A).
- As time passes and they become subacute, or if the subdural blood is mixed with lower attenuating CSF, they may appear isointense (isodense) to the remainder of brain, in which case you should look for **sulci displaced away from the inner table** (Fig. 25-6B).
- May see a **fluid-fluid level after 1 week** (cells settle under serum)
- **Chronic subdural hematoma**
  - More than 3 weeks after injury
  - Chronic subdural hematomas are usually **low density** (Fig. 25-6C).

INTRACEREBRAL HEMATOMA

- Injuries occurring at the **point of impact (coup)** and injuries occurring **opposite the point of impact (contrecoup)** are most common following trauma.
  - **Coup** injuries are most often due to **shearing** of small intracerebral vessels.
  - **Contrecoup** injuries are acceleration/deceleration injuries that occur when the brain is **propelled in the**

Table 25-2

THE MENINGES

Layer	Comments
Dura mater	Composed of two layers—an **outer periosteal layer,** which cannot be separated from the skull, and an **inner meningeal layer,** which forms the tentorium and falx
Arachnoid	The avascular middle layer, it is separated from the dura by a potential space known as the **subdural space**
Pia mater	Closely applied to the brain and spinal cord, it carries blood vessels that supply both; separating the arachnoid from the pia is the **subarachnoid space;** together the pia and arachnoid are called the **leptomeninges**

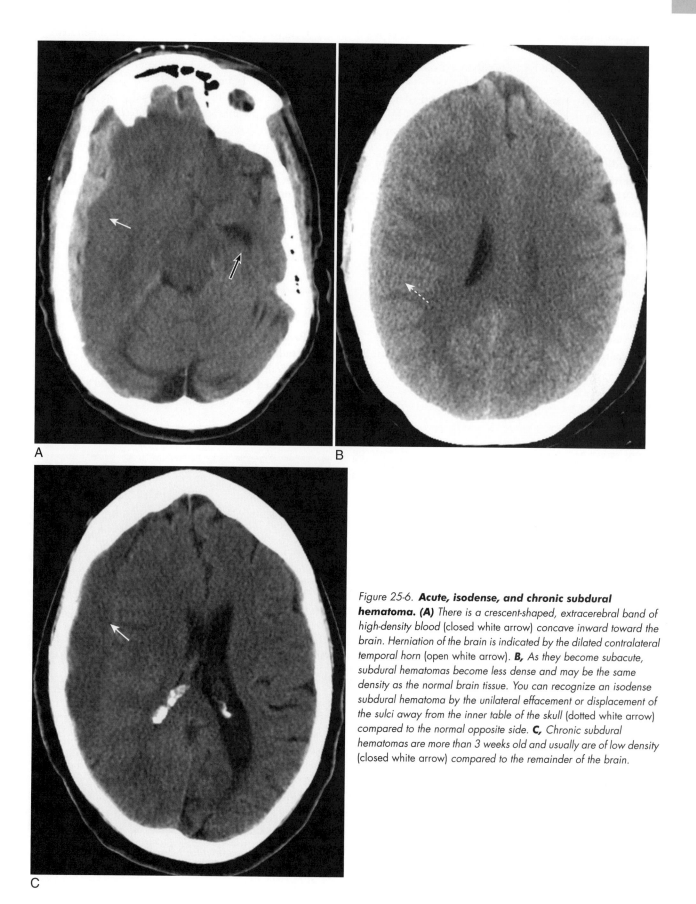

Figure 25-6. **Acute, isodense, and chronic subdural hematoma. (A)** There is a crescent-shaped, extracerebral band of high-density blood (closed white arrow) concave inward toward the brain. Herniation of the brain is indicated by the dilated contralateral temporal horn (open white arrow). **B,** As they become subacute, subdural hematomas become less dense and may be the same density as the normal brain tissue. You can recognize an isodense subdural hematoma by the unilateral effacement or displacement of the sulci away from the inner table of the skull (dotted white arrow) compared to the normal opposite side. **C,** Chronic subdural hematomas are more than 3 weeks old and usually are of low density (closed white arrow) compared to the remainder of the brain.

opposite direction and strikes the inner surface of the skull.

- Either of these mechanisms can produce a **cerebral contusion.**
- **Contusions** are **hemorrhages** with **associated edema** usually found in the **inferior frontal lobes and temporal lobes on or near the surface of the brain** (Fig. 25-7).
- **CT findings change over time** and **may not be evident on the initial scan.**
  - MRI typically demonstrates the lesions from the time of injury, but is frequently not available on an emergency basis.
- **Recognizing traumatic intracerebral hemorrhage on CT**
  - Multiple, small, well-demarcated areas of **high attenuation** within the brain parenchyma on CT.
  - Surrounded by a **rim of** hypoattenuation from **edema** (see Fig. 25-7)
  - **Mass effect is common.**
    - **Compression** of the **ventricles, shift of the third ventricle and septum pellucidum** to the opposite side

- At risk for subtentorial and subfalcine brain herniation and death
- **Intraventricular blood** may be present (Fig. 25-8).

DIFFUSE AXONAL INJURY

- The injury responsible for prolonged coma following head trauma and the injury with the poorest prognosis.
- Acceleration/deceleration forces **diffusely injure axons deep to the cortex,** producing unconsciousness from the moment of injury.
  - Most often the result of a motor vehicle accident
- The **corpus callosum is most commonly affected** and the initial CT scan may underestimate the degree of injury.
  - CT findings may be similar to those described for intracerebral hemorrhage following head trauma.
- **MR is the study of choice in identifying diffuse axonal injury.**

Increased Intracranial Pressure

- Some of the clinical signs of **increased intracranial pressure:**
  - **Papilledema**
  - **Headache and diplopia**
- In general, increased intracranial pressure is due to either
  - **Increased volume of the brain (cerebral edema)** or
  - **Increased size of the ventricles**

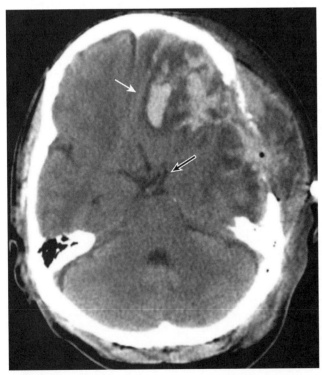

Figure 25-7. **Cerebral contusion, left frontal lobe.** *Cerebral contusions are usually the result of trauma and are manifest by multiple areas of high attenuation blood (closed white arrow) within the brain parenchyma on CT. They are frequently surrounded by a rim of hypoattenuation from edema and mass effect is common, as is demonstrated here by amputation of the ipsilateral basilar cisterns (open white arrow) and midline displacement. A portion of the left side of the skull has been surgically removed.*

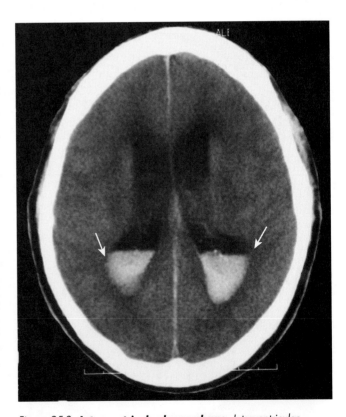

Figure 25-8. **Intraventricular hemorrhage.** *Intraventricular hemorrhage (closed white arrows) is common in premature infants but rare in adults. It usually results from breakthrough bleeding from a brain contusion or subarachnoid hemorrhage and requires a considerable amount of force to produce. Therefore, it is typically associated with severe brain damage and has a poor prognosis.*

CEREBRAL EDEMA

- In adults, trauma, **hypertension** (associated as it is with **intracerebral bleeds** and **stroke**)**,** and **masses** are the most common causes of diffuse brain edema.
- There are **two types** of cerebral edema: **vasogenic** and **cytotoxic.**
  - **Vasogenic edema** represents extracellular accumulation of fluid and is the type that is associated with **malignancy** and **infection.**
    - It is due to **abnormal permeability of the blood-brain barrier.**
    - It predominantly affects the **white matter** (Fig. 25-9A).
  - **Cytotoxic edema** represents cellular edema and is associated with **cerebral ischemia.**
    - It is due to **cell death.**
    - It **affects both the gray and white matter** (Fig. 25-9B).
- Recognizing cerebral edema
  - **Loss of normal differentiation between gray and white matter**

- **Effacement** (narrowing or obliteration) of the normal **sulci**
- **Ventricular compression** (Fig. 25-10)
- **Herniation** of the brain, which is manifest, in part, by **effacement of the basilar cisterns** (see Fig. 25-7)
- **Subfalcine herniation**
  - The lateral ventricle and septum pellucidum herniate beneath the falx and shift across the midline toward the opposite side (see Fig. 25-9B).
- **Transtentorial herniation**
  - The cerebral hemispheres are displaced downward beneath the tentorium compressing the ipsilateral temporal horn and causing **dilatation of the contralateral temporal horn** (see Fig. 25-6A).
- Increased intracranial pressure secondary to increase in the size of the ventricles is discussed under "Hydrocephalus."

Stroke

GENERAL CONSIDERATIONS

- Stroke is not a medical term, but usually denotes an acute loss of neurologic function that occurs when blood supply to an area of the brain is lost or compromised.

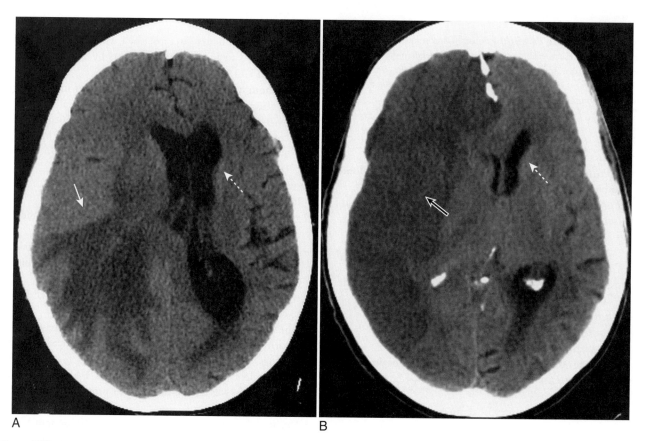

A

B

Figure 25-9. ***Vasogenic and cytotoxic edema.*** *There are two major categories of cerebral edema: vasogenic **(A)** and cytotoxic **(B).*** ***A,*** *Vasogenic edema (closed white arrow) represents extracellular accumulation of fluid and is the type that occurs with infection and malignancy, as in this unenhanced scan of a patient with a glioma. It predominantly affects the white matter.* ***B,*** *Cytotoxic edema (open white arrow) represents cellular edema and affects both the gray and white matter. Cytotoxic edema is associated with cerebral ischemia, as in this patient with a large ischemic infarct on the right. In both of these patients, there is increased intracranial pressure as manifested by the herniation of brain to the contralateral side (dotted white arrows).*

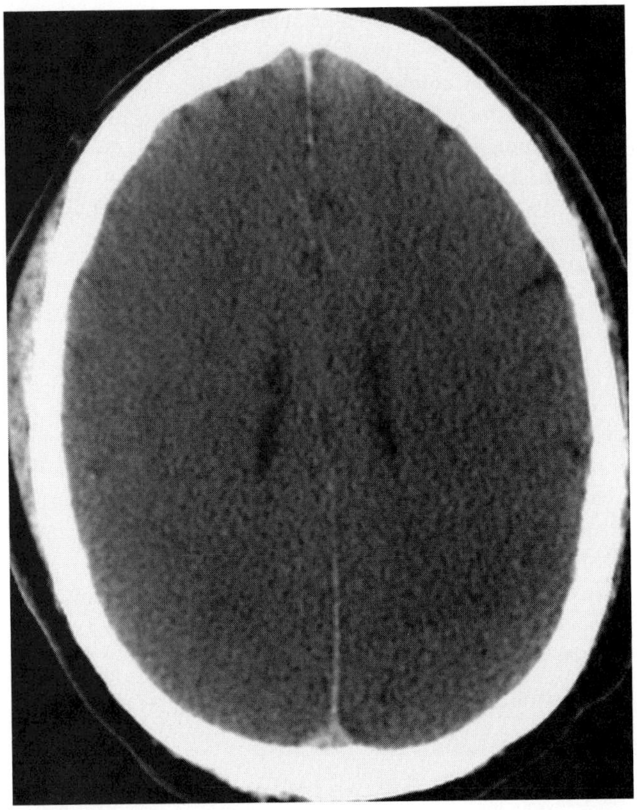

Figure 25-10. **Diffuse cerebral edema.** *Cerebral edema produces loss of normal differentiation between gray and white matter, effacement (narrowing or obliteration) of the normal sulci, and ventricular compression, all of which are present in this patient with anoxic encephalopathy.*

- **Uses for imaging in strokes**
  - To determine if there is **another cause of the neurologic impairment** besides a stroke, e.g., a brain tumor
  - To **identify the presence of blood** so as to distinguish **ischemic** from **hemorrhagic** stroke
    - This differentiation may determine whether or not thrombolytic therapy will be instituted.
  - Lastly, to **identify** the **infarct** and **characterize it.**
- Most strokes are **embolic** in origin, the emboli arising from the internal carotid artery or the common carotid bifurcation.
  - Another common cause of stroke is **thrombosis,** particularly of the middle cerebral artery.
- Most **acute strokes are initially imaged by obtaining a non-contrast-enhanced CT scan** (within 24 hours of the onset of symptoms).
  - CT findings may be present about 6 hours after the onset for ischemic stroke.
  - **Diffusion-weighted MRI** is more sensitive in detecting early infarction with the capacity to detect changes within a few minutes of the onset of the event.
    - It will become more widely used for early diagnosis, but CT is still the most widely used initial study for suspected stroke.

ISCHEMIC STROKE

- **Thromboembolic disease** consequent to **atherosclerosis** is the **most common cause.**
  - The **source of the emboli** can be from atheromatous debris, arterial stenosis and occlusion, or from emboli arising from the left side of the heart (as in atrial fibrillation).
- *Vascular watershed* areas are the distal arterial territories that represent the **junctions between areas served by the major intracerebral vessels,** such as the region between the anterior cerebral artery distribution and the middle cerebral artery distribution.
  - Reduction in blood flow, for whatever reason, affects these sensitive watershed areas the most.
- **The most common finding of an acute, nonhemorrhagic stroke is a normal CT scan (less than 6 hours old).**
  - If multiple vascular distributions are involved, emboli or vasculitis should be thought of as the cause.
  - If the stroke crosses or falls between vascular territories, then hypoperfusion due to hypotension *(watershed infarcts)* should be considered.
- **Recognizing ischemic stroke**
  - The findings will depend on the amount of time that has elapsed since the original event:
  - **12 to 24 hours:** indistinct area of low attenuation in a vascular distribution
  - **>24 hours:** better circumscribed with mass effect that peaks at 3 to 5 days and disappears by 2 to 4 weeks (Fig. 25-11A)
  - **72 hours:** although contrast is rarely used in the setting of acute stroke, contrast enhancement typically occurs when the mass effect is waning or has disappeared.
  - **>4 weeks:** no mass effect; well-circumscribed low attenuation lesion with no contrast enhancement (Fig. 25-11B)

HEMORRHAGIC STROKE

- Hemorrhage **occurs in about 15%** of strokes.
  - Hemorrhage is associated with higher morbidity and mortality rates than ischemic stroke.
- In the majority of cases, there is **associated hypertension.**
  - **About 60% of hypertensive hemorrhages occur in the basal ganglia.**
  - Other areas involved are the thalamus, pons, and cerebellum (Fig. 25-12).
- The decision to utilize thrombolytic therapy is based on algorithms formulated by the initial nonenhanced CT scan findings.
  - Treatment should be initiated **within 1 hour after the patient arrives at the hospital** to provide its maximum benefit.
- **Recognizing intracerebral hemorrhage (in general)**
  - Freshly extravasated whole blood with a normal hematocrit will be visible as **increased density** (hyperdensity, hyperattenuation) on nonenhanced CT scans of the brain (see Fig. 25-12).
    - This is due to the protein in the blood (mostly hemoglobin).

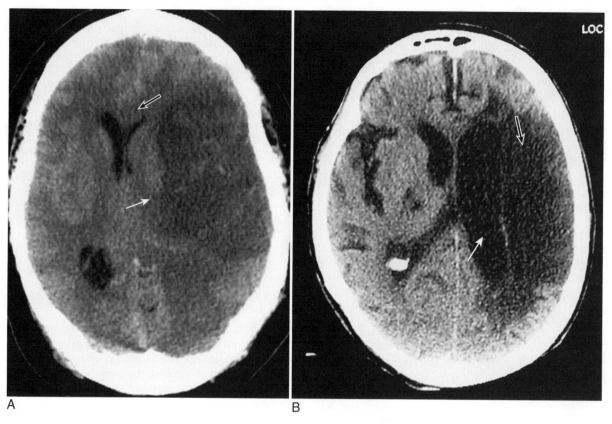

A   B

Figure 25-11. **Ischemic stroke, newer and older.** *The findings in ischemic stroke will depend on the amount of time that has elapsed since the original event.* **A,** *At about 24 hours, the lesion becomes relatively well circumscribed* (closed white arrow) *with mass effect shown here by shift of ventricles* (open white arrow) *that peaks at 3 to 5 days and disappears by 2 to 4 weeks.* **B,** *As the stroke matures, it loses its mass effect, tends to become an even more sharply marginated low attenuation lesion* (open white arrow), *and may be associated with enlargement of the adjacent ventricles due to loss of brain substance in the infarcted area* (closed white arrow).

- **Dissection** of blood into the **ventricular system** can occur in hypertensive intracerebral bleeds (see Fig. 25-8).
- As the clot begins to form, the **blood becomes denser for about 3 days** because of dehydration of the clot.
- **After the 3rd day,** the **clot decreases in density** and becomes invisible over the next several weeks.
  - The clot loses density from the **outside in** so that it **appears to shrink.**
- After about 2 months, only a small hypodensity may remain (Fig. 25-13) (Box 25-1).

Ruptured Aneurysms

- The most frequent central nervous system aneurysm is the **berry aneurysm,** which develops from a **congenital weakening in the arterial wall,** usually at the sites of vessel branching in the **circle of Willis.**
  - **Hypertension** and **aging** play a role in the growth of aneurysms.
  - **Larger aneurysms bleed more frequently** than do smaller ones.
- The goal is to discover and treat the aneurysm before it has undergone a major bleed.

- The classical history a patient offers with a ruptured aneurysm is "the worst headache" of their life.
- When aneurysms rupture, the **blood usually enters the subarachnoid space.**
  - Rupture of an aneurysm is the **most common cause of a subarachnoid hemorrhage** (50–70%), but it is not the only cause, as trauma, arteriovenous malformations, and breakthrough of an intraparenchymal bleed can also produce subarachnoid hemorrhage.
- Today, most aneurysms are detected by **either CT angiography or MR angiography.**
  - **CT angiography** is performed using a power injector to deliver a rapid bolus intravenous injection of iodinated contrast; it uses a CT scanner capable of rapid acquisition of data and special computer algorithms and postprocessing techniques that can highlight the vessels and, if desired, display them three-dimensionally.
  - **MR angiography** can be done without any contrast, but is usually performed with the intravenous injection of MR contrast (gadolinium), using an MR scanner and specialized computer applications that allow for highlighting the blood vessels being studied.

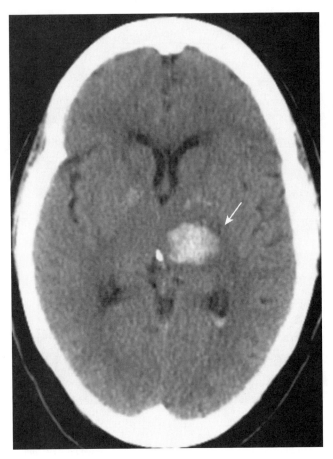

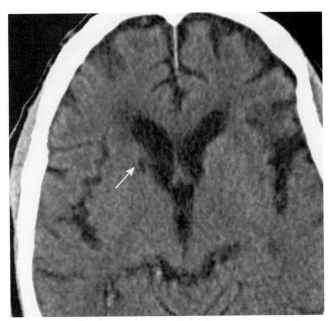

Figure 25-13. **Lacunar infarct.** A lacunar infarct, or **lacune,** is a small cerebral infarct produced by occlusion of an end artery. Lacunar infarcts have a predilection for the basal ganglia, internal capsule, and pons and are primarily related to hypertension and atherosclerosis. The term lacunar infarct is reserved for low-density, cystic lesions 5 to 15 mm in size (closed white arrow).

Figure 25-12. **Intracerebral hemorrhage, acute.** Freshly extravasated whole blood, as in this bleed into the thalamus (closed white arrow), will be visible as increased density on nonenhanced CT scans of the brain due primarily to the protein in the blood (mostly hemoglobin). As the clot begins to form, the blood becomes denser for about 3 days because of dehydration of the clot. After the third day, the clot gradually decreases in density from the outside in and becomes invisible over the next several weeks.

Box 25-1

Lacunar Infarcts
Small cerebral infarct produced by occlusion of an end artery
Predilection for the basal ganglia, internal capsule, and pons primarily related to hypertension and atherosclerosis
The term lacunar infarct is reserved for low-density, cystic lesions 5–15 mm

- Recognizing a **subarachnoid hemorrhage (from a ruptured aneurysm).**
  - **CT is the initial study of choice.**
  - **Blood is hyperdense and may be visualized within the sulci and basal cisterns** (Fig. 25-14).
  - The region of the **falx may become hyperdense,** widened, and irregularly marginated.
  - Generally, the **greatest concentration of blood indicates the most likely site of the ruptured aneurysm.**
- Other causes of intracerebral hemorrhage besides aneurysms include arteriovenous malformations, tumors, mycotic aneurysms, and amyloid angiopathy (Box 25-2).

Hydrocephalus

- **Expansion of the ventricular system** on the basis of an increase in the volume of cerebrospinal fluid (CSF) contained within them (Box 25-3).
  - May be due to
    - **Overproduction of cerebrospinal fluid** (rare)

- **Underabsorption of cerebrospinal fluid** (at the level of the arachnoid villi)
- **Obstruction of the outflow of cerebrospinal fluid from the ventricles**
- In general, the **ventricles** are **disproportionately dilated** compared to the **sulci** in **hydrocephalus,** whereas **both the ventricles and sulci** are **proportionately enlarged** in **atrophy.**
- The **temporal horns are particularly sensitive** to increases in CSF pressure.
  - The size of the temporal horns in hydrocephalus is greater than 2 mm (Fig. 25-15A).
  - In the absence of hydrocephalus, the **temporal horns are barely visible.**

OBSTRUCTIVE HYDROCEPHALUS

- Obstructive hydrocephalus is divided into two major categories: **communicating** *(extraventricular*

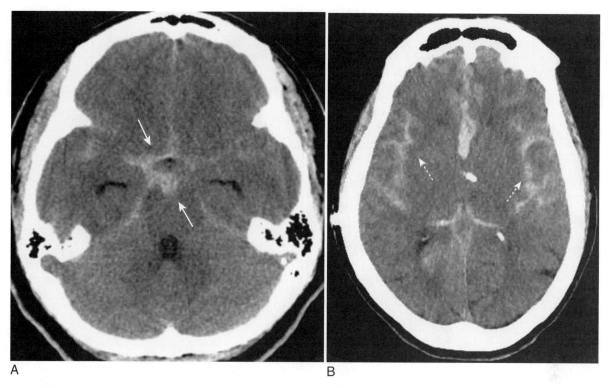

A   B

Figure 25-14. **Subarachnoid hemorrhage.** *Subarachnoid hemorrhage is frequently the result of a ruptured aneurysm. Blood may be most easily visualized within the basal cisterns (closed white arrows in* **A)** *and interdigitated in the subarachnoid spaces of the sulci (dotted white arrows in* **B).** *Generally, the greatest concentration of blood indicates the most likely site of the ruptured aneurysm. Other causes of intracerebral hemorrhage include arteriovenous malformations, tumors, mycotic aneurysms, and amyloid angiopathy.*

Box 25-2

Amyloid Angiopathy

Amyloid is a proteinaceous material that can be deposited with increasing age in the media and adventitia of small and medium-sized intracranial vessels, mostly involving the frontal and parietal lobes.

This deposit produces a loss of elasticity of the vessels and increases their fragility.

Hemorrhages from amyloid angiopathy are usually large, involving an entire lobe; they may be multiple and occur in several areas simultaneously.

There is no association with hypertension, and it is not associated with amyloid elsewhere.

Box 25-3

Normal Flow of Cerebrospinal Fluid

Most cerebrospinal fluid is produced by the choroid plexuses in the ventricles, primarily the lateral and fourth ventricles.

The direction of flow is from the lateral ventricles through the foramen of Monro to the third ventricle through the aqueduct of Sylvius to the fourth ventricle and then into the basilar subarachnoid cisterns through the two lateral foramina of Luschka and the medial foramen of Magendie.

CSF then passes either upward over the convexities to be reabsorbed into the bloodstream at the arachnoid villi, or inferiorly down the spinal subarachnoid space where it is either reabsorbed directly or ascends back to the brain to the arachnoid villi.

obstruction) and **noncommunicating *(intraventricular obstruction).***

- **Communicating hydrocephalus** is due to abnormalities that **inhibit the resorption of cerebrospinal fluid,** most often at the level of the arachnoid villi (see Fig. 25-15).
  - **CSF flow** through the **ventricles** and **over the convexities** is **unimpeded.**

- Reabsorption through the arachnoid villi can become obstructed by such things as **subarachnoid hemorrhage** and **meningitis.**
- Classically, the fourth ventricle is **dilated** in **communicating hydrocephalus** and **normal** in size in **noncommunicating** hydrocephalus.
- Communicating hydrocephalus is **usually treated with a ventricular shunt** tube.

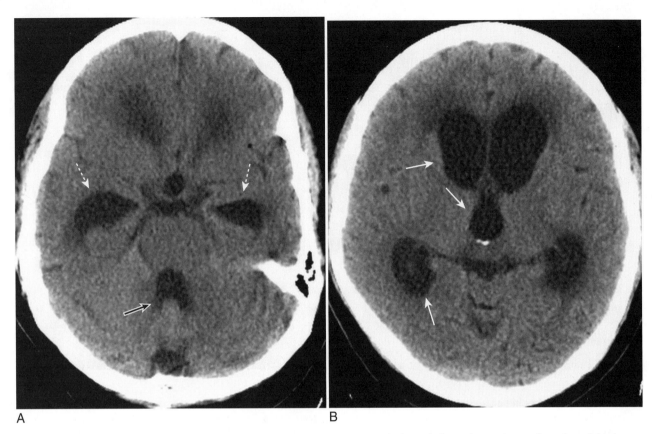

A   B

Figure 25-15. **Communicating hydrocephalus, two examples.** *Communicating hydrocephalus is due to abnormalities that inhibit the resorption of cerebrospinal fluid, most often at the level of the arachnoid villi. Classically, the fourth ventricle is dilated in communicating hydrocephalus (open white arrow in* **A***) but normal in size in noncommunicating hydrocephalus. The temporal horns are particularly sensitive to increases in intraventricular volume or pressure (dotted white arrows).* **B,** *The frontal horns, occipital horns, and third ventricle are markedly dilated (closed white arrows). There is a disproportionate dilatation of the ventricles compared to the sulci (which are normal to small here). Communicating hydrocephalus is usually treated with a ventricular shunt tube.*

- **Noncommunicating hydrocephalus** occurs as result of **tumors, cysts,** or other physically obstructing lesions that **do not allow cerebrospinal fluid to exit from the ventricles** (Fig. 25-16).
  - In congenital hydrocephalus, it is often produced by a blockage between the third and fourth ventricles at the level of the **aqueduct of Sylvius *(aqueductal obstruction).***
  - When the obstruction is caused by a tumor or a cyst, noncommunicating hydrocephalus is **usually treated by surgically** removing the obstructing lesion.
- **Nonobstructive hydrocephalus** from overproduction of CSF is rare and can occur with a *choroid plexus papilloma.*

NORMAL-PRESSURE HYDROCEPHALUS (NPH)

- NPH is a form of communicating hydrocephalus characterized by a classical triad of clinical symptoms including **abnormalities of gait, dementia,** and **urinary incontinence.**
- Age of onset is typically between 50 and 70 years old.
- Imaging findings are similar to other forms of communicating hydrocephalus and include **enlarged ventricles,** particularly the temporal horns, with **normal or flattened sulci.**
- Usual treatment is insertion of a one-way *ventriculoperitoneal shunt,* which allows the CSF to exit the ventricles and drain into the peritoneal cavity where the CSF is reabsorbed.

CEREBRAL ATROPHY

- Disorders associated with **gross cerebral atrophy** are also associated with **dementia, Alzheimer's disease being one of the most common.**
  - The major finding in patients with Alzheimer's disease (though not specific) is **diffuse cortical atrophy,** especially in the **temporal lobes** (Fig. 25-17).
- Alcoholism is the most common cause of **cerebellar** atrophy.
- Atrophy implies a loss of both gray and white matter.
- Like hydrocephalus, the **ventricles dilate** in cerebral atrophy but do so because a loss of normal cerebral tissue produces a vacant space that is filled passively with CSF.
  - Unlike hydrocephalus, the **dynamics of CSF** production and absorption are **normal in atrophy.**

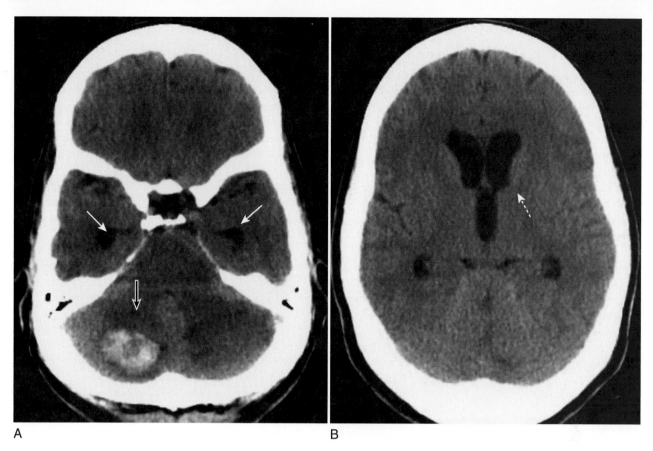

A   B

Figure 25-16. **Noncommunicating hydrocephalus.** There is dilatation of the temporal horns (closed white arrows in **A**) and the frontal horns and third ventricle (dotted white arrow in **B**), but the sulci are not dilated. There is a hemorrhagic metastatic lesion (open white arrow in **A**) that is obstructing the fourth ventricle. This form of hydrocephalus is the result of obstruction to the outflow of cerebrospinal fluid from the ventricles.

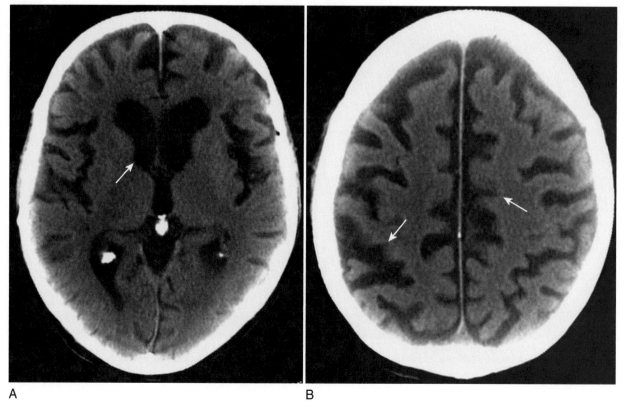

A   B

Figure 25-17. **Diffuse cortical atrophy.** In general, cerebral atrophy produces enlargement of the sulci and the ventricles secondarily. CSF dynamics are normal in atrophy, as compared to hydrocephalus. Disorders associated with gross cerebral atrophy are also associated with dementia, Alzheimer's disease being one of the most common. The major finding in patients with Alzheimer's disease (though not specific) is diffuse cortical atrophy manifest by enlargement of the ventricles and the sulci (closed white arrows).

- In general, cerebral atrophy produces **proportionate enlargement of both the ventricles and the sulci.**

Brain Tumors

GLIOMAS OF THE BRAIN

- **Most common primary supratentorial, intra-axial mass in adults**
- **Gliomas account for 35 to 45% of all intracranial tumors,** and *glioblastoma multiforme* accounts for more than half of them, astrocytomas about 20%, and the remainder are split between *ependymomas, medulloblastoma,* and *oligodendroglioma.*
- Glioblastoma multiforme has the **worst prognosis** of all gliomas.
  - Occurs **more commonly in males** between 65 and 75 years of age, especially in the **frontal and temporal lobes.**
- **Recognizing glioblastoma multiforme**
  - As the most aggressive of tumors, glioblastoma multiforme frequently demonstrates **necrosis** within the tumor.

- The tumor **infiltrates** the surrounding brain tissue, frequently **crossing** the white matter tracts of **the corpus callosum** to the opposite cerebral hemisphere, producing a pattern called a *butterfly glioma* (Fig. 25-18).
- It tends to **produce considerable vasogenic edema** and **mass effect** and **contrast enhances,** at least in part.

METASTASES

- Solitary intra-axial masses are about evenly split between **solitary metastases** and **primary brain tumors.**
- About **40% of all intracranial neoplasms** are metastases.
  - Metastases to the brain are frequently **well-defined, round masses near the gray-white junction.**
  - They are **usually multiple, but can be solitary** (up to 50%).
  - They are **typically hypodense or isodense on nonenhanced CT.**
  - With intravenous contrast, they can sometimes **enhance** in a pattern of **ring-enhancement** (Fig. 25-19).
  - Most evoke some **vasogenic edema,** frequently out of proportion to the size of the mass.
- **Lung cancer, breast cancer, and melanoma** are the most common primary malignancies to produce brain metastases.

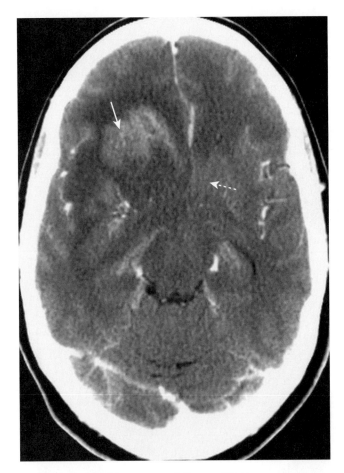

Figure 25-18. **Glioblastoma multiforme.** *Glioblastoma multiforme has the worst prognosis of all gliomas. It most commonly occurs in the frontal and temporal lobes, as is seen in this patient's contrast-enhanced CT. The tumor infiltrates the surrounding brain tissue (dotted white arrow), may contrast enhance (closed white arrow), and frequently crosses the corpus callosum to the opposite cerebral hemisphere, producing a pattern called a* **butterfly glioma.**

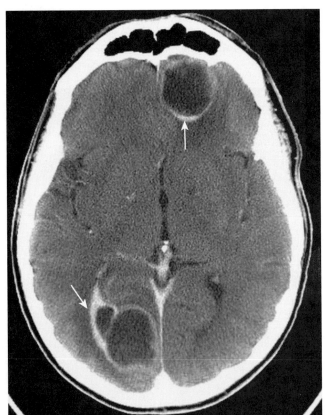

Figure 25-19. **Metastases.** *About 40% of all intracranial neoplasms are metastases. They typically produce well-defined, round masses near the gray-white junction and are usually multiple. With intravenous contrast, they can enhance and show ring enhancement (closed white arrows). Lung cancer, breast cancer, and melanoma are the most common primary malignancies that produce brain metastases. This patient had a lung cancer.*

MENINGIOMA

- The **most common extra-axial mass,** meningiomas usually occur in middle-aged women.
- Most common locations are **parasagittal, over the convexities,** the sphenoid wing, and the cerebellopontine angle cistern, in decreasing frequency.
- When **multiple,** they may have an association with *neurofibromatosis type 2.*
- They tend to be **slow-growing** with an **excellent prognosis** if surgically excised.
- **Recognizing a meningioma on CT scan of the brain**
  - **On unenhanced CT,** over **half are hyperdense** to normal brain and about **20% contain calcification** (Fig. 25-20).
  - On contrast-enhanced studies, **meningiomas enhance markedly.**
  - They **may have edema** surrounding them.

ACOUSTIC NEUROMA (SCHWANNOMA)

- Most common symptom is **hearing loss.**
- They are actually *schwannomas* and occur most commonly along the **course of the eighth cranial nerve** within the internal auditory canal at the **cerebellopontine angle** (Fig. 25-21).
- MRI is the most sensitive imaging study for detecting acoustic neuromas.

Multiple Sclerosis

- **Most common demyelinating disease**
- Characterized by a **relapsing and remitting course,** there are specific clinical criteria that need to be met for drawing this diagnosis, such as two or more white matter lesions at least 1 month apart in different locations of the brain.
- Lesions of multiple sclerosis have a **predilection for the periventricular area, corpus callosum, and optic nerves** (Fig. 25-22).
- **MRI is the study of choice** in imaging multiple sclerosis because of its greater sensitivity than CT in demonstrating plaques both in the brain and spinal cord.
  - The lesions produce **discrete, globular foci of high signal intensity (white) on T_2-weighted images** and enhance with gadolinium on T_1-weighted images.

Terminology

- Table 25-3 summarizes important terminology used in this chapter.

WebLink

More information on recognizing abnormalities on head CT is available to registered users on StudentConsult.com.

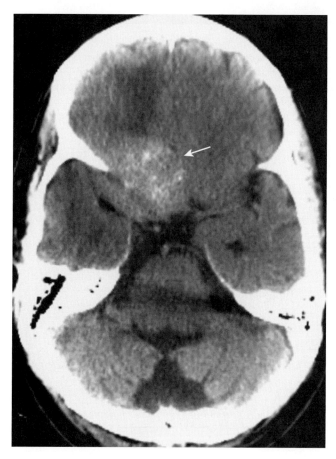

Figure 25-20. **Meningioma.** *The most common extra-axial mass, meningiomas usually occur in middle-aged women. This meningioma is arising along the right sphenoid wing, a relatively common site of origin. On unenhanced CT, over half are hyperdense to normal brain and about 20% contain calcification, as does this lesion, that appears as a dense mass (closed white arrow). On contrast-enhanced studies, meningiomas markedly enhance.*

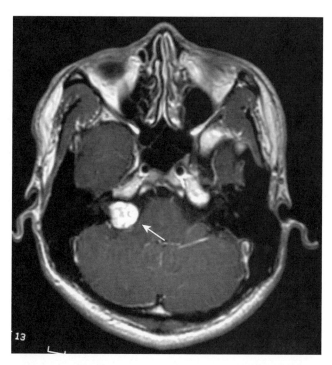

Figure 25-21. **Acoustic neuroma (schwannomas), T_1-weighted MRI with contrast.** *Acoustic neuromas occur most commonly along the course of the eighth cranial nerve within the internal auditory canal at the cerebellopontine angle (closed white arrow). Hearing loss is the most common presenting symptom.*

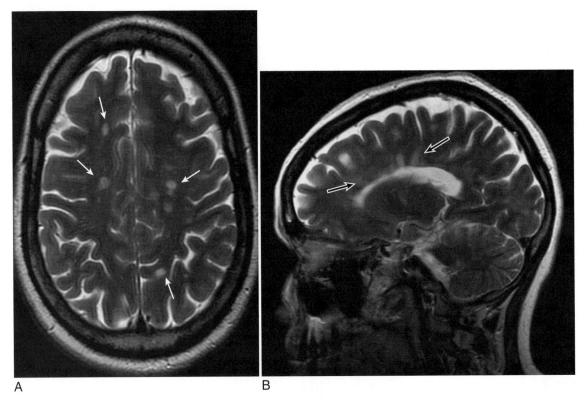

Figure 25-22. **Multiple sclerosis, axial and sagittal MRI.** *Lesions of multiple sclerosis have a predilection for the periventricular area, corpus callosum, and optic nerves (closed white arrows).* **A,** *The lesions produce discrete, globular foci of high signal intensity (white) on T$_2$-weighted images.* **B,** *Ovoid lesions with their long axis perpendicular to the ventricular surface are called* **Dawson's fingers** *(open white arrows). MRI is the study of choice in imaging multiple sclerosis because of its greater sensitivity than CT in demonstrating plaques both in the brain and spinal cord.*

Table 25-3

TERMINOLOGY USED IN THIS CHAPTER

Intra-axial/extra-axial	Intra-axial lesions originate in the brain parenchyma, and extra-axial lesions originate outside the brain substance (meninges, intraventricular)
Infratentorial	Beneath the tentorium cerebelli, which includes the cerebellum, brain stem, fourth ventricle, and cerebellopontine angles
Supratentorial	Above the tentorium cerebelli, which includes the cerebral hemispheres (frontal, parietal, occipital, and temporal lobes) and the sella
Transient ischemic attack (TIA)	Sudden neurologic loss that persists for a short time and resolves within 24 hours
Completed stroke	Deficit lasts for > 21 days
Open versus closed head injuries	**Open**—communication of intracranial material outside the skull; **closed**—no external communication
Increased attenuation/hyperattenuation/ hyperdense/hyperintense	On CT, tissue that is of increased attenuation, that hyperattenuates, is hyperdense, or is hyperintense is whiter than surrounding tissues
Decreased attenuation/hypoattenuation/ hypodense/hypointense	On CT, tissues that these terms apply to are darker than surrounding tissues
Diffusion-weighted imaging (DWI)	An MRI sequence that can be rapidly acquired and which is extremely sensitive to detecting abnormalities in normal water movement in the brain so that it can identify a stroke within minutes after the event; also helps differentiate acute infarction from more chronic infarction

TAKE-HOME POINTS: Recognzing Abnormal Head CT Findings

Linear skull fractures are important mainly for the intracranial abnormalities that may have occurred at the time of the fracture; **depressed skull fractures** can be associated with underlying brain injury and may require elevation of the fragment.

Blow-out fractures of the orbit result from a direct blow and may present with orbital emphysema, fracture through either the floor or medial wall of the orbit, and entrapment of fat or extraocular muscles in the fracture.

Epidural hematomas represent hemorrhage into the potential space between the dura mater and the inner table of the skull and are usually due to injuries to the middle meningeal artery or vein from blunt head trauma; almost all (95%) have an associated skull fracture.

When acute, epidural hematomas appear as hyperintense collections of blood that typically have a lenticular shape; as they age, they become hypodense to normal brain.

Subdural hematomas most commonly result from deceleration injuries or falls; they represent hemorrhage into the potential space between the dura mater and the arachnoid; acute subdural hematomas portend the presence of more severe brain injury.

Subdural hematomas are crescent-shaped bands of blood that may cross suture lines and enter the interhemispheric fissure, although they do not cross the midline; they are typically concave inward to the brain and may appear isointense (isodense) to remainder of brain as they become subacute and hypodense when chronic.

Traumatic intracerebral hematomas are frequently associated with shearing injuries and present as petechial or larger hemorrhages in the frontal or temporal lobes; they may be associated with increased intracranial pressure.

Diffuse axonal injury is a serious consequence of trauma in which the corpus callosum is most commonly affected; CT findings are similar to those for intracerebral hemorrhage following head trauma; MRI is the study of choice in identifying diffuse axonal injury.

In general, increased intracranial pressure is due to either increased volume of the brain (brain swelling) or increased size of the ventricles.

There are two major categories of cerebral edema: vasogenic and cytotoxic.

Vasogenic edema represents extracellular accumulation of fluid and is the type that occurs with malignancy and infection and affects the white matter more.

Cytotoxic edema represents cellular edema, is due to cell death, and affects both the gray and white matter; cytotoxic edema is associated with cerebral ischemia.

Strokes are usually due to embolic or thrombotic events and are typically divided into ischemic (more common) and hemorrhagic varieties (poorer prognosis); hypertension is frequently associated.

Intracerebral hemorrhage, when visible, will have increased density on nonenhanced CT scans of the brain; as the clot begins to form, the blood becomes denser for about 3 days because of dehydration of the clot and then decreases in density, becoming invisible over the next several weeks; after about 2 months, only a small hypodensity may remain.

Berry aneurysms are formed from congenital weakening in the arterial wall; when they rupture the blood typically enters the subarachnoid space, presenting in the basilar cisterns and in the sulci.

Hydrocephalus represents an increased volume of cerebrospinal fluid (CSF) in the ventricular system and may be due to overproduction of CSF (rare), underabsorption of CSF at the level of the arachnoid villi (communicating), or obstruction of the outflow of CSF from the ventricles (noncommunicating).

Normal-pressure hydrocephalus is a form of communicating hydrocephalus characterized by a classical triad of clinical symptoms including abnormalities of gait, dementia, and urinary incontinence, all of which may be improved by insertion of a shunt.

Cerebral atrophy is a loss of both gray and white matter that may resemble hydrocephalus except that the fluid dynamics of the CSF are normal in atrophy and, in general, cerebral atrophy produces proportionate enlargement of both the ventricles and the sulci; there is diffuse cerebral atrophy associated with Alzheimer's disease.

Glioblastoma multiforme is a highly malignant glioma that occurs most commonly in the frontal and temporal lobes, producing a very aggressive, infiltrating, sometimes necrotic, partially enhancing mass that may cross the corpus callosum to the opposite cerebral hemisphere.

Metastases to the brain are frequently well-defined, round masses near the gray-white junction, usually multiple, typically hypodense or isodense on nonenhanced CT and enhancing with contrast; they can provoke vasogenic edema out of proportion to the size of the mass; lung cancer, breast cancer, and melanoma are the most frequent causes of brain metastases.

Meningiomas usually occur in middle-aged women in a parasagittal location; they tend to be slow-growing with an excellent prognosis if surgically excised; on CT, they characteristically can be dense without contrast because of calcification within the tumor; they may enhance dramatically.

Acoustic neuromas occur most commonly along the course of the eighth nerve within the internal auditory canal at the cerebellopontine angle and are best identified on MRI.

Multiple sclerosis is the most common demyelinating disease, characterized by a relapsing and remitting course and predilection for the periventricular area, corpus callosum, and optic nerves; it is best visualized on MRI and produces discrete, globular foci of high-signal intensity (white) on T_2-weighted images.

Bibliography

Texts

Blickman H: Pediatric Radiology: The Requisites, 2nd ed. St. Louis, The Mosby Company, 1998.

Fraser RS, Pare P, Fraser R, Pare PD: Synopsis of Diseases of the Chest, 2nd ed. Philadelphia, W.B. Saunders, 1994.

Greenspan A: Orthopedic Radiology: A Practical Approach, 3rd ed. Philadelphia, Lippincott Williams and Wilkins, 2000.

Grossman RL, Yousem DM: Neuroradiology: The Requisites. St. Louis, Mosby, 1994.

Guyton AC, Hall J: Textbook of Medical Physiology, 11th ed. Philadelphia, W.B. Saunders, 2005.

McCloud T: Thoracic Radiology: The Requisites, 1st edition, St. Louis, Mosby, 1998.

Meyers MA: Dynamic Radiology of the Abdomen: Normal and Pathological Anatomy, 2nd ed. New York, Springer-Verlag, 1982.

Resnick D: Diagnosis of Bone and Joint Disorders, 4th ed. Philadelphia, W.B. Saunders, 1981.

Resnick D: Diagnosis of Bone and Joint Disorders, 2nd ed. Philadelphia, W.B. Saunders, 2002.

Schultz RJ: The Language of Fractures. Huntington, NY, Robert E. Krieger, 1972.

Webb WR, Brant WE, Helms CA: Fundamentals of Body CT. Philadelphia, W.B. Saunders, 1991.

Weissleder R, Wittenberg J, Harisinghani MG: Primer of Diagnostic Imaging, 3rd ed. St. Louis, Mosby, 2003.

Journal Articles

Aberle DR, Wiener-Kronish JP, Webb WR, Matthay MA: Hydrostatic versus increased permeability pulmonary edema: Diagnosis based on radiographic data in critically ill patients. Radiology 168:73–79, 1988.

Bates D, Ruggieri P: Imaging modalities for evaluation of the spine. Radiol Clin North Am 29(4):675–690, 1991.

Burney K, Burchard F, Papouchado M, Wilde P: Cardiac pacing systems and implantable cardiac defibrillators (ICDs): A radiological perspective of equipment, anatomy, and complications. Clin Radiol 59(8):699–708, 2004.

Dalinka MK, Reginato AJ, Golden DA: Calcium deposition disease. Semin Roentgenol 17(1):39–47, 1982.

Edeiken J: Radiologic approach to arthritis. Semin Roentgenol 17(1):8–15, 1982.

Garcia MJ: Could cardiac CT revolutionize the practice of cardiology? Cleve Clin J Med 72(2):88–89, 2005.

Gaskill MF, Lukin R, Wiot JG: Lumbar disc disease and stenosis. Radiol Clin North Am 29(4):75–764, 1991.

Haus BM, Stark P, Shofer SL, Kuschner WG: Massive pulmonary pseudotumor. Chest 124(2):758–760, 2003.

Hendrix RW, Rogers LF: Diagnostic imaging of fracture complications. Radiol Clin North Am 27(5):1023–1033, 1989.

Henschke CI, Yankelevitz DF, Wand A, Davis SD, Shiau M: Accuracy and efficacy of chest radiography in the intensive care unit. Radiol Clin North Am 34(1):21–31, 1996.

Henry M, Arnold T, Harvey J: British Thoracic Society's guidelines for the management of spontaneous pneumothorax. Thorax 58(Suppl 2):39–52, 2003.

Indrajit IK, Shreeram MN, d'Souza JD: Multislice CT: A quantum leap in whole body imaging. Indian J Radiol Imaging 14(2):209–216, 2004.

Johnson JL: Pleural effusions in cardiovascular disease. Postgrad Med 107(4):95–101, 2000.

Kundel HL, Wright DJ: The influence of prior knowledge on visual search strategies during the viewing of chest radiographs. Radiology 93:315–320, 1969.

Lingawi SS: The naked facet sign. Radiology 219:366–367, 2001.

Old JL, Calvert M: Vertebral compression fractures in the elderly. Am Fam Physician 69(1):111–116, 2004.

Pathria MN, Petersilge CA: Spinal trauma. Radiol Clin North Am 29(4):847–865, 1991.

Riddervold HO: Easily missed fractures. Radiol Clin North Am 30(2):475–494, 1992.

Shifrin RY, Choplin RH: Aspiration in patients in critical care units. Radiol Clin North Am 34(1):83–95, 1996.

Thomas EL, Lansdown EL: Visual search patterns of radiologists in training. Radiology 81:288–292, 1963.

Tie MLH: Basic head CT for intensivists. Crit Care Res 3:35–44, 2001.

Tocino I, Westcott JL: Barotrauma. Radiol Clin North Am 34(1):59–81, 1996.

Yu S, Haughton VM, Rosenbaum AE: Magnetic resonance imaging and anatomy of the spine. Radiol Clin North Am 29(4):675–690, 1991.

Yuh W, Quets J, Lee H, Simonson TM, Michalson LS, Nguyen PT, Sato Y, Mayr NA, Berbaum KS: Anatomic distribution of metastases in the vertebral body and modes of hematogenous spread. Spine 21(19):2243–2250, 1996.

Index

Note: Page numbers followed by b indicate boxed material; those followed by f indicate figures; those followed by n indicate footnotes; those followed by t indicate tables.